Since it was first described by Kanner in 1943, autism has been the focus of sustained interest from clinicians and researchers, although the precise neurobiological basis of the disorder has yet to be established. This volume reflects recent progress in the understanding of autism and related conditions, with contributions from leading authorities in the clinical and social sciences, and offers an international perspective on current thinking. In common with earlier volumes in this influential series, it brings together developmental studies with the latest information on psychopathology and management.

Chapters cover current approaches to definition and diagnosis, prevalence and planning for service delivery, cognitive, genetic and neurobiological features, and pathophysiological mechanisms. Interventions reviewed include the pharmacological, behavioural and educational, and a thoughtful final chapter addresses the nature of the fundamental social disturbance that characterizes autism.

As a summary of what is now known about autism and related disorders, and an indicator of what is still poorly understood, this book will be an essential resource for clinicians, researchers, and carers. In describing areas of progress, and targets for future research, it carries an informed and hopeful message to those concerned with these perplexing conditions.

FRED VOLKMAR is Professor at the Child Study Center, Yale University. He is an Associate Editor of the *Journal of Autism* and the *Journal of Child Psychology and Psychiatry*. In 1997 he was awarded the Ittelson Prize of the American Psychiatric Association.

Autism and Pervasive Developmental Disorders

MONOGRAPHS IN CHILD AND ADOLESCENT PSYCHIATRY

Child and adolescent psychiatry is an important and growing area of clinical psychiatry. Recent years have seen a rapid expansion of scientific knowledge in this field and a new understanding of the underlying pathology of mental disorders in these age groups. This series is aimed at practitioners and researchers both in child and adolescent mental health services and developmental and clinical neuroscience. Focusing on psychopathology, it highlights those topics where the growth of knowledge has had the greatest impact on clinical practice and on the treatment and understanding of mental illness. Individual volumes benefit both from the international expertise of their contributors and a coherency generated through a uniform style and structure for the series. While each volume is complete in its own right, volumes also relate to each other to create a flexible and collectable series that should appeal to students as well as experienced scientists and practitioners.

Executive Editors

The late William Ll. Parry-Jones
Department of Child and Adolescent Psychiatry, Glasgow University, UK.

Ian M. Goodyer
Section of Developmental Psychiatry, Cambridge University, UK.

Associate Editors

Donald J. Cohen
Yale Child Study Center, New Haven, USA.

Helmut Remschmidt,
Klinik für Kinder und Jugendpsychiatrie, Klinikum der Philipps-Universität, Marburg, Germany.

Already published in this series:
The Depressed Child and Adolescent edited by Ian M. Goodyer
ISBN 0 521 43326 6
Hyperactivity Disorders of Childhood edited by Seija Sandberg
ISBN 0 521 432502

CAMBRIDGE MONOGRAPHS IN CHILD AND
ADOLESCENT PSYCHIATRY

Autism and Pervasive Developmental Disorders

Edited by

FRED R. VOLKMAR

Child Study Center, Yale University

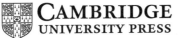
CAMBRIDGE
UNIVERSITY PRESS

PUBLISHED BY THE PRESS SYNDICATE OF THE UNIVERSITY OF CAMBRIDGE
The Pitt Building, Trumpington Street, Cambridge, United Kingdom

CAMBRIDGE UNIVERSITY PRESS
The Edinburgh Building, Cambridge CB2 2RU, UK   www.cup.cam.ac.uk
40 West 20th Street, New York, NY 10011–4211, USA   www.cup.org
10 Stamford Road, Oakleigh, Melbourne 3166, Australia
Ruiz de Alarcón 13, 28014 Madrid, Spain

First published 1998
Reprinted 1999

Printed in the United Kingdom at the University Press, Cambridge

Typeset in Times 10/13pt [VN]

A catalogue record for this book is available from the British Library

Library of Congress Cataloguing in Publication data

Autism and pervasive developmental disorders / edited by Fred R.
   Volkmar.
      p. cm. – (Cambridge monographs in child and adolescent
psychiatry)
   ISBN 0 521 55386 5 (hardback)
   1. Autism in children.   2. Developmental disabilities.
   I. Volkmar, Fred. R.   II. Series.
   [DNLM: 1. Autism, Infantile.   2. Child Development Disorders,
Pervasive.   WM 203.5 A9369 1998]
RJ506.A9A8928   1998
618.92′8982 – dc21   97-35997 CIP
DNLM/DLC
for Library of Congress

ISBN 0 521 55386 5 hardback

Every effort has been made in preparing this book to provide accurate and up-to-date
information which is in accord with accepted standards and practice at the time of
publication. Nevertheless, the authors, editors and publisher can make no warranties that
the information contained herein is totally free from error, not least because clinical
standards are constantly changing through research and regulation. The authors, editors
and publisher therefore disclaim all liability for direct or consequential damages resulting
from the use of material contained in this book. Readers are strongly advised to pay careful
attention to information provided by the manufacturer of any drugs or equipment that they
plan to use.

Contents

Contents

Contributors

Deborah Fein
>Psychology Department U-20
>University of Connecticut
>406 Babbidge Road
>Storrs, CT 06269-1020
>USA

Eric Fombonne
>MRC Child Psychiatry Unit
>Institute of Psychiatry
>Denmark Hill
>De Crespigny Park
>London SE5 8AF
>UK

Susan Goode
>Department of Psychology
>Institute of Psychiatry
>Denmark Hill
>De Crespigny Park
>London SE5 8AF
>UK

Sandra L. Harris
Graduate School of Applied and Professional Psychology
PO Box 819
Rutgers University
Piscataway, NJ08855-0819
USA

Patricia Howlin
Department of Psychology
St George's Hospital Medical School
Hunter Wing, Cranmer Terrace
London SW17 0RE
UK

Marshall B. Jones
Department of Behavioral Sciences
The Pennsylvania State University
Hershey Medical Center
500 University Drive
Hershey, PA 17033
USA

Catherine Lord
Department of Psychiatry
University of Chicago
5841 South Maryland
MC 3037
Chicago, IL 60637
US

Christopher J. McDougle
Department of Psychiatry and Child Study Center
Yale University School of Medicine
New Haven, CT 06519
USA

Sally Ozonoff
Department of Psychology
University of Utah
Salt Lake City, UT 84112
USA

Contributors

Margot Prior
Department of Psychology
Melbourne University
Parkville, Victoria 3052
Australia

Fritz Poustka
Department of Child and Adolescent Psychiatry
J.W. Goethe University
Deutschordenstrasse 50
D-60590 Frankfurt am Main
Germany

Peter Szatmari
Department of Psychiatry
McMaster University
Faculty of Health Sciences
1200 Main Street West
Hamilton, Ontario L8N 3S5
Canada

Fred R. Volkmar
Child Study Center
Yale University
PO Box 207900
New Haven, CT 06520
USA

Lynn Waterhouse
Child Behavior Study
226 Bray Hall
The College of New Jersey
Trenton, NJ 08650-4700
USA

Preface

Interest in what are now recognized as the pervasive developmental disorders can be traced to the middle of the nineteenth century with the first descriptions of childhood 'psychosis' (Volkmar, 1996). This interest stemmed from an increasing awareness of the importance of the factors of both experience and endowment in child development. Early descriptions of childhood 'insanity' were followed by descriptions of childhood schizophrenia (DeSanctis, 1906). The latter term became synonymous with all forms of severe mental disorder in children. The particular genius of Leo Kanner was reflected in his description in 1943 of the syndrome of infantile autism which he initially believed to be quite different from the forms of childhood 'psychosis' then recognized. In the subsequent five decades autism has been the focus of considerable interest from clinicians and researchers alike.

Autism has been the topic of a very substantial body of work. While major advances have been made (Bristol et al., 1996) precise pathophysiological models have yet to be specified. In an attempt to specify such models essentially all the theories of psychology and neurobiology have been utilized. While specification of such mechanisms remains an important, if as yet unrealized, goal considerable accomplishments have been made.

A substantial body of research has established the validity of autism as a diagnostic concept, e.g. on the basis of its characteristic clinical features and course. The neurobiological basis of the disorder has been established and better and more effective treatment methods have been developed. Recent attention has focused on genetic mechanisms in autism as well as on the spectrum of conditions which share some similarities with autism and which are now included in the pervasive developmental disorder category. Some of these conditions, such as Asperger's and Rett's syndromes, were proposed after Kanner's classic description of autism whereas others, notably childhood disintegrative disorder, were proposed many years before Kanner's work.

This volume reflects the considerable progress that has been made in recent years in our understanding of autism and related conditions. The authors have summarized current knowledge in various areas. The contributors represent various disciplines and provide truly international perspectives on current research in autism and related conditions.

The first chapter provides an overview of current approaches to the diagnosis and definition of autism and related conditions. Catherine Lord and Fred Volkmar review the development of diagnostic concepts and the rational for the definitions presently employed in both ICD-10 (1993) and DSM-IV (1994). While these definitions have retained important historical continuity with earlier ones they also reflect advances in knowledge and are based on a large body of empirical data (Volkmar et al., 1994). More importantly, the international (ICD-10) and American (DSM-IV) depictions are now conceptually convergent.

Advances in diagnosis have improved methods of case detection and are reflected in the results of more recent epidemiological studies. Such research tells us about the prevalence of a disorder and helps in planning for service delivery. Eric Fombonne provides a helpful summary of the present knowledge in this area. As he notes, an even larger group of children have impairments in social interaction and the characterization of their difficulties remains an important area for future research.

Studies of the cognitive and neurocognitive development of individuals with autism have made it clear that it is necessary to carefully study individuals with different levels of cognitive ability using various approaches. Margot Prior and Sally Ozonoff have summarized the literature on this topic with particular emphasis on those findings most specific to autism. Their chapter is a masterful summary of a large and diverse literature and outlines areas of work that are presently of particular interest, e.g. in executive functioning.

The importance of genetic factors in the pathogenesis of autism was relatively underappreciated until quite recently. Somewhat paradoxically the field has gone from a situation in which it was believed that genetic factors had little importance for syndrome pathogenesis to the present situation where it appears that such factors have major importance and where specific genetic mechanisms may indeed be identified in the relatively near future. Peter Szatmari's chapter reviews this work and notes the major changes in our understanding of genetic factors in recent years; as he observes the issue today is not whether autism has a genetic basis but what that basis is.

The relevance of neurobiological factors in the pathogenesis of autism has undergone a similar transformation. At the time of his original description Kanner (1943) minimized the importance of such factors. Now it appears that such factors may be present in 10% or more of cases (Rutter et al. 1994). While the nature of such associations has been debated (Gillberg & Coleman, 1996) these do suggest important areas for research in underlying pathophysiological mechanisms. Fritz Poutska provides a critical summary of this work and notes areas in which knowledge is still lacking.

Given the severity of autism and associated conditions it is probably not surprising that essentially every conceivable intervention has been attempted. Christopher McDougle reviews the literature on pharmacological treatments. As noted in his chapter recent work suggests important potential benefits of drug treatments in selected cases.

Over the past 50 years a considerable body of data has established the centrality of intensive, structured educational intervention as the bedrock of intervention in autism. This work has its origins both in behavioural psychology and special education. As Sandra Harris notes, progress continues to be made in behavioural and educational interventions that have improved the outcome of autism and related conditions. Patricia Howlin summarizes these changes in her review of outcome studies. The child with autism or a related condition presents major challenges for parents, siblings and other family members. The improvement in outcome, however, is a major accomplishment of the past 50 years of clinical work and reflects the substantial gains in implementation of remedial programmes.

In the final chapter Lynn Waterhouse and Deborah Fein address the nature of the fundament social disturbance that characterizes autism. The centrality of social deficits in the definition of this and related conditions has repeatedly been emphasized in depictions of the disorder beginning with Kanner's initial description. Despite this we continue to have a rather limited understanding of the nature of social deficits in syndrome pathogenesis. Waterhouse and Fein provide an interesting synthesis of work in this area.

This volume provides a summary of what is known as well as what remains poorly understood. While researchers and clinicians have learned much over the past five decades of work on autism we continue to have little understanding of the nature of the autistic social dysfunction or, for that matter, of its underlying neurobiological basis. There are, however, reasons to be hopeful. Advances in treatment (both behavioural and pharmacological) have led to improved outcomes. Current work underscores the possibility that at least some form or forms of autism may have a strong genetic component and it is possible that some genetic mechanism may be described in the relatively near future, such a finding will advance research in other areas as well, as we begin to understand pathogenic mechanisms more fully. The chapters in this monograph are a testament to the advances that have been made as well as to the continuing need for research and treatment of these perplexing conditions.

I am grateful to all the chapter authors for their contributions to this volume. In addition I thank the series editors, Professors Goodyer and Parry-Jones, as well as Dr Richard Barling of Cambridge University Press, for their help and support.

Fred Volkmar MD   New Haven, CT, USA

REFERENCES

American Psychiatric Association. *Diagnostic and Statistical Manual of Mental Disorders.* Washington, DC. American Psychiatric Association, 3rd edn (DSM III), 1980, 3rd edn, revised (DSM-III-R), 1987; 4th edn (DSM-IV), 1994.

Bristol, M. M., Cohen, D. J., Costello, E. J., Denckla, M., Eckberg, T. J., Kallen, R., Kraemer, H. C., Lord, C., Maurer, R., McIlvane, W. J., Minshew, N., Sigman, M. & Spence, M. A. (1996). State of the science in autism: report to the National Institutes Health. *Journal of Autism and Developmental Disorders,* 26, 121–54.

De Sanctis, S (1906) Sopra alcune varieta della demenzi precoce. *Revista Sperimentale De Feniatria E. Di Medicina Legale,* 32, 141–65.

Gillberg, C. & Coleman, M. (1996). Autism and medical disorders: a review of the literature. *Developmental Medicine and Child Neurology,* 38, 191–202.

Kanner, L. (1943) Autistic disturbances of affective contact. *Nervous Child,* 2, 217–50.

Rutter, M., Bailey, A., Bolton, P. & Le Couter, A. (1994). Autism and known medical conditions: myth and substance. *Journal of Child Psychology and Psychiatry and Allied Disciplines,* 35, 311–22.

Volkmar, F. R. (1996), Childhood and adolescent psychosis: a review of the past 10 years. *Journal of the American Academy of Child and Adolescent Psychiatry,* 35, 843–51.

Volkmar, F. R., Klin, A., Siegel, B., Szatmari, P. et al. (1994). Field trial for autistic disorder in DSM-IV. *American Journal of Psychiatry,* 151, 1361–7.

World Health Organization. *International Statistical Classification of Diseases and Related Health Problems.* Diagnostic Criteria for Research, 10th edn (ICD-10), 1993. Geneva: World Health Organization.

1

Diagnosis and definition of autism and other pervasive developmental disorders

Fred R. Volkmar and Catherine Lord

INTRODUCTION

Autism and other pervasive developmental disorders (PDDs) are a phe-nomenologically related set of neuropsychiatric disorders. These condi-tions are characterized by patterns of both delay and deviance in multiple areas of development, typically their onset is in the first months of life. Although often associated with some degree of mental retardation, the pattern of developmental and behavioural features differs from that seen in children with mental retardation not associated with PDD in that certain sectors of development, such as social interaction and communication, are most severely effected whereas other areas, such as nonverbal cognitive abilities, may be within normal limits. While the validity of autism has been relatively well established, issues of syndrome boundaries remain the topic of some debate. In this chapter, the development of autism as a diagnostic concept, current definitions of the condition and of related diagnostic concepts, and their differentiation from other disorders will be reviewed.

DEVELOPMENT OF DIAGNOSTIC CONCEPTS

Over the past 150 years, a major point of controversy has been the continuity, or discontinuity, of the severe psychiatric disorders of child-hood with the adult psychoses. For example, the great British psychiatrist, Maudsley, suggested that children, like adults, could exhibit 'insanity' (1867). Similarly Kraepelin's concept of dementia praecox, or what we would now term schizophrenia, was extended to children (dementia praecocissima) (DeSanctis, 1906). While some investigators like Potter (1933) urged the use of more stringent definitions for childhood schizophrenia, there was a general assumption of a fundamental continuity of child and adult 'psychosis'. The presumption of continuity was based largely on the severity of these conditions with rather little appreciation of the importance of developmental factors in children's understanding of reality. These issues contributed to the confusion and controversy which surrounded Kanner's (1943) initial description of the autistic syndrome.

Kanner's description of autism

Kanner's description of 11 children with 'autistic disturbances of affective contact' was atheoretical and quite lucid. This description reflected his remarkable clinical acumen and present day definitions of the autistic syndrome remain profoundly influenced by it. Kanner noted that his patients exhibited a disorder characterized by a profound lack of social engagement from, or shortly after, their birth. Kanner noted his cases also exhibited a range of communication problems and unusual responses to the inanimate environment as well. These children might, for example, not be particularly responsive to their parents but be exquisitely sensitive to some sounds or they might have major difficulties with transitions or changes in routine. Three of the 11 children were mute, but the language of those who did speak was remarkable for echolalia, literalness and pronoun reversal.

Although not amenable to formal psychometric assessment, these children sometimes could be engaged on certain subtests of cognitive or developmental tests and might do well; because of this, and because of their usually attractive appearance, Kanner speculated that they probably had good intellectual potential. In his original report, he suggested that the disorder was different from other psychiatric conditions and not associated with specific medical conditions. Kanner also mentioned that in many instances parents, usually the fathers, were remarkably successful and that interactions with the child often seemed strange or odd; on the other hand, his emphasis on the apparently congenital nature of the problem made it difficult to attribute the disorder exclusively to parent–child disturbance.

In Kanner's view, the essential feature of autism was the children's inability to relate. He put this observation within a developmental context and also cited the work of Gessel which had shown that normally developing infants exhibit marked interest in social interaction from very early in life. Kanner's use of Bleuler's (1911/1950) term 'autism' for the idiosyncratic, self-centred thinking observed in schizophrenia was intended by Kanner to suggest the notion of the child's living in his or her own world. His use of this word and certain aspects of his original report proved to be false leads for research which impeded subsequent research.

Early studies and false leads for research

Kanner's use of the term 'autism' immediately suggested schizophrenia; this was consistent with the very broad and inclusive views of schizophrenia which then were dominant. Clinicians and researchers did not have to question long standing assumptions about severe psychiatric disturbance in children. Unfortunately, this meant that there was considerable confusion about autism with some investigators, e.g. Bender (1947), assuming continuity of 'psychotic' conditions in younger children with more typical adult forms of schizophrenia. This has proved not to be the case which makes it difficult to interpret much of the early work on autism. The issue of continuity of autism and schizophrenia was resolved only in the 1970s as the work of Kolvin (1971) and Rutter (1970) suggested important differences between the condition, e.g. in course, family history and clinical features.

As cases of autism were followed for a decade it became apparent that Kanner's original assumption that autism was not associated with any medical condition was not correct. Many children with autism exhibit signs of overt central nervous system dysfunction including, most strikingly, seizures. As many as 25% of cases developed seizures, particularly during adolescence (Rutter, 1970). Other signs of neurological function were also often observed. Some reports associated autism with diverse medical conditions including chromosomal abnormalities, prenatal infections, various brain abnormalities, and so forth. When taken together with the data on neurological dysfunction, they seemed to suggest the importance of multiple potential insults which acted through one or more mechanisms to cause autism (Rutter et al., 1994).

Similarly, Kanner's assumption that children with autism had normal intellectual potential proved mistaken. This notion was based on the accurate observation that some 'splinter skills' were often present and that the occasional individual with autism had truly unusual (and usually very isolated) abilities in one area (Treffert, 1988). It took over two decades

3

before clinicians and investigators realized that if all aspects of a test of intelligence were administered the child with autism usually scored in the mentally retarded range in terms of overall IQ. For many years, low IQ scores were mistakenly attributed to 'poor test taking' skills or willful noncompliance. In any case, the notion of preserved intellectual skills in autism endures to the present and is sometimes the basis for unproven and sometimes fraudulent treatments or the application of treatments that would be appropriate if indeed the individual functioned at a higher level.

Probably most unfortunately Kanner's's observation of high levels of parental achievement and problems in parent–child interaction led some clinicians to attribute the source of autism to problems in parent–child interaction or deficits in child care (e.g. Desperet, 1956; Bettelheim, 1967). This view was congruent with the ethos of the time which tended to minimize the importance of biological factors in psychiatric conditions. Their ideas seemed superficially consistent with the nature of the disorder, i.e. should it not be the case that a problem characterized by deficits in social interaction is caused by deficits in social interaction. As controlled studies were conducted, however, it became clear that the parents of autistic children did not exhibit greater psychopathology (Cox et al., 1975), unusual personality traits (McAdoo & DeMyer, 1978), nor were specific deficits in infant–child care noted (Cantwell et al., 1978). Similarly, studies of children reared in horribly deprived settings, e.g. in orphanages, did not reveal associations with autism. A growing appreciation of the role of the child in the parent–child interaction also suggested that it was just as reasonable to assume that deviance in such interaction might sometimes be a function of a basic disturbance in the child rather than in the parent, i.e. interactions with a child who produces highly deviant social behaviours will differ from interactions with children who do not have this disability. Similarly, the idea that parents of autistic children tended to have much higher levels of occupational and educational achievement proved mistaken. Careful studies which controlled for possible bias in case detection and referral (Schopler et al., 1980; Wing, 1980) make it clear that children with autism come from families of all backgrounds and do not show any particular social class preponderance. In retrospect, it seems quite reasonable to assume that the high levels of education in parents of Kanner's original cases resulted from an understandable referral bias, i.e. the parents who were able to locate Kanner were just those who had access to a greater array of resources.

'Nonautistic' pervasive developmental disorders

As noted above the issue of continuity of adult and child forms of schizo-phrenia was, until quite recently, a major source of confusion. Over the past century, various diagnostic concepts other than autism have been proposed for patterns of disturbance in children with severe developmental disorders. Three of these conditions are now officially recognized in both the *Diagnostic and Statistical Manual of Mental Disorders* (DSM-IV) and the *International Classification of Diseases* (ICD-10).

CHILDHOOD DISINTEGRATIVE DISORDER

Heller (1908, 1930/1969) proposed the term dementia infantilis, or what now would be termed childhood disintegrative disorder, to account for children who develop normally for some period prior to profound develop-mental regression and the development of many 'autistic like' features. This condition (also sometimes referred to as Heller's syndrome or disinte-grative psychosis), appears to be very uncommon; slightly over 100 cases have been reported since Heller's original (1908) report (Volkmar, 1997). It is, however, likely that cases have frequently been misdiagnosed (Volkmar and Rutter, 1995).

Childhood disintegrative disorder is now included in both DSM-IV and ICD-10 (Appendix 1). The condition is difficult to distinguish from autism once it develops. The pattern of onset with a dramatic developmental deterioration and the onset of various 'autistic like' behaviours in a previ-ously apparently normal child is very highly distinctive. The outcome appears to be worse than that in autism (Volkmar et al., 1997). The presumption in DSM-III and III-R had been that such cases typically resulted from the presence of a significant neuropathological process, e.g. a childhood 'dementia'; however, review of the published cases suggests that this is not the case. There is an increased rate of electroencephalographic (EEG) abnormalities and seizure disorder similar to that in autism but specific medical conditions which might account for the regression are not usually identified.

ASPERGER'S SYNDROME

In 1944, Hans Asperger, a Viennese medical student unaware of Kanner's earlier report, suggested the concept of autistic psychopathy or what is now

5

usually termed Asperger's syndrome. Asperger's description resembled that of Kanner (1943) in some ways, e.g. in the use of the word autism/ autistic, to describe marked problems in social interaction. Asperger suggested that the condition he described was seen only in males, was observed in the face of relatively strong language and cognitive skills, and tended to run in families. Unusual, idiosyncratic interests were common, e.g. affected children would have marked interests in acquiring certain kinds of knowledge. Early research on the condition was largely confined to non-English speaking Europe until Wing's (1981) influential literature review and case series. Subsequent work has yielded somewhat contradictory results (e.g. Szatmari et al., 1990; Pomeroy, 1991; Tantam, 1991); however, this may be a function of the absence, until recently, of generally recognized definitions. While the continuity of Asperger's syndrome with autism remains the topic of debate (Klin et al., 1995; Schopler, 1985) the condition has now been included in DSM-IV and ICD-10 (Appendix 1).

The overlap of Asperger's syndrome with other diagnostic concepts remains an important topic for research (e.g. Wolff & Barlow, 1979; Denckla, 1983; Klin et al., 1995). One set of issues has to do with the validity of the diagnostic concept as different from 'higher functioning autism'. Available data on this question remain somewhat contradictory, again reflecting, at least in part, the inconsistencies in approaches to diagnosis (for a review, see Klin and Volkmar, 1997). Careful reading of the original reports of Kanner (1943) and Asperger (1944; reprinted 1991) suggests several points of differentiation.

Kanner suggested that in autism the condition was congenital, Asperger thought that the syndrome he identified came to attention only after age 3 or 4 years. In Asperger's disorder language skills are usually an area of strength. In contrast even in higher functioning individuals with autism verbal skills tend not to be advanced over nonverbal ones. Several studies have suggested that different IQ profiles characterize the two conditions. Asperger's syndrome is associated with higher, often much higher, verbal IQ whereas in autism verbal IQ is either lower or roughly on a par with nonverbal IQ (Klin et al., 1995; Volkmar et al., 1994). Asperger's syndrome may also be associated with a characteristic profile on neuropsychological testing referred to as a nonverbal learning disability (Rourke, 1989; Klin et al., 1995). In the long term the question will be whether it is scientifically or clinically helpful to classify individuals with these patterns into separate categories of autism and Asperger's syndrome or whether it would be better to treat them as part of a greater continuum.

A final source of controversy and confusion arises from the numerous other concepts, developed in diverse disciplines, to characterize the nature of complex problems of social interaction and development in higher functioning individuals. Thus, terms like semantic-pragmatic processing disorder (Bishop, 1989), right hemisphere learning problems (Ellis et al., 1994), and schizoid disorder (Wolff and McGuire, 1995) have called attention to specific features that overlap with those of pervasive developmental disorders. The degree to which they represent truly separate syndromes is also an important area of study.

RETT'S SYNDROME

Rett (1966) reported an unusual syndrome, observed only in girls, where a very brief period of normal development is followed by decelerated head growth, loss of purposeful hand movements and development of severe psychomotor retardation. Although the condition differs from autism in important ways (Tsai, 1992), there is some potential for confusion with autism, particularly during the preschool years. Usually, however, the diagnosis is relatively straightforward (Hagberg et al., 1983). It was the potential for confusion with autism that led to the inclusion of Rett's syndrome in the PDD class in both ICD-10 and DSM-IV. Criteria for the condition are provided in Appendix 1.

To date, this condition has been observed only in girls. The course of the condition is quite characteristic. Various unusual behaviours (e.g. breath-holding, air swallowing) and motor problems (ataxia, apraxia) are observed and the individual becomes severely or profoundly mentally retarded (Tsai, 1992).

PERVASIVE DEVELOPMENTAL DISORDER NOT OTHERWISE SPECIFIED: ATYPICAL AUTISM

The term pervasive developmental disorder–not otherwise specified (PDD-NOS) (also referred to as atypical personality development, atypical PDD, or atypical autism) was included in DSM-IV to encompass 'sub-threshold' cases. It is intended to describe individuals who have a marked impairment of social interaction, communication and/or stereotyped behaviour patterns or interest suggestive of a pervasive developmental disorder but who do not meet the criteria for any of the formally defined disorders in that class. ICD-10 (Appendix 1) adopts a somewhat different approach in that the term can be used when a case meets behavioural criteria for autism but fails the onset criteria, or when the onset criteria are met but the behavioural criteria are not, or when individuals appear to have an 'autistic like' illness but meet neither the onset nor behavioural criteria. It seems likely that many possible subtypes are encompassed within this category (Towbin, 1997b).

The limited available evidence suggest that children with PDD-NOS probably come to professional attention rather later than is usually the case in autism but this may reflect the fact that intellectual and language skills tend to be more preserved. Some have argued that PDD-NOS and Asperger's syndrome are synonymous terms. More research on continuities of all these conditions is needed. In the DSM-IV field trial, cases with a clinical diagnosis of Asperger's differed significantly from cases with clinical diagnoses of autism and PDD-NOS/atypical autism.

APPROACHES TO THE DIAGNOSIS OF AUTISM

Definitions of autism subsequent to Kanner

The controversy surrounding the nature of autism and the dearth of careful research studies impeded progress for many years. Starting in the 1970s, however, there was a growing appreciation that autism was indeed a distinctive condition, not simply the earliest manifestation of childhood schizophrenia. For example, in a classic series of clinical studies Kolvin (1971) demonstrated that autism and childhood schizophrenia differed in clinical features, course and family history. Rutter (1970) and others also noted the high frequency of seizures and the considerable evidence for some degree of organic involvement. In addition, there was a growing tendency to de-emphasize the role of theory and establish reliable description of the syndrome in research. As a result of these developments, there were various efforts to develop guidelines for the diagnosis of autism which would facilitate research; this approach also had its parallel in the attempts in adult psychiatry to develop precise definitions of syndromes for research purposes (e.g. Spitzer et al., 1978).

Of these early attempts to develop more precise categorical definitions that of Rutter (1978) is undoubtedly the most important. This definition was fundamentally grounded in Kanner's early phenomenological description of the condition but also recognized the importance of subsequent research. Rutter suggested that there were four features essential for the diagnosis of autism: (1) an onset prior to 30 months of age, (2) impaired social development of a distinctive type which did not simply reflect any associated mental retardation, (3) impaired communicative development which again was distinctive and not simply the result of an overall cognitive delay, and (4) the presence of unusual behaviours subsumed under the concept of 'insistence on sameness', i.e. resistance to change, idiosyncratic responses to the environment, and so forth. This definition particularly shaped the first official categorical definition of autism.

Categorical definition of autism

DSM-III

In DSM-III (American Psychiatric Association, 1980), autism was accorded diagnostic status for the first time. This inclusion reflected the body of work on autism which had accumulated over the previous decade. In DSM-III, the condition, termed infantile autism, was included in a new class of disorders, the pervasive developmental disorders. Several other conditions, including a separate category for childhood onset pervasive developmental disorder and another category, termed 'residual' autism, were included in this class as well. Although the term PDD was rather cumbersome, it achieved relatively wide acceptance. The DSM-III definition of infantile autism was much influenced by Rutter's earlier work and emphasized the early onset of serious disturbances in social and communicative development and unusual patterns of environmental responsiveness. The recognition of autism in DSM-III was a major advance, as was the availability of an officially recognized definition of the condition.

Unfortunately, the other categories proposed and some of the decisions made were less constructive. Partly in response to the early confusion about autism and schizophrenia, the two conditions were made mutually exclusive. While the available data suggested that the two conditions are not, in fact, commonly associated there seems no reason why having autism would necessarily act to protect a person from subsequently developing schizophrenia. A few such cases, i.e. of individuals with autism who then also develop schizophrenia, have, in fact, been observed (Volkmar & Cohen, 1991). Similarly, the term 'residual autism' was used in cases where the individual's disorder had once met criteria for infantile autism but no longer did so. In essence, this approach reflected the fact that the criteria proposed for infantile autism did indeed emphasize the way the condition presented in early childhood, e.g. with more 'pervasive' social deficits. The system did not adequately address the fact that older children and adults continued to exhibit autism which changed somewhat in its expression over the course of development. The term 'residual' also had the most unfortunate effect of suggesting that somehow children 'outgrew' autism; this clearly is NOT the case (Cohen et al., 1987; Rumsey et al., 1985). As a result of these concerns relatively major changes were made in the definition of autism in DSM-III-R (American Psychiatric Association, 1987).

DSM-III-R

In DSM-III-R, the term pervasive developmental disorders was retained to describe the overarching diagnostic class to which autism was assigned. The more problematic diagnostic concepts, e.g. childhood onset PDD and residual autism, were eliminated. The DSM-III-R definition was specifically designed to be more developmentally oriented and to be appropriate to the entire range of syndrome expression over both age and developmental level. This was reflected in the new name 'autistic disorder' rather than the DSM-III term 'infantile autism'. DSM-III-R included more criteria and a polythetic definition; because of various concerns, age of onset was not included as an essential diagnostic features although age of onset could be specified. Criteria in DSM-III-R were arranged developmentally and grouped into three broad categories relating to: (1) social development, (2) communication and play, and (3) restricted activities and interests. This last category reflects the earlier concept of 'insistence on sameness' included in previous diagnostic schemes, e.g. Rutter (1978). For a diagnosis of autism, an individual was required to exhibit at least eight of the sixteen criteria with at least two from the social and one from each of the two remaining groups. In DSM-III-R, only autism and the 'subthreshold' category PDD-NOS were included in the PDD class.

The strong developmental orientation of DSM-III-R was a major improvement. Unfortunately, it was quickly apparent that the new scheme had resulted in a significantly broadened diagnostic concept (Volkmar et al., 1988; Factor et al., 1989; Hertzig et al., 1990). This broadening was a source of considerable concern for many reasons. The task of interpreting research using DSM-III-R would be complicated (for a discussion, see Rutter & Schopler, 1992). Differences from the pending revision of the international diagnostic system, the International Classification of Diseases (10th edition) (ICD-10; World Health Organization, 1990) were also marked.

ICD-10

The ICD-10 system provided separate clinical descriptions and research criteria. Major differences in both criteria for autism and disorders from previous diagnostic systems were noteworthy. The draft ICD-10 research definition included age of onset as an essential diagnostic feature and included more detailed and numerous criteria for autism. In addition, other disorders in the PDD class included Rett's syndrome, Asperger's syndrome, childhood disintegrative disorder (Heller's syndrome) and atypical autism, as well as the subthreshold PDD-NOS category (Rutter & Schopler, 1992).

DSM-IV

As a result of concerns about the DSM-III-R definition of autism and an awareness of the categories and criteria pending in ICD-10, a large multi-site field trial was undertaken for DSM-IV. This field trial (Volkmar et al., 1994) included ratings of nearly 1000 cases by over 100 clinicians of varying backgrounds and experience. Consistent with previous research, the DSM-III-R system was noted to have a high false positive rate, particularly in individuals with high levels of mental handicap. This was true regardless of whether DSM-III-R was compared with the clinician's best judgement (clinical diagnosis) or clinician ratings of other diagnostic criteria (e.g. for DSM-III and ICD-10), and when alternative methods of judging the probability of 'caseness' were employed. While the DSM-III definition (in its 'lifetime' sense) had some advantages, it was much less developmentally oriented than DSM-III-R. The ICD-10 system worked reasonably well but tended to err on the side of over stringency. The large number and detail of the research criteria were of concern for a system like DSM-IV which was meant for both clinical and research use. Together, recent research and data collected in the field trial indicated reductions in the number and details of the ICD-10 criteria which still yielded good results even when less experienced clinicians were using the criteria (Lord et al., 1994; Volkmar et al., 1994). Thus a modified version of the original ICD-10 draft criteria for autism was proposed for both the American (DSM-IV) and International (ICD-10) systems. Although primarily focused on the definition of autism, the results of the field trial also provided some support for the inclusion, as in ICD-10, of Rett's syndrome, childhood disintegrative disorder (Heller's syndrome) and Asperger's syndrome in the PDD class in DSM-IV.

11

The ICD-10 research definitions of autism and other pervasive developmental disorders are provided in Appendix 1. For a diagnosis of autism, a total of at least six criteria (from impairments in social interaction, communication, and restricted interests and activities) is required, with at least two social impairment criteria present. By definition, the condition must have its onset before age 3 years and not be due to either Rett's syndrome or childhood disintegrative disorder. The choice of 3 years as an arbitrary cut-off point for the onset was consistent with previous research (e.g. Harper & Williams, 1975; Rogers & DiLalla 1990) and the results of the field trial for autism (Volkmar et al., 1994) which suggested that only very rarely does a behavioural syndrome resembling autism have its onset after age 3 years. The convergence of the USA and international definitions of autism should enhance clinical work as well as research.

Dimensional approaches to diagnosis

As an alternative, and sometimes as a complement to, categorical diagnoses various diagnostic instruments, rating scales and diagnostic checklists have been devised relative to autism. These approaches have been concerned with aspects of diagnosis, assessment and behavioural characterization and have been used for both research and clinical purposes. In some instances the results of dimensional assessments can be operationalized into categorical diagnoses with some instruments, e.g. the Autism Diagnostic Interview-Revised (ADI-R) (Lord et al., 1994) explicitly 'keyed' to categorical diagnostic criteria.

Deficits in the three areas that characterize autism are affected by many factors, other than the presence of the disorder. These include chronological age, developmental level, specific language functioning and comorbidity with other disorders, such as hyperactivity or oppositional behaviour (Lord, 1991). The ability to quantify the severity of autism would be helpful both for research and for clinical communication (Lord, 1991). Often parents ask 'How severe is my child's autism?' Similarly, many questions in genetic research are dependent on an estimate of the severity of a disorder (Bolton et al., 1994); however, such estimates become very complex because of the developmental nature of autism. For example, restricted and repetitive behaviours are less common in very young (i.e. under age 3 years) autistic children, probably in part because of their mobility, access to certain events and objects and cognitive level (Lord, 1995). These behaviours appear to increase in frequency for at least a few years in preschool and then often decrease or change in nature from fascination with particular objects (e.g. stir sticks) and repetitive behaviours (e.g. lining them up) to more complicated interests and activities (e.g. an interest in astronomy or Scottish clans). Comparing the severity of these deficits becomes problematic, even if a metric of impairment of family life is used, given that families usually adjust to and have different expectations for children who are 2 years of age than for those who are 16. Choosing a particular chronological age as a standard, such as the use of the period between 4 and 5 years of age in the ADI-R (Lord et al., 1994) and having different metrics for verbal and nonverbal individuals can minimize these problems to some degree (Lord et al., 1994), but still does not control for differences in cognitive functioning. In almost every empirical study of dimensional instruments, severity of quantitative measures is highly correlated with severity of mental handicap (Lord, 1991). It is important for clinicians and researchers to be aware of this relationship in interpreting dimensional scales. This finding also implies that it is very important in interpreting psychometric data from dimensional scales to be certain that autistic and nonautistic groups are equivalent on measures such as cognitive level, language ability and chronological age before statements about the validity of cut-offs can be made. Finding such groups is not always easy.

The one clear improvement that multidimensional scales such as the ADI-R and ADOS/PL-ADOS/ADOS-G (Lord et al., 1989, 1997; Di-Lavore et al., 1995) can offer is separate documentation of the presence of abnormalities in each of the three areas that define autism: social reciprocity, communication and restricted, repetitive behaviours. With scales that produce a single score, it is possible that severe deficits in one area or two areas (e.g. sensory abnormalities and expressive language) may heighten scores sufficiently to reach a cut-off for autism, even though deficits in other areas are not marked. Having separate scores in the three areas that comprise DSM-IV and ICD-10 diagnoses allows confirmation that an individual has the specific pattern of deficits defined as autism.

There are some important issues in the development and use of dimensional assessment instruments and parent interviews. As the individual with autism may not always be amenable to direct interview, dimensional assessment instruments usually rely either on behavioural observation (in structured or unstructured situations) or parent or carer report. As aspects of syndrome expression change with age, some instruments have focused particularly on the preschool period; when the person being evaluated is older such an approach entails potential problems with the reliability of

13

parental retrospection. Some behaviours, e.g. self-injurious behaviours, may be important because of severity but may be low in frequency; this is a problem for instruments which rely exclusively on behavioural observation. Teacher reports bring other questions of reliability particularly when teachers are asked to rate behaviours which they encounter only very rarely. Unfortunately aspects of reliability and validity have not always been adequately addressed (Parks, 1983).

Rimland's (1964) diagnostic checklist for the diagnosis of autism is of considerable interest historically. It represents one of the earliest attempt to provide a more truly operational approach to diagnosis. The checklist is completed by parents and contains a set of questions about the development of the child in the first years of life. The total score is used to provide an indication of the likelihood that the person exhibits autism (Rimland, 1971). There has been concern that the questionnaire results in diagnoses that are not equivalent to standard criteria or other measures, but it was an important first step in the creation of standardized instruments in autism (Parks, 1983).

The Behaviour Rating Instrument of Autistic and Atypical Children (BRIAAC) (Ruttenberg et al., 1977) was based on observations of children with autism enrolled in a day treatment programme. Scales in this instrument are behaviourally defined and examine various domains of functioning, e.g. relationship to adult, communication, drive for mastery, vocalization and expressive speech, sound and speech reception, social responsiveness, body movement and psychobiological development. Scores on each scale range from normal to severely autistic. BRIAAC scores appear to be related to some important aspects of clinical diagnosis (Cohen et al., 1978) but are not directly comparable to current diagnostic frameworks.

The Behaviour Observation Scale for Autism (BOS) (Freeman et al., 1980) has been used for behavioural assessment and monitoring of behavioural response to intervention. A series of behaviours are evaluated during a structured period of observation. Another observational method, the Autism Diagnostic Observation Schedule (ADOS) has been developed by Lord and colleagues (Lord et al., 1989). General ratings provided better discrimination between groups of children and adolescents with autism and mild mental retardation than did coding related to specific tasks.

The Childhood Autism Rating Scale (CARS; Schopler et al., 1980) is based on observation of behaviour. A trained rater observes the child during a structured situation. Various scales are included with scores ranging on a continuum from normal to severely abnormal. It is possible to operationalize the ratings into an estimate of the severity of autism. This scale has the advantage of encompassing the age of the child and the intensity of specific behaviours that are present. Reliability and discriminant validity are good (Teal & Wiebe, 1986).

The Autism Behaviour Checklist (ABC; Krug et al., 1979, 1980) is designed for completion by teachers. It is comprised of a series of dichotomous items with items weighted relative to how strongly they predict a diagnosis of autism. The weighted items are then summed across five symptom areas and the probability that the individual exhibits autism can then be estimated. Sums of item weights within an area can also be plotted and compared with children of similar chronological age. Volkmar et al. (1987) noted that while individual item reliability was not high, the instrument had reasonable sensitivity but rather poor specificity (i.e. it accurately identifies autism in autistic individual but tends to overdiagnosis autism in individuals who do not otherwise appear to have autism).

More recently instruments have been developed which have been specifically 'keyed' to categorical diagnostic systems, e.g. the Autism Diagnostic Interview-Revised (ADI-R) (Lord et al., 1994). This instrument is a semi-structured investigator based interview. It is applicable for individuals with mental ages from 18 months to adulthood and is specifically linked to ICD-10 and DSM-IV diagnostic criteria. Data on reliability and validity of individual items has been presented and is generally very good to excellent (Lord et al., 1994). This instrument is particularly useful for research purposes and as is true for several of the dimensional instruments described here. Specific training in its administration and scoring is required.

In addition to rating scales specifically designed for individuals with autism, well-standardized assessments applicable in the general population can be used in the assessment of persons with autism. The social disability associated with autism is highly distinctive (Fein et al., 1986); there have been some attempts, using the Vineland Adaptive Behaviour Scales (Sparrow et al., 1984) to provide more dimensional assessments of social dysfunction. Volkmar et al. (1993) noted that levels of social skills could be predicted on the basis of a series of regression equations using mental or chronological age as the predictor variable; individuals with autism were much more likely to exhibit lower actual levels of social skill than would otherwise be predicted on the basis of their age or cognitive development. This approach may have particular utility for screening purposes as it relies on a well-standardized, semi-structured interview and is concerned with the acquisition of developmentally expected skills; the development of

15

supplementary norms specific to autism will also add to the usefulness of the Vineland in this population.

DIFFERENTIAL DIAGNOSIS OF AUTISM AND RELATED CONDITIONS

Autism and related pervasive developmental disorders must be differentiated from other developmental disorders such as mental retardation and language disorders as well as from sensory impairments such as deafness and, less frequently, from other conditions. The use of a developmentally oriented, multiaxial approach is always indicated as behavioural features and diagnostic criteria and guidelines are best interpreted within a developmental context. Assessments of both cognitive (verbal and nonverbal) and communicative skills are helpful and should be chosen as appropriate to the individual case. Similarly, measures of adaptive skills may provide information, such as about social skills, relevant to diagnosis and help in the formulation of remedial programmes. Any associated medical conditions should be identified. Additional medical and other investigators should usually be guided by history and examination, e.g. Fragile-X screening, neurological consultation and other assessments may be indicated. Audiological evaluation should be obtained if there is concern about the child's ability to hear. Assessment procedures are summarized in Table 1.1.

A careful history from parents significantly facilitates the diagnostic process. In taking a history, it is often helpful to frame questions about specific skills or developmental abilities around certain well-remembered times, e.g. the child's first birthday. The use of videotapes and home movies may also be helpful. The diagnosis of autism is most straightforward in instances where parents report severe problems in social interaction and communication, dating from early in the child's life. Many parents report that socially their autistic children were not obviously unusual until some time in the second year of life (Le Couteur et al., 1989). Sometimes parents give clear descriptions of marked changes in children's social behaviour sometime in their second year (such as children who spend increasing amounts of time alone or stop participating in infant social games), but many report what seems to be more a gradual stagnation of social insolvent beyond physical contact (i.e. many children continue to enjoy being tickled and roughhoused with), once their children are walking and more independently mobile.

In addition, about one-quarter of parents report that their autistic

Table 1.1. *Evaluation procedures*

1. Historical information
   Early development and characteristics of development
   Age and nature of onset
   Medical and family history

2. Psychological/communicative examination
   Estimate(s) of intellectual level (particularly nonverbal)
   Communicative assessment
     Receptive and expressive vocabulary
     Language skills
     Use of nonverbal skills and pragmatic communication
   Adaptive behaviour
   (Evaluate social and communicative skills relative to nonverbal intellectual abilities)

3. Psychiatric examination
   Nature of social relatedness
     eye contact, attachment behaviours, interest in peers
     imitation skills, style of interacting
   Behavioural features
     stereotypy/self-stimulation, resistance to change, unusual interests
     unusual sensitivities to the environment, etc.
   Play skills
     nonfunctional use of play materials
     developmental level of play activities

4. Medical evaluation
   Note associated medical conditions and risk factors including infectious, genetic, pre- and perinatal risk
   Genetic screen (chromosome analysis for fragile X) and genetic consultation if indicated
   Hearing or vision tests (if indicated)
   Consultation (neurological, occupational or physical therapy) as indicated by history and current examination
   Additional evaluations as needed (e.g. electroencephalogram, computed tomography/magnetic resonance imaging scan)

children had some words, using fewer than ten, up to the age of 12–18 months, which faded out after only a few months or sometimes weeks of appearance (Kurita, 1985; Shulman et al., 1996). In some cases, these reports may be due to parents' overly enthusiastic interpretation of their children's early babble, but in other cases, it has been possible to verify the presence of a few meaningful words around the first birthday in children who are not speaking at the time of diagnosis (at 2 or 3 years). Generally, the number of words is very small and they are present for only a period of weeks or months. Often the words are used in appropriate context (e.g. saying 'buh-buh' for bottle); sometimes they also appear to be intentional and sometimes they appear to be part of a general action routine without necessarily being used by the child for communication.

When parents report that a child loses more language than just a few words (including a larger vocabulary or some spontaneous, nonroutinized sentences) or experiences a loss closer to his or her second birthday, then consideration of the diagnosis of childhood disintegrative disorder should be made. In that condition development up to at least 2 years must be perfectly normal. This is then followed by a marked developmental regression, in multiple areas, and the gradual development of an 'autistic like' clinical picture. The regression in this condition is, however, very dramatic and understandably typically causes parents to quickly begin a search for possible medical explanations (which usually are not found). Similarly in Rett's syndrome parents will report a very early and unusual regression in their daughters; this will be associated with the loss of purposeful hand movements and head growth deceleration. While there may be some confusion with autism in the preschool years, the usual course of Rett's is quite distinctive (Tsai, 1992).

Mental retardation is present in about 75% of individuals with autism, if the results of formal assessments of nonverbal intelligence are used; if full scale scores (which include language skills) are employed the proportion of mental handicap is even higher. The frequency of autistic like symptoms (particularly stereotyped behaviours) increases with more severe retardation and may be the source of some confusion. For a diagnosis of autism to be made in an individual with profound or severe mental retardation, the clinician should be careful to evaluate the presence of social and communicative deficits relative to the person's overall intellectual level. Although these behaviours are highly associated with autism in persons who are not mentally handicapped they are much more common in individuals with severe to profound mental retardation. Thus the presence of only motor mannerisms or stereotyped behaviours does not establish a diagnosis of autism.

In childhood schizophrenia, in most instances, early and subsequent development well into the primary school years is reasonably normal (Werry, 1992). In a smaller group of cases, a longer standing pattern of neurodevelopmental disability may be present; however, in contrast to autism, marked deficits and deviance in social interaction and communication are not typical. Although differing in some respects from schizophrenia in adults, the main clinical features of schizophrenia in children and adults are quite similar, i.e. delusions, disorganized thinking, hallucinations and so forth (Werry, 1992). The onset of schizophrenia in childhood is extremely rare. Very occasionally an individual with autism, particularly during adolescence or young adulthood, may also then develop schizophrenia; in such cases, both diagnoses are made.

The differential diagnosis of Asperger's syndrome and higher functioning autism remains an area of controversy. The lack, at least until very
recently, of official guidelines for diagnosis has contributed to difficulties in
interpreting available research. Some clinicians have used the term Asperger's syndrome in ways that are essentially either synonymous with higher
functioning autism, with PDD-NOS or even with reference to adults with
autism; none of these uses add particularly to a classification system. The
use of more stringent definitions of Asperger's syndrome may help to
resolve these issues. Consistent with ICD-10 and DSM-IV, criteria cases
with Asperger's syndrome would be expected to have better language skills
than are typically observed in autism. Preliminary work (Klin et al., 1995)
does suggest that strictly defined cases of higher functioning autism and
Asperger's syndrome do differ in important respects. Cases of Asperger's
syndrome also appear to be at risk for exhibiting a particular profile of
learning disability on psychological testing. This profile of nonverbal
learning disability (Rourke, 1989) include deficits in tactile perception,
psychomotor coordination and nonverbal problem solving in the face of
well-developed rote verbal and verbal memory skills; problems in social
interaction are noted. The neuropsychological pattern associated with this
condition differs from that usually seen in autism and individuals with
autism who have higher cognitive abilities.

The PDD-NOS category's definition by exclusion is problematic (Towbin, 1997a). Essentially this category should be used when an individual
fails to meet specific criteria for autism or another explicitly defined pervasive developmental disorder but has difficulties of similar quality. Research
on this heterogeneous condition(s) has been impeded by the need for a so-
called 'subthreshold' category and its consequent intrinsic limitations.
Attempts to define and validate possible subgroups are needed.

Certain other disorders should also be considered in the differential
diagnosis of autism. In attachment disorder, children exhibit deficits in
capacities for social interaction which, by definition, arise through markedly deviant caretaking experiences, e.g. institutional rearing or severe ne-
glect. These deficits do, however, typically remit with provision of an
appropriately supportive environment. Other features typical of autism are
not present. In selective mutism, a child will speak but only in certain
situations, e.g. at home. In this condition the characteristic social disturbance observed in autism is not present and the child exhibits a wider range
of social communicative functioning than would be expected in autism.

Fred R. Volkmar and Catherine Lord

SUMMARY

Considerable progress in the diagnosis and classification of autism has occurred in the 50 years which have passed since Kanner's description of the syndrome of infantile autism. It is now clear that autism and other pervasive developmental disorders are very distinctive conditions which differ in various ways from other serious disorders of childhood. With the publication of DSM-IV and ICD-10 there has been a move towards greater uniformity in diagnostic practice which should simplify the lives of clinicians and researchers.

On the other hand the inclusion of 'new' disorders in the PDD category has been somewhat more controversial. Many of these conditions, e.g. childhood disintegrative disorder and Asperger's syndrome, have a long tradition of clinical interest and/or research as long or nearly as long as that on autism. They have, however, been more difficult to study partly because they have not been as well defined. For childhood disintegrative disorder the rational for inclusion of this condition has less to do with the frequency of the disorder and more to do with its possible implication for research. For Rett's syndrome the various differences from autism are clear but inclusion in the PDD class has seemed justified given the potential for confusion with autism in the preschool years. While some have argued that Rett's might best be thought of as a 'neurological' (i.e. as opposed to a psychiatric) disorder the same argument could just as reasonably be made for autism, i.e. nearly a quarter of cases will develop seizures, various (if usually nonspecific) neurological signs are present, and so forth.

The inclusion of Asperger's in both DSM-IV and ICD-10 has been more controversial. Particularly in the USA the tendency has been to equate this condition either with higher functioning autism, with the 'subthreshold' category of PDD-NOS, or sometimes with adult autism. From the point of view of nomenclature these uses of the term are not particularly relevant or interesting, i.e. only if the condition differs in some important ways (other than those central to the definition) is the disorder of interest from the point of view of clinical work and research. While preliminary work suggests this is the case the final word is not yet in and it indeed may be that the concept will undergo further refinement or even that it may eventually be abandoned if it does not significantly add to our nomenclature.

For PDD-NOS there is a striking paradox that this condition is probably much more common than the other conditions included in the PDD class but the condition is much less frequently studied. The dearth of studies reflects, at least in part, the 'nondefinition' definition which has been employed as well as the vicissitudes, in these days of tight research funding, of gaining support for the study of a very poorly defined condition. Indeed it is likely that multiple conditions are presently subsumed within this unitary term and a major goal for the next decade will be to identify meaningful subgroups within it.

REFERENCES

American Psychiatric Association. (1980). *Diagnostic and Statistical Manual of Mental Disorders*, 3rd edn. Washington, DC: APA.

American Psychiatric Association. (1987). *Diagnostic and Statistical Manual of Mental Disorders*, 3rd edn. revised. Washington, DC: APA.

American Psychiatric Association. (1994). *Diagnostic and Statistical Manual of Mental Disorders*, 4th edn. Washington, DC: APA.

Asperger, H. (1944/1991). Autistic psychopathy in childhood (translated by Uta Frith). In *Autism and Asperger's syndrome*, ed. Cambridge: U. Frith, Cambridge University Press.

Bettelheim, B. (1967). *The Empty Fortress*. New York: Free Press.

Bender, L. (1947). Childhood schizophrenia: clinical study of one hundred schizophrenic children. *American Journal of Orthopsychiatry*, **17**, 40–56.

Bishop, D. V. (1989). Autism, Asperger's syndrome, and semantic-pragmatic disorder: where are the boundaries? Special issue on autism. *British Journal of Communication*, **24**, 102–21.

Bleuler, E. (1911/1950). *Dementia praecox oder Gruppe der Schizophrenien* (J. Zinkin, Trans.). New York: International Universities Press (originally published 1911).

Bolton, P., Macdonald, H., Pickles, A., Rios, P., Goode, S., Crowson, M., Bailey, A. & Rutter, M. (1994). A case-control family history study of autism. *Journal of Child Psychology and Psychiatry*, **35**, 877–900.

Cantwell, D., Rutter, M. & Baker, L. (1978) Family factors. In *Autism: a Reappraisal of Concepts and Treatment*, ed. M. Rutter and E. Schopler. New York: Plenum.

Cohen, D. J., Caparulo, B., Gold, J., Waldo, M., Shaywitz, B., Ruttenberg, B. & Rimland, B. (1978). Agreement in diagnosis: clinical assessment and behaviour rating scales for pervasively disturbed children. *Journal of the American Academy of Child Psychiatry*, **17**, 689–95.

Cohen, D. J., Paul, R. & Volkmar, F. R. (1987). Issues in the classification of pervasive developmental disorders and associated conditions. In *Handbook of Autism and Pervasive Developmental Disorders*. ed. D. Cohen and A. Connellan. New York: Wiley.

Cox, A., Rutter, M., Newman, S. & Bartak, L. A. (1975). A comparative study of infantile autism and specific developmental receptive language disorder. I. Parental characteristics. *British Journal of Psychiatry*, **126**, 146–59.

Denckla, M. (1983). The neuropsychology of social-emotional learning disabilities. *Archives of Neurology*, **40**, 461–2.

DeSanctis, S. (1906). Sopra alcune varieta della demenza precoce. *Rivista Sperimentale De Feniantria E. Di Medicina Legale*, **32**, 141–65.

Desperet, J. (1956). Some considerations relating to the genesis of autistic behaviour in children. *American Journal of Orthopsychiatry*, **20**, 335–50.

DiLavore, P., Lord, C. & Rutter, M. (1995). Pre-linguistic Autism Diagnostic Observation Schedule (PL-ADOS). *Journal of Autism and Developmental Disorders*, **25**, 355–79.

21

Ellis, H. D., Ellis, D. M., Fraser, W. & Deb, S. (1994). A preliminary study of right hemisphere cognitive deficits and impaired social judgements among young people with Asperger syndrome. *European Child & Adolescent Psychiatry*, **3**, 255–66.

Factor, D. C., Freeman, N. L. and Kardash, A. (1989). A comparison of DSM-III and DSM-III-R criteria for autism. *Journal of Autism and Developmental Disorders*, **19**, 637–40.

Fein, D., Pennington, B., Markowitz, P., Braverman, M. & Waterhouse, L. (1986). Towards a neuropsychological model of infantile autism: are the social deficits primary? *Journal of the American Academy of Child Psychiatry*, **25**, 198–212.

Freeman, B. J., Schroth, P., Ritvo, E., Guthrie, D. & Wake, L. (1980). The behaviour observation scale for autism (BOS): Initial results of factor analyses. *Journal of Autism and Developmental Disorders*, **10**, 343–6.

Hagberg, B., Aicardi, J., Dias, K. & Ramos, O. (1983). A progressive syndrome of autism, dementia, ataxia and loss of purposeful hand use in girls: Rett's syndrome: report of 35 cases. *Annals of Neurology*, **14**, 471–9.

Harper, J. & Williams, S. (1975). Age and type of onset as critical variables in early infantile autism. *Journal of Autism and Childhood Schizophrenia*, **5**, 25–35.

Heller, T. (1908). Dementia infantilis. *Zeitschrift fur die Erforschung und Behandlung des Jungenlichen Schwachsinns*, **2**, 141–65.

Heller, T. (1930). Uber Dementia infantalis. *Zeitschrift fur Kinderforschung*, **37**, 661–7. Reprinted in *Modern Perspective in International Child Psychiatry*, ed. J. G. Howells. Edinburgh: Oliver & Boyd, 1969.

Hertzig, M., Snow, M., New, E. & Shapiro, T. (1990). DSM-III and DSM-III-R diagnosis of autism and PDD in nursery school children. *Journal of the American Academy of Child Psychiatry*, **29**, 123–6.

Kanner, L. (1943). Autistic disturbances of affective contact. *Nervous Child*, **2**, 217–50.

Klin, A. & Volkmar, F. R. (1997). Asperger syndrome. In *Handbook of Autism and Pervasive Developmental Disorders*, ed. D. J. Cohen & F. R. Volkmar, 2nd edn, pp. 94–122. New York: Wiley & Sons.

Klin, A., Volkmar, F. R., Sparrow, S. S., Cicchetti, D. V. & Rourke, B. P. (1995). Validity and neuropsychological characterization of Asperger's syndrome. *Journal of Child Psychology and Psychiatry*, **36**, 1127–40.

Kolvin, I. (1971). Studies in childhood psychoses. I. Diagnostic criteria and classification. *British Journal of Psychiatry*, **118**, 381–4.

Krug, D. A., Arick, J. R. & Almond, P. J. (1979). Autism screening instrument for educational planning: background and development. In *Autism: Diagnosis Instruction, Management and Research*, ed. J. Gilliam. Austin: University of Texas at Austin Press, 1979.

Krug, D. A., Arick, J. & Almond, P. (1980). Behaviour checklist for identifying severely handicapped individuals with high levels of autistic behaviour. *Journal of Child Psychology and Psychiatry*, **21**, 221–9.

Kurita, H. (1985). Infantile autism with speech loss before the age of 30 months. *Journal of the American Academy of Child and Adolescent Psychiatry*, **24**, 191–6.

Le Couteur, A., Rutter, M., Lord, C. & Rios, P. E. A. (1989). Autism Diagnostic Interview: a standardized investigator-based. *Journal of Autism and Developmental Disorders*, **19**, 363–87.

Lord, C. (1991). Methods and measures of behaviour in the diagnosis of autism and related disorders. *Psychiatric Clinics of North America*, **14**, 69–80.

Lord, C. (1995). Follow-up of two-year-olds referred for possible autism. *Journal of Child Psychology and Psychiatry*, **36**, 1365–82.

Lord, C., Rutter, M., Goode, S., Hemmsbergen, J., Jordan, H., Mawhood, L. & Schopler, E. (1989). Autism Diagnostic Observation Schedule: a standardized observation of communicative and social behaviour. *Journal of Autism and Developmental Disorders,* **19**, 185–212.

Lord, C., Rutter, M., Goode, S., Heemesbergen, J. (1989). Autism Diagnostic Observation Schedule: a standardized observation of communicative and social behaviour. *Journal of Autism and Developmental Disorder,* **19**, 185–212.

Lord, C., Rutter, M. & Le Couteur, A. (1994). Autism Diagnostic Interview-Revised: a revised version of a diagnostic interview for caregivers of individuals with possible pervasive developmental disorder. *Journal of Autism and Developmental Disorders,* **24**, 659–85.

Lord, C., Rutter, M. & DiLavore, P. (1997). *Autism Diagnostic Observation Schedule-Generic (ADOS-G)*. The Psychological Corporation.

McAdoo, W. G. & DeMyer, M. K. (1978). Personality characteristics of parents. In *Autism: a Reappraisal of Concepts and Treatment,* ed. M. Rutter & E. Schopler. New York: Plenum.

Maudsley, H. (1867) *The Physiology and Pathology of the Mind.* Macmillan: London.

Parks, S. L. (1983). The assessment of autistic children: a selective review of available instruments. *Journal of Autism and Developmental Disorders,* **13**, 255–67.

Pomeroy, J. D. (1991). Autism and Asperger's: same or different? *Journal of the American Academy of Child and Adolescent Psychiatry,* **30**, 152–3.

Potter, H. W. (1933). Schizophrenia in children. *American Journal of Psychiatry,* **89**, 1253–70.

Rett, A. (1966). Uber ein eigenartiges hirntophisces Syndrome bei Hyperammonie im Kindersalter. *Wein Medizinische Wochenschrift,* **118**, 723–6.

Rimland, B. (1964). *Infantile Autism: the Syndrome and its Implications for a Neural Theory of Behaviour.* New York: Appleton-Century-Crofts.

Rimland, B. (1971). The differentiation of childhood psychoses: an analysis of checklists for 2218 psychotic children. *Journal of Autism and Childhood Schizophrenia,* **1**, 161–74.

Rogers, S. J. & DiLalla, D. L. (1990). Age of symptom onset in young children with pervasive developmental disorder. *Journal of the American Academy of Child and Adolescent Psychiatry,* **29**, 863–72.

Rourke, B. P. (1989). *Nonverbal Learning Disabilities: The Syndrome and the Model.* New York: Guilford.

Rumsey, J. M., Rapoport, J. L. & Scerry, W. R. (1985). Autistic children as adults: psychiatric, social and behavioural outcomes. *Journal of the American Academy of Child Psychiatry,* **24**, 465–73.

Ruttenberg, B. A., Kalish, B. I., Wenar, C. & Wolf, E. G. (1977). *Behaviour rating instrument of autistic and other atypical children* (Revised edn.) Philadelphia: Developmental Center for Autistic Children.

Rutter, M. (1970). Autistic children: infancy to adulthood. *Seminars in Psychiatry,* **2**, 435–50.

Rutter, M. (1972). Childhood schizophrenia reconsidered. *Journal of Autism and Childhood Schizophrenia,* **2**, 315–38.

Rutter, M. (1978). Diagnosis and definition. In *Autism: a Reappraisal of Concepts and Treatment,* ed. M. Rutter and E. Schopler. New York: Plenum Press.

Rutter M., Bailey, A., Bolton, P. & Le Couteur, A. (1994). Autism and known medical conditions: myth and substance. *Journal of Child Psychology and Psychiatry,* **35**, 311–22.

Rutter, M. & Schopler, E. (1992). Classification of pervasive developmental disorders: some concepts and practical considerations. *Journal of Autism and Developmental Disorders,* **22**, 459–82.

Schopler, E. (1985). Convergence of learning disability, higher-level autism, and Asperger's syndrome. *Journal of Autism and Developmental Disorders*, **15**, 359.

Schopler, E., Andrews, C. E. & Strupp, K. (1980). Do autistic children come from upper middle-class parents? *Journal of Autism and Developmental Disorders*, **10**, 91–103.

Schopler, E., Reichler, R. J., DeVellis, R. F. & Daly, K. (1980). Toward objective classification of childhood autism: childhood autism rating scale (CARS). *Journal of Autism and Developmental Disorders*, **10**, 91–103.

Shulman, C., Lord, C. & DiLavore, P. (1996). Early loss of language in the autism spectrum. *Poster presented at the meeting of the International Society for the Study of Behaviour Development*, Quebec City.

Sparrow, S., Balla, D & Ciccheti, D. (1984). *Vineland Adaptive Behaviour Scales*. Circle Pines, Minnesota: American Guidance Service.

Spitzer, R. L., Endicott, J. R. & Robins, E. (1978). Research diagnostic criteria. *Archives of General Psychiatry*, **25**, 773–82.

Spitzer, R. & Williams, J. B. W. (1988). Having a dream: a research strategy for DSM-IV. *Archives of General Psychiatry*, **45**, 871–4.

Szatmari, P., Tuff, L., Finlayson, M. A. J. & Bartolucci, G. (1990). Asperger's syndrome and autism: neurocognitive aspects. *Journal of the American Academy of Child and Adolescent Psychiatry*, **29**, 130–6.

Tantam, D. (1991). *Asperger's syndrome in adulthood*. In *Autism and Asperger's Syndrome*, ed. U. Frith. Cambridge: Cambridge University Press.

Teal, M. B. & Wiebe, M. J. (1986). A validity analysis of selected instruments used to assess autism. *Journal of Autism & Developmental Disorders*, **16**, 485–94.

Towbin, K. E. (1997a). Pervasive developmental disorder not otherwise specified: a review and guidelines for clinical care. *Child and Adolescent Psychiatric Clinics of North America*, **3**, 149–60.

Towbin, K. E. (1997b). Pervasive developmental disorder not otherwise specified. In *Handbook of Autism and Pervasive Developmental Disorders*, ed. D. J. Cohen & F. R. Volkmar, 2nd edn. pp. 123–147. New York: John Wiley.

Treffert, D. A. (1988). The idiot savant: a review of the syndrome. *American Journal of Psychiatry*, **145**, 565–72.

Tsai, L. (1992). Is Rett's syndrome a subtype of pervasive developmental disorder? *Journal of Autism and Developmental Disorders*, **22**, 551–62.

Volkmar, F. R. (1997). Childhood disintegrative disorders. In *DSM-IV Source Book*, ed. A. J. F. T. A. Widiger, H. A. Pincus, R. Ross, M. B. First, W. Davis, vol. 3, pp. 35–42. Washington, DC: American Psychiatric Association Press.

Volkmar, F. R., Cohen, D. J., Hoshino, Y. & Rende, R. D. E. A. (1988). Phenomenology and classification of the childhood psychoses. *Psychological Medicine*, **18**, 191–201.

Volkmar, F. R. & Cohen, D. J. (1991). Co-morbid association of autism and schizophrenia. *American Journal of Psychiatry*, **148**, 1705–7.

Volkmar, F. R., Cicchetti, D. V., Dykens, E., Sparrow, S., Leckman, J. F. & Cohen, D. J. (1987). An evaluation of the Autism Behaviour Checklist. *Journal of Autism and Developmental Disorders*, **18**, 81–97.

Volkmar, F. R., Carter, A., Sparrow, S. S. & Cicchetti, D. V. (1993). Quantifying social development in autism. *Journal of the American Academy of Child and Adolescent Psychiatry*, **32**, 627–32.

Volkmar, F. R., Klin, A., Marans, W. & Cohen, D. J. (1997). Childhood disintegrative disorder. In *Handbook of Autism and Pervasive Developmental Disorders*, 2nd edn, pp. 47–59). New York: John Wiley.

Volkmar, F. R., Klin, A., Siegel, B., et al. (1994). Field Trial for Autistic Disorder in DSM-IV. *American Journal of Psychiatry*, **151**, 1361–7.

Volkmar, F. R. & Rutter, M. (1995). Childhood disintegrative disorder: results of the DSM-IV Autism Field Trial. *Journal of the American Academy of Child and Adoles-*

cent Psychiatry, **34**, 1092–5.

Werry, J. (1992). Child and adolescent (early onset) schizophrenia: a review in light of DSM-III-R. *Journal of Autism and Developmental Disorders*, **22**, 601–24.

Wing, L. (1980). Childhood autism and social class: a question of selection? *British Journal of Psychiatry*, **137**, 410–17.

Wing, L. (1981). Asperger's syndrome: a clinical account. *Psychological Medicine*, **11**, 115–29.

Wolff, S. & Barlow, A. (1979). Schizoid personality in childhood: a comparative study of schizoid, autistic, and normal children. *Journal of Child Psychology and Psychiatry*, **20**, 29–46.

Wolff, S. & McGuire, R. J. (1995). Schizoid personality in girls: a follow-up study: What are the links with Asperger's syndrome? *Journal of Child Psychology and Psychiatry and Allied Disciplines*, **36**, 793–817.

World Health Organization. (1990). *International Classification of Diseases, 10th edn.* Diagnostic Criteria for Research (draft). Geneva: WHO.

25

Appendix

ICD-10 Research Diagnostic Criteria*

PERVASIVE DEVELOPMENTAL DISORDERS

Childhood Autism (F84.0)

A. Abnormal or impaired development is evident before the age of 3 years in at least one of the following areas:
    (1) receptive or expressive language as used in social communication,
    (2) the development of selective social attachments or of reciprocal social interaction,
    (3) functional or symbolic play.

B. A total of at least six symptoms from (1), (2) and (3) must be present, with at least two from (1) and at least one from each of (2) and (3)
    (1) Qualitative impairment in social interaction are manifest in at least two of the following areas:
        (a) failure adequately to use eye-to-eye gaze, facial expression, body postures and gestures to regulate social interaction,
        (b) failure to develop (in a manner appropriate to mental age, and despite ample opportunities) peer relationships that involve a mutual sharing of interests, activities and emotions,
        (c) lack of socioemotional reciprocity as shown by an impaired or deviant response to other people's emotions; or lack of modulation of behaviour according to social context; or a weak integration of social, emotional, and communicative behaviours.
        (d) lack of spontaneous seeking to share enjoyment, interests or achievements with other people (e.g. a lack of showing, bringing or pointing out to other people objects of interest to the individual).
    (2) Qualitative abnormalities communication as manifest in at least one of the following areas:

* Reprinted, with permission, from World Health Organization, *Disorders of Psychological Development* (*Criteria for Research*) (1993). Geneva: WHO, pp. 154–5.

    (a) delay in or total lack of, development of spoken language that is *not* accompanied by an attempt to compensate through the use of gestures or mime as an alternative mode of communication (often preceded by a lack of communicative babbling);

    (b) relative failure to initiate or sustain conversational interchange (at whatever level of language skill is present), in which there is reciprocal responsiveness to the communications of the other person;

    (c) stereotyped and repetitive use of language or idiosyncratic use of words or phrases;

    (d) lack of varied spontaneous make-believe play or (when young) social imitative play.

(3) Restricted, repetitive, and stereotyped patterns of behaviour, interests and activities are manifested in at least one of the following:

    (a) an encompassing preoccupation with one or more stereotyped and restricted patterns of interest that are abnormal in content or focus; or one or more interests that are abnormal in their intensity and circumscribed nature though not in their content or focus;

    (b) apparently compulsive adherence to specific, nonfunctional routines or rituals;

    (c) stereotyped and repetitive motor mannerisms that involve either hand or finger flapping or twisting or complex whole body movements:

    (d) preoccupations with part-objects or non-functional elements of play materials (such as their odour, the feel of their surface, or the noise or vibration they generate).

    (e) The clinical picture is not attributable to the other varieties of pervasive developmental disorders; specific development disorder of receptive language (F80.2) with secondary socioemotional problems' reactive attachment disorder (F94.1) or disinhibited attachment disorder (F94.2); mental retardation (F70-F72) with some associated emotional or behavioural disorders; schizophrenia (F20.-) of unusually early onset; and Rett's syndrome (F84.12).

F84.1 Atypical autism

A.   Abnormal or impaired development is evident at or after the age of 3 years (criteria as for autism except for age of manifestation).

B.   There are qualitative abnormalities in reciprocal social interaction or in communication, or restricted, repetitive and stereotyped patterns of behaviour, interests and activities. (Criteria as for autism except that it is unnecessary to meet the criteria for number of areas of abnormality.)

C.   The disorder does not meet the diagnostic criteria for autism (F84.0). Autism may be atypical in either age of onset (F84.10) or symptomatology (F84.11); the two types are differentiated with a fifth character for research purposes. Syndromes that are typical in both respects should be coded F84.12.

F84.10 Atypicality in age of onset

A. The disorder does not meet criterion A for autism (F84.0); i.e. abnormal or impaired development is evident only at or after age 3 years.
B. The disorder meets criteria B and C for autism (F84.0).

F84.11 Atypicality in symptomatology

A. The disorder meets criterion A for autism (F84.0); that is abnormal or impaired development is evident before age 3 years.
B. There are qualitative abnormalities in reciprocal social interactions or in communication, or restricted, repetitive and stereotyped patterns of behaviour, interests and activities. (Criteria as for autism except that it is unnecessary to meet the criteria for number of areas of abnormality.)
C. The disorder meets criterion C for autism (F84.0).
D. The disorder does not fully meet criterion B for autism (F84.0).

F84.12 Atypicality in both age of onset and symptomatology

A. The disorder does not meet criterion A for autism (F84.0); i.e. abnormal or impaired development is evident only at or after age 3 years.
B. There are qualitative abnormalities in reciprocal social interactions or in communication, or restricted, repetitive and stereotyped patterns of behaviour, interests and activities. (Criteria as for autism except that it is unnecessary to meet the criteria for number of areas of abnormality.)
C. The disorder meets criterion C for autism (F84.0).
D. The disorder does not fully meet criterion B for autism (F84.0).

Rett's syndrome

A. There is an apparently normal prenatal and perinatal period *and* apparently normal psychomotor development through the first 5 months *and* normal head circumference at birth.
B. There is deceleration of head growth between 5 months and 4 years *and* loss of acquired purposeful hand skills between 5 and 30 months of age that is associated with concurrent communication dysfunction and impaired social interactions and the appearance of poorly coordinated/unstable gait and/or trunk movements.

C.   There is severe impairment of expressive and receptive language, together with severe psychomotor retardation.

D.   There are stereotyped midline hand movements (such as hand-wringing or 'hand-washing') with an onset at or after the time when purposeful hand movements are lost.

F84.3 Other childhood disintegrative disorder

A.   Development is apparently normal up to the age of at least 2 years. The presence of normal age-appropriate skills in communication, social relationships, play and adaptive behaviour at age 2 years or later is required for diagnosis.

B.   There is a definite loss of previously acquired skills at about the time of onset of the disorder. The diagnosis requires a clinically significant loss of skills (not just a failure to use them in certain situations) in at least two of the following areas:
   (1) expressive or receptive language;
   (2) play;
   (3) social skills or adaptive behaviour;
   (4) bowel or bladder control;
   (5) motor skills.

C.   Qualitatively abnormal social functioning is manifest in at least two of the following areas:
   (1) qualitative abnormalities in reciprocal social interaction (of the type defined for autism);
   (2) qualitative abnormalities in communication (of the type defined for autism);

F84.4 Asperger's syndrome

A.   There is no clinically significant general delay in spoken or receptive language or cognitive development. Diagnosis requires that single words should have developed by 2 years of age or earlier and that communicative phrases be used by 3 years of age or earlier. Self-help skills, adaptive behaviour and curiosity about the environment during the first 3 years should be at a level consistent with normal intellectual development. However, motor milestones may be somewhat delayed and motor clumsiness is usual (although not a necessary diagnostic feature). Isolated special skills, often related to abnormal preoccupations, are common, but are not required for the diagnosis.

B.   There are qualitative abnormalities in reciprocal social interaction (criteria as for autism).

C.   The individual exhibits an unusual intense, circumscribed interest or restricted, repetitive and stereotyped patterns of behaviour interests and activities (criteria as for autism;* however it would be less usual for these to include either motor mannerisms or preoccupations with part-objects or nonfunctional elements of play materials).

D.   The disorder is not attributable to other varieties of pervasive developmental disorder; simple schizophrenia schizotypal disorder; obsessive-compulsive disorder; anakastic personality disorder; reactive and disinhibited attachment disorders of childhood.

DSM-IV CRITERIA FOR AUTISTIC DISORDER (299.0)*

A.   A total of at least six items from (1), (2) and (3), with at least two from (1), and one each from (2) and (3):

(1) Qualitative impairment in social interaction, as manifested by at least two of the following:
    (a) marked impairment in the use of multiple nonverbal behaviours such as eye-to-eye gaze, facial expression, body postures, and gestures to regulate social interaction,
    (b) failure to develop peer relationships appropriate to developmental level,
    (c) markedly impaired expression of pleasure in other people's happiness,
    (d) lack of social or emotional reciprocity,

(2) Qualitative impairments in communication as manifested by at least one of the following:
    (a) delay in or total lack of the development of spoken language (not accompanied by an attempt to compensate through alternative modes of communication such as gestures or mime)
    (b) in individuals with adequate speech, marked impairment in the ability to initiate or sustain a conversation with others
    (c) stereotyped and repetitive use of language or idiosyncratic language
    (d) lack of varied spontaneous make-believe play or social imitative play appropriate to developmental level

(3) Restricted repetitive and stereotyped patterns of behaviour, interests and activities, as manifested by at least one of the following:
    (a) encompassing preoccupation with one or more stereotyped and restricted patterns of interest that is abnormal either in intensity or focus.
    (b) apparently compulsive adherence to specific, nonfunctional routines or rituals
    (c) stereotyped and repetitive motor mannerisms (e.g. hand or finger flapping or twisting, or complex whole body movements)
    (d) persistent preoccupation with parts of objects

B.   Delays or abnormal functioning in at least one of the following areas, with onset prior to age three: (1) social interaction, (2) language as used in social communication, or (3) symbolic or imaginative play.

C.   Not better accounted for by Rett's disorder or childhood disintegrative disorder.

*Reprinted with permission from the *Diagnostic and Statistical Manual of Mental Disorders*, Fourth Edition. Copyright 1994 American Psychiatric Association.

2

Epidemiological surveys of autism

Eric Fombonne

INTRODUCTION

Epidemiology is the discipline which is concerned with patterns of disease occurrence in human populations and by the factors which influence these patterns of occurrence. Typical study designs are the follow-up study and the case control study depending upon whether subjects are ascertained according to their exposure or disease status. Cross-sectional or prevalence studies are based on general population samples and characterized by the fact that both disease and exposure status are determined contemporaneously. Epidemiological investigations of psychiatric disorders have often started with cross-sectional surveys which provide useful information on the patterns of risk factors or correlates of the disorder among representative samples. In addition, these surveys are relevant to public health and services planning in portraying the needs that various professional groups have to meet. In autism, epidemiological surveys started in the mid-1960s in England (Lotter, 1966) and have since been conducted in many countries. This chapter provides an up to date review of the methodological features and substantive results of these studies.

SELECTION OF STUDIES

The studies were identified through systematic searches from the major scientific literature databases and from prior reviews (Zahner & Pauls, 1987; Wing, 1993). Only studies published in the English language were included in this review. This led to the exclusion of several questionnaire based studies or of small scale investigations published in the national literature of the relevant countries (Haga and Miyamoya, 1971; Nakai, 1971; Ishii and Takahashi, 1983; Aussilloux et al., 1989; Herder, 1993) and, most certainly, of other studies unknown to the author. Overall, 19 studies published over a 30 year period were selected which surveyed autism in clearly demarcated, nonoverlapping samples. They are listed in Table 2.1 by order of their appearance in the literature. Studies are numbered from one to 19, and these numbers are subsequently used in Tables 2.2 to 2.7, as well as in the text, to index each study. For several studies, the publication listed in Table 2.1 is the most detailed account or the earliest one; however, other published articles were used to extract relevant information from the same study, when appropriate. In the particular case of studies conducted in Göteborg by Gillberg and colleagues (Gillberg, 1984; Steffenburg and Gillberg, 1986; Gillberg et al., 1991), the examination of the samples studied in each of these three reports showed that there was a partial sample overlap between the first and the second report, and that the sample of the second report was included in the sample of the third report. Accordingly, only the last report (Gillberg et al., 1991) was taken into consideration for this review. It is worth noting that the prevalence estimate from this last report is both the highest and the most recent.

The surveys were conducted in ten countries and half of the results have been published during the last decade. Details on the precise sociodemographic composition and economical activities of the area surveyed in each study were generally lacking, as for example the exact proportion of children from immigrant families. The age range of the population included in the surveys is spread from birth to early adult life although the median age of 17 samples was comprised between 5 and 12 years, with an overall median age of 9 years across studies. Similarly, there is huge variation in the size of the populations surveyed with a median population size of 78 106 subjects (mean = 210 694) and about half of the studies relying on targeted populations ranging in size from 40 000 to 275 000. The total number of children surveyed is just above four million.

STUDY DESIGNS

The case finding techniques and case definition adopted in each study are presented in Table 2.2. Most investigations have relied on a two stage or multistage approach to identify cases in underlying populations. The first

Table 2.1. Description of the studies

No.	Year of publication	Authors	Country	Region/State province	Area	Year of data collection	Age group (years)	Size of target population	Proportion of immigrants
1.	1966	Lotter	UK	Middlesex	Mainly urban	1964	8–10	78 000	DK
2.	1970	Brask	Denmark	Aarhus county	Mostly urban	1962	2–14	46 500	DK
3.	1970	Treffert	USA	Wisconsin	Rural (36%) + urban (64%)	1962–67	3–12	899 750	DK
4.	1976	Wing et al.	UK	Camberwell	Urban	1970–72	5–14	25 000	Substantial minority of West Indian families
5.	1982	Hoshino et al.	Japan	Fukushima-Ken	Mixed	1977–79	0–18	609 848	DK
6.	1983	Bohman et al.	Sweden	County of Västerborren	Rural	1979	0–20	69 000	DK
7.	1984	McCarthy et al.	Ireland	East	—	1978	8–10	65 000	DK
8.	1986	Steinhausen et al.	Germany	West Berlin	Urban	1982	0–14	279 616	DK
9.	1987	Burd et al.	USA	North Dakota	—	DK	2–18	180 986	DK
10.	1987	Matsuishi et al.	Japan	Kurume City	—	1983	4–12	32 834	DK
11.	1988	Tanoue et al.	Japan	Southern Ibaraki	Rural	1977–85	7	95 394	Very low
12.	1988	Bryson et al.	Canada	Part of Nova Scotia	Suburban and rural	1985	6–14	20 800	Very low
13.	1989	Sugiyama & Abe	Japan	Nagoya	Urban	1979–84	3	12 263	DK
14.	1989	Cialdella & Mamelle	France	One department (Rhône)	Urban	1986	3–9	135 180	DK
15.	1989	Ritvo et al.	USA	Utah	Mixed	1984–88	3–27	769 620	DK
16.	1991	Gillberg et al.	Sweden	Southwest Gothenburg + Bohuslän county	Mixed	1984–88	4–13	78 106	DK

17.	1992	Fombonne & du Mazaubrun	France	Four regions 14 departments	Mixed	1985	9 and 13 year olds	274 816	DK
18.	1992	Wignyosumarto et al.	Indonesia	Yogyakarita (southeast of Jakarta)	—	1991	4–7	5120	DK
19.	1997	Fombonne et al.	France	Three 'départements'	Mixed	1992–93	8–16	325 347	DK

DK: do not know

Table 2.2. *Case identification and case definition methods*

	Screening					Intensive assessment					
No. Instrument	Informants	Refusal rate (%)	Reliability (%)	Number Selected	Number Assessed	Participation rate (%)	Informants	Instruments	Diagnostic criteria	Reliability
1. 22 items behaviour questionnaire	All sources (teachers + child guidance clinics) + systematic screening of records of handicapped children	3[b] 23.7[b]	>87	135	124	92.5	Prof Ch Rec Par	Multistage (children interview + tests) + parent interview + records	Rating scale	No
2. Inspection of case notes	Psychiatric hospital, institutions, medical wards	—	—	—	60	—	Rec Prof	Review of all records + interview of professionals	Clinical	No
3. Computer search of clinical attenders with a DSM-III diagnosis of childhood schizophrenia	Administrative data from clinics and hospitals	—	—	280	69	—	Rec	Review of diagnostic notes	Kanner	No

4. 15 items interview[c]	Teachers, speech therapists, observations	—	—	—	108	108	—	Rec Prof Par Ch	Interview of professionals or parents, psychological tests	24 items rating scale of Lotter	90
5. Questionnaire requesting behavioural descriptions	Normal and special schools, medical and welfare institutions	No	27.4	No	397	386	97.2	Par Ch	Parent and child interview	Kanner's criteria	No
6. Two-stage screening questionnaire + follow-up telephone interview	716 professionals	No	25	No	72	?	?	Par Ch Rec	Clinical	Rutter criteria[a]	No
7. Letter + follow-up telephone calls	Psychiatrists + special schools	No	—	No	—	28	—	Ch Rec Pro	Observation + review of all data	Kanner	No
8. Direct identification of children already known to child psychiatry clinics, or attending an Autistic Society educational programme	Local professionals	No	—	No	53	52	98	Rec	Review of available data	Rutter	No

Table 2.2. (cont.)

No. Instrument	Screening			Number		Participation rate (%)	Intensive assessment			
	Informants	Refusal rate (%)	Reliability (%)	Selected	Assessed		Informants	Instruments	Diagnostic criteria	Reliability
9. Letter with behavioural descriptors derived from DSM-III + telephone calls	All schools and health professionals + parent association	<1	No	—	>200	?	Par Ch Rec	Structured parental interview + review all data available	DSM-III	No
10. Screening of records	All schools and medical institutions	—	No	—	51	NA	Rec Ch	Direct clinical examination	DSM-III	No
11. Children referred to local child guidance centre	—	—	—	—	132	NA	Ch	?	DSM-III	No
12. 19 items questionnaire	Teachers/counsellors	<0.27	No	46	35	76.1	Par Prof Ch Rec	WISC-R M-PV PPVT-R RDLS VABS WRAT-R ABC	New RDC	No

13. Routine developmental checks at 18 months, with repeat follow-up investigations up to the age of 3 years	Paediatricians + nurses + parents + children	—	—	168	139	82.7	Ch	Gesell test + direct assessment + review of records	DSM-III	87.5
14. Completion of an open ended questionnaire for children with 'infantile psychosis'	Mental health professionals + special schools	18.7	No	220	—	NA	Prof	Psychiatric diagnosis based on analysis of questionnaire information	DSM-III like	Agreement 63.9% (Kappa = 0.41)
15. Screening through media campaigns and advertising to a range of professionals	Review and quantative rating of records by two 'blind' psychiatrists	—	—	489	423	87.2	Prof Par Ch Rec	Parent and child assessment + record review	DSM-III	No
16. Mailed questionnaire + register search	Doctors + teachers in institutions + associated professions	—	No	—	74	—	Ch Rec Pro Par	Psychiatric assessment + review of all records. VABS Griffiths + WISC-R ABC interview schedule	DSM-III-R	100

Table 2.2. (*cont.*)

| | Screening | | | | | | Intensive assessment | | | |
No. Instrument	Informants	Refusal rate (%)	Reliability (%)	Number Selected	Assessed	Participation rate (%)	Informants	Instruments	Diagnostic criteria	Reliability
17. Systematic survey of special education local authorities + survey of psychiatric hospitals	Child psychiatrists + parents + records	—	No	—	154	—	Rec	Review of all relevant information	Clinical	No
18. 19 items Bryson's screening scale	Professionals trained to the screening instrument	—	No	66	—	—	Par Ch	Psychiatric interview + WISC-R + Merrill-Palmer	CARS	No
19. Systematic survey of special education local authorites + survey of psychiatric hospitals	Child psychiatrists	6[d]	No	—	174	NA	Rec	Review of all information	Clinical	No

Ch: child; Par: parents; Rec: records (medical, etc. . . .); Pro: professionals (i.e. teachers, paediatricians, . . .). WISC-R: Wechsler Intelligence Scale for Children – Revised (Wechsler, 1974); ABC: Autism Behaviour Check List (Krug, Ariek and Almond, 1980); CARS: Childhood Autism Rating Scale (Schopler et al. (1986); M-P: Merrill-Palmer Scale of Mental Tests (Stutsman, 1984); PPVT-R: Peabody Picture Vocabulary Test – Revised (Dunn and Dunn, 1981); RDC: Research Diagnostic Criteria; RDLS: Reynell Developmental Language Scales (Reynell, 1978); VABS: Vineland Adaptive Behaviour Scales (Sparrow, Balla and Cicchetti, 1984); WRAT-R: Wide Range Achievement Test – Revised (Jastak and Wilkinson, 1984); NA: Does not apply.

[a]Relaxed for the age of onset.

[b]3% is the refusal rate for normal schools. 23.7% is the rate of questionnaires not returned for the handicapped group.

[c]Findings for this study were also extracted from other references (Wing & Gould, 1979; Wing, 1980).

[d]This refusal rate is that from parents.

screening stage of these studies often consisted in sending letters or brief screening scales requesting professionals to identify possible cases of autism. Each investigation varied in several key aspects of this screening stage. First, the coverage of the population varies enormously from one study to another. In some (i.e. studies 3, 17 and 19), only cases already known from educational or medical authorities could be identified whereas in other surveys an extensive coverage of the entire population, including children attending normal schools (study 1) or children undergoing systematic developmental checks (study 13) was achieved. In addition, the surveyed areas varied in terms of service development as a function of the specific educational or health care systems of each country and of the year of the study. Second, the type of information sent out to professionals inviting them to identify children varied from simple letters including a few clinical descriptors of autism-related syndromes to more systematic screening based on questionnaires or rating scales. Third, participation rates in the first screening stages provide another source of variation in the screening efficiency of surveys. Few studies could examine the extent to which refusal to participate or uncooperativeness in surveys is associated with the likelihood that the corresponding children have autism. Bryson et al. (1988), however, provided some evidence that those families who refused cooperation in the intensive assessment phase had children with ABC scores similar to other false positives in their study, thereby suggesting that these children were unlikely to have autism. By contrast, in a Japanese study (Sugiyama & Abe, 1989) where 17.3% of parents refused further investigations for their 18-month children who had failed a developmental check, the authors obtained follow-up data at age 3 years, which suggested that half of the children still displayed developmental problems. Whether these problems were connected to autism is unknown, but this study points to higher rates of developmental disorders among nonparticipants in surveys. In Lotter's study (1966), 58 questionnaires covering schools for handicapped children were returned out of 76 forms sent out, and independent review of the records showed that four of the 18 missing forms corresponded to autistic children. It is difficult, therefore, to draw firm conclusions from these accounts. Moreover, refusal rates for the screening stage were not available for the majority of studies. Among studies where they were available, refusal rates varied from less than 1% to 27.4%. Thus, although there is no consistent evidence that refusal to cooperate is associated with autism, it appears that a small proportion of cases may be missed surveys as a consequence of nonparticipation in screening.

Few studies provide estimates of the reliability of their screening procedures (Table 2.2). The sensitivity of the screening procedure is also difficult to gauge. The usual method which consists of sampling at random screened negative subjects in order to estimate the proportion of false negatives has not been used in surveys of autism for the obvious reason that, due to the rare frequency of the disorder, it would be both imprecise and costly to undertake such estimations. The consequence of these remarks is that prevalence estimates must be seen as underestimates of 'true' prevalence rates because cases are being missed due either to lack of cooperation or to imperfect sensitivity of the screening procedure. The magnitude of this underestimation is unknown in each survey but it is unlikely to be substantial.

Similar considerations about the variability across studies apply to the phases of intensive assessment of surveys (Table 2.2). Participation rates in these second stage assessments were in general very high although they were not always available or were simply not calculated as the design and/or method of data collection did not lead easily to their estimation. The number of subjects involved in intensive assessments varied from 28 to 423 (mean 135), with a median number of 108 subjects per investigation. The source of information used to determine caseness usually involved a combination of informants and data sources with a direct assessment of the person with autism in 13 studies.

The assessments were conducted with various diagnostic instruments, ranging from a classical clinical examination to the use of batteries of standardized measures. The precise diagnostic criteria retained to define caseness vary according to the study and, to a large extent, reflect historical changes in classification systems. Thus, Kanner's criteria, Lotter's & Rutter's definitions were used in the first eight surveys whereas *Diagnostic and Statistical Manual of Mental Disorders* (DSM) based definitions took over thereafter. Some studies have partially relaxed some diagnostic criteria such as the requirement of an age of onset before 30 months (study 6) or that of the absence of schizophrenic like symptoms (studies 13 and 14). It is however impossible to assess the impact of a specific diagnostic scheme or of a particular diagnostic criterion on the estimate of prevalence because other powerful methodological factors confound between studies comparisons of rates. Surprisingly, few studies have a built-in reliability assessment of the diagnostic procedure. All these methodological differences should be borne in mind for between studies comparisons as these factors are likely to account for most of the variation in rates.

Table 2.3. Surveys of autism: main characteristics of identified samples

No.	No. with autism	Positive predictive value	With no speech (%)	In residential school/home (%)	IQ distribution			Sex ratio (M:F)		
					Normal range (%)	Mild/moderate retardation (%)	Severe/profound retardation (%)	Overall	Normal IQ range	Moderate to profound retardation
1.	32	25.8	28	—	15.6	15.6	68.8	2.6 (23/9)	∞ (10/0)	1.3 (12/9)
2.	20	33.3						1.4 (12/7)	Higher proportion of boys	—
3.	69	24.6						3.06 (52/17)		—
4.	17[b]	15.7	59		30	35.0	35.0	16 (16/1)		—
5.	142	36.8						9.9 (129/13)		—
6.	39	54		8.1	20.5	30.8	48.7	1.6 (24/15)		Higher proportion of girls 0.6 (3/5)
7.	28		54					1.33 (16/12)		
8.	52				55.8	44.2[a]	(see previous column)	2.25 (36/16)		
9.	59	<29.5						2.7 (43/16)	2.22 (20/9)	—
10.	51							4.7 (42/9)		—
11.	132							4.07 (106/26)		—
12.	21	60	19	19	23.8	33.3	42.8	2.5 (15/6)	∞ (5/0)	1.25 (5/4)

No.										
13.	16	11.5	—	—	—	—	—	—	—	—
14.	61	27.7	—	—	—	—	—	2.3	—	—
15.	241	49	—	—	34	25.1	40.9	3.73 (190/51)	6.3 (69/11)	2.7 (70/26)
16.	74	—	—	—	18	28	54	2.7 (54/20)	2.2 (9/4)	1.9 (26/14)
17.	154	—	32.9	—	13.3	181.1	68.6	2.1 (105/49)	6.0 (12/2)	1.9 (47/25)
18.	6	9.1	—	50	0	100.0	0	2.0 (4/2)	—	—
19.	174	—	34.5	—	12.1	6.6	81.3	1.81 (112/62)	—	—

[a]Rate for combined levels of mental retardation (IQ < 70).
[b]This corresponds to the sample described in Wing and Gould (1979) and has been used for Tables 2.3, 2.5 and 2.6.

CHARACTERISTICS OF IDENTIFIED SAMPLES

A total number of 1388 subjects assessed in the second stage of the 19 surveys were considered to suffer from autism, this number ranging from 6 to 241 across studies (median 52). As indicated in Table 2.3 (third column), the positive predictive value, or proportion of screened positive children who turned out to have autism, never exceeded 60%, with a median value of 28.5% (range 9.1–60%). Thus, two to three nonautistic children were assessed intensively for each autistic child. These features highlight the costs of conducting surveys on such rare conditions and also reflect the relative lack of specificity of the screening procedures used in epidemiological surveys of a rare disorder such as autism.

The assessment of intellectual function was obtained in ten studies. These assessments were conducted with various approaches; furthermore, results were pooled together in broad bands of intellectual level which do not share the same boundaries. As a consequence, differences in rates of cognitive impairment across and between studies should be interpreted with caution. With these caveats in mind, some general conclusions can nevertheless be reached. The median proportion of subjects without intellectual impairment is 19.2% (range 0–55.8%). The corresponding figures are 29.4% (range 6.6–100%) for mild to moderate intellectual impairments and 45.7% (range 0–81.3%) for severe to profound level of mental retardation. In order to control for differences in sample sizes, these proportions were weighted by each study sample size. The three weighted averages were in close correspondence with the aforementioned median values (respectively, 23.5%, 22.3% and 54.9%).

Sex repartition among subjects with autism was reported in 18 studies and the male/female sex ratio varied from 1.33 (study 7) to 16.0 (study 4), with a median ratio of 2.55 (mean 3.7). Thus, no epidemiological study ever identified more girls than boys, a finding which parallels the sex differences found in clinically referred samples. Weighting each sex ratio by the sample size, an average weighted estimate of 3.68 could be derived for an overall sample of 1372 subjects. The association between sex and intellectual functioning was assessed within subgroups with either normal or severely impaired intellectual function in nine studies. The overall pattern supported the notion that sex differences are more pronounced when autism is not associated with mental retardation. In seven studies (representing a total sample of 748 subjects) where the sex difference was quantitatively estimated, the median sex ratio was 6.0 within the normal band of intellectual functioning. Conversely, in six studies including a total number of 696 subjects, the median sex ratio was 1.68 in the group of moderately to severely mentally retarded persons with autism.

PREVALENCE ESTIMATIONS

The findings on prevalence estimates are presented in Table 2.4. Prevalence estimates range from 0.7 per 10 000 to 15.5 per 10 000, with a median value of 4.8. Confidence intervals were computed for each estimate and the width of these intervals (range 0.3–18.8; mean 4.5) indicates the variation in the sample sizes and in the precision achieved in each study. Prevalence rates are negatively correlated with sample size (Spearman $r = -0.68$; $P < 0.01$). The weighted average estimate for 18 studies (excluding study 3 which had both a poorly sensitive case finding method and a high sample size) yielded an estimate of 4.01 per 10 000. Population values between 4.6 to 5.5 per 10 000 would be included in about half the confidence intervals (nine studies). The six surveys with prevalence rates over 6 per 10 000 were all published since 1987; the correlation between prevalence rate and year of publication was however nonsignificant (Spearman $r = 0.49$; n.s.).

Age specific rates were available in some studies for the preschool period (four studies), the school age period (ten studies) and the teenage years (six studies) (Table 2.4). A ratio of each of these age specific rates to the overall study prevalence rate was computed for these studies. The average values were 0.78, 1.34 and 0.95 for preschool, school and teenage years, respectively. Thus, within studies comparisons suggest that rates for the school age period are on average 34% higher than unadjusted prevalence rates; conversely, rates for the very young or for adolescents are typically lower, probably reflecting difficulties in identifying and diagnosing cases in these age groups, developmental changes in autistic symptomatology and variations with age in patterns of medical care and educational services. For the ten studies which provided separate estimates for the school age period, the median rate was 5.0 per 10 000.

In six studies, the sample was broken down according to typical or atypical forms of autism, the precise meaning and reliability of this differentiation being somewhat questionable. Thus, atypical autism has been defined as either presentations departing from Kanner's original descriptions or as autism associated with neurological features (as in study 14). For these six studies (studies 1, 4, 6, 7, 9 and 16), the mean prevalence rate ratio of typical to atypical forms was 1.20 (median 0.93) thereby suggesting about equal frequency of both presentations.

47

Table 2.4. *Prevalence rates estimates per 10 000*

No.	Overall	95% CI[a]	Age group (years)			Type	
			Preschool	School age	Teenage period	Typical	Atypical
1.	4.1	2.7; 5.5	—	—	—	1.9	2.2
2.	4.3	2.4; 6.2	—	—	—	—	—
3.	0.7	0.6; 0.9	—	—	—	—	—
4.	4.8[b]	2.1; 7.5	—	—	—	2.0	2.8
5.	2.33	1.9; 2.7	—	4.96 (4–10)	1.1[a] (11–16)	—	—
6.	5.6	3.9; 7.4	1.7 (0–3)	12.6 (7–9)	4.6 (13–15)	3.04[a]	2.6[a]
7.	4.3	2.7; 5.9	—	2.37[a] (3–14)	—	2.15	2.15
8.	1.9	1.4; 2.4	—	—	—	1.9	—
9.	3.26	2.4; 4.1	—	4.04 (5–14)	—	1.16	2.10
10.	15.5	11.3; 19.8	17.1 (4–6)	14.7 (7–12)	—	—	—
11.	13.8	11.5; 16.2	—	—	—	—	—
12.	10.1	5.8; 14.4	—	—	—	—	—
13.	13.0	6.7; 19.4	—	—	—	—	—
14.	4.5	3.4; 5.6	—	5.1 (5–9)	—	—	—
15.	2.47	2.1; 2.8	2.17 (3–7)	3.57 (8–12)	3.16 (13–17)	—	—
16.	9.5	7.3; 11.6	7.8 (4–7)	10.8 (8–10)	10.0 (11–13)	7.0	2.4
17.	4.9	4.1; 5.7	—	4.7 (9)	5.1 (13)	—	—

18.	11.7	2.3; 21.1	—	—	5.02 (8–12)	—
19.	5.35	4.6; 6.1	—	—	5.68 (13–16)	—

[a]CI: confidence interval. Computed by the author.
[b]This rate corresponds to the first report on this study and is based on 12 subjects among the 5–14 year olds.

Eric Fombonne

ASSOCIATED MEDICAL CONDITIONS

Rates of medical conditions associated with autism were reported in 11 surveys (Table 2.5). It will be appreciated that these medical conditions were investigated by very different means ranging from questionnaires to full medical workups; however, some consistent findings derive from epidemiological samples. The median rates and range for each disorder were 16.7% for epilepsy (eight studies, range 4.8–26.4%), 2.75% for cerebral palsy (four studies; range 1.4–4.8%), 2% for fragile X (five studies; range 0–6%), 1.1% for tuberous sclerosis (seven studies; range 0–3.1%), 0% for phenylketonuria (five studies; range 0–0%), 0.3% for neurofibromatosis (four studies; range 0–1.4%), 1.1% for Down's syndrome (six studies; range 0–2.6%), 0.9% for congenital rubella (seven studies; range 0–5.9%), 3.1% for hearing impairments (five studies; range 0.9–5.9%) and 1.3% for visual impairments (three studies; range 0–2.9%). The number of studies from which these summary statistics derive is sometimes small, and the findings should also be checked against the characteristics of the samples included in each survey, particularly regarding the rate of mental retardation.

Nevertheless, the results consolidate scientific knowledge on the association between autism and known medical conditions. Thus, conditions such as congenital rubella, phenylketonuria and neurofibromatosis appear to have no association with autism. Thus, our estimate of 0.3% for autism and neurofibromatosis is in keeping with that found in a large series of 341 referred cases (Mouridsen et al., 1992) and does not exceed the rate expected under the assumption of independence of the two disorders. Similarly, bearing in mind the high rate of mental retardation among samples of autistic subjects, the rates found for cerebral palsy and Down's syndrome equally suggest no particular association. The recognition that Down's syndrome and autism co-occur in some individuals has been the focus of attention in recent reports (Bregman & Volkmar, 1988; Ghazziudin et al., 1992; Howlin et al., 1995); the epidemiological findings give further support to the validity of these clinical descriptions although they do not suggest the rate of comorbidity is higher than that expected by chance. For fragile X, the low rate available in epidemiological studies is most certainly an underestimate because fragile X was not recognized until relatively recently and in the most recent surveys systematic screening for fragile X was very rarely undertaken. In line with prior reports (Smalley et al., 1992), tuberous sclerosis has a consistently high frequency among autistic samples. Assuming a population prevalence of 1 per 10 000 for tuberous sclerosis, it appears that the rate of tuberous sclerosis is about 100 times higher than that expected under the hypothesis of no association. The rate of tuberous sclerosis in autistic samples is however much lower in these epidemiological studies than the 9% minimum rate claimed in a recent study (Gillberg et al., 1994). Whether the association between tuberous sclerosis and autism is mediated by epilepsy, localized brain lesions or direct genetic effects is a currently active direction of research. The proportion of cases of autism attributable to known medical disorders remains low therefore. From the eight surveys where rates of one of seven clearcut medical disorders (cerebral palsy, fragile X, tuberous sclerosis, phenylketonuria, neurofibromatosis, congenital rubella and Down's syndrome) were available in most studies, we computed the proportion of subjects with at least one of these recognizable disorders. As the overlap between these conditions is typically low and information was not available, this overall rate was obtained by summing directly the rates for each individual condition for each study; the resulting rate might therefore be an overestimate. The fraction of cases of autism with a known medical condition ranged from 0 to 12.3%, with a median and mean values of 6.1 and 6.2%, respectively. Even if some adjustment were made to account for the underestimation of the rate of fragile X in epidemiological surveys of autism, the attributable proportion of cases of autism would be around the 10% figure for any medical disorder (excluding epilepsy). Although this figure does not incorporate other medical events such as encephalitis, congenital anomalies and other rare medical syndromes, it is similar to that reported in a recent review of the question (Rutter et al., 1994). It is worth noting that autism epidemiological surveys of very large samples (i.e. studies 15, 17 and 19) provided estimates in line with our conservative summary statistics. By contrast, claims of average rates of medical conditions as high as 24% appear to apply to studies of smaller size and relying on a broadened definition of autism (Gillberg & Coleman, 1996).

Rates of epilepsy are high among autism samples. The proportion suffering from epilepsy tends also to be higher in those studies which have higher rates of severe mental retardation (as in studies 16, 17 and 19). Age specific rates for the prevalence of epilepsy are not available. The samples where high rates of epilepsy were reported tend to have a higher median age although these rates seem mostly to apply to school age children. Thus, in light of the increased incidence of seizures during adolescence among subjects with autism (Rutter, 1970; Deykin & McMahon, 1979), the epidemiological rates should be regarded as underestimates of the lifetime risk of epilepsy. These rates are nonetheless high and support the findings of a bimodal peak of incidence of epilepsy in autistic samples

Table 2.5. *Rates of associated medical characteristics*

Study number[d]	Epilepsy		Cerebral palsy		Abnormal physical feature or congenital abnormalities		Associated syndromes	Fragile X anomaly		Tuberous sclerosis	
	n	%	n	%	n	%		n	%	n	%
1.	4	12.5	—	—	—	—	—	—	—	1[f]	3.1
2.	2	16.6	—	—	—	—	Abnormal EEGs in 5.8%	—	—	—	—
3.	—	—	—	—	—	—	2 encephalopathies	—	—	0	—
4.	3	16.8	—	—	1	5.9	28.2% with unspecified CNS impairments	—	—	—	—
6.	—	—	—	—	—	—					
10.	—	—	—	—	—	—	—	0	—	0	—
12.	1	4.8	1[c]	4.8	3	14.3	1 Coffin-Lowry[a] 1 Mucopolysaccharidosis[b]	—	—	—	—
15[e]	34	14.6	—	—	1 Spina bifida		3 Chromosomal abnormalities 6 Viral/bacterial infections 7 Metabolic disorders 4 Rett's syndromes 2 Tourette's syndromes	2	0.9	1	0.4
16.	17	23.0	1	1.4	—	—	3 Moebius' syndrome 1 Laurence–Moon–Biedl syndrome 1 hydrocephalus 1 Williams' syndrome 3 Chromosomal abnormalities	6	8.1	1	1.4
17.	34	22.0	4	2.6	—	—		1	0.6	2	1.3
19.	46	26.4	5	2.9	—	—	2 Chromosomal abnormalities (other than Down's syndrome)	3	1.7	2	1.1

Table 2.5 (*cont.*)

| No. | Phenylketonuria | | Neurofibromatosis | | Down's syndrome | | Congenital rubella | | Sensory impairments | | | | | |
| | | | | | | | | | Hearing | | Visual | | Both | |
	n	%	n	%	n	%	n	%	n	%	n	%	n	%
1.	—	—	—	—	—	—	1	3.1	1	3.1	—	—	—	—
2.	—	—	—	—	—	—	—	—	—	—	—	—	—	—
3.	—	—	—	—	—	—	—	—	—	—	—	—	—	—
4.	0	—	0	—	0^g	—	1	5.9	1	5.9	0	—	—	—
6.	0	—	—	—	—	—	0	—	—	—	—	—	—	—
10.	0	—	—	—	0	—	—	—	—	—	—	—	—	—
12.	—	—	—	—	—	—	—	—	—	—	—	—	—	—
15^e	—	—	1	1.4	6	2.6	2	0.9	2	0.9	3	1.3	—	—
16.	0	—	—	—	0	—	0	—	3	4.1	—	—	9	5.8
17.	0	—	0	—	2	1.3	2	1.3	—	—	—	—	9	5.8
19.	0	—	1	0.6	3	1.7	1	0.6	3	1.7	5	2.9	8	4.6

[a]Provisional diagnosis.
[b]Tentative diagnosis.
[c]Acquired hemiplegia.
[d]Findings from study 11 were not included in this Table since they applied to a broad definition including DSM-III like autism and other pervasive developmental disorders (results for the subgroup of children meeting stricter DSM-III criteria were not available).
[e]Based on 233 subjects whose medical records were available.
[f]Based on a post-mortem examination at follow-up (Lotter, 1974).
[g]Children with Down's syndrome and autistic features were, however, excluded from this study (Wing et al., 1976: 95).

Table 2.6. *Informative studies on rates on nonautism pervasive developmental disorders*

No.	Study	Rates of autism	Prevalence rate of other PDD	Combined rate autism + other PDDs	Prevalence rate ratio[a]	Case definition for other PDDs
1.	Lotter (1966, 1967)	4.1	3.3	7.8	1.90	Children with some behaviour similar to autistic children
2.	Brask (1970)	4.3	1.9	6.2	1.44	Children with 'other psychoses' or 'borderline psychotic'
4.	Wing et al. (1976)	4.9	16.3	21.2	4.33	Socially impaired (triad of impairments)
5.	Hoshino et al. (1982)	2.33	2.92	5.25	2.25	Autistic mental retardation
9.	Burd et al. (1987)	3.26	>7.79[b]	>11.05[b]	3.39	Children referred by professionals with 'autistic like' symptoms, not meeting DSM-III criteria for IA, COPDD or atypical PDD
14.	Cialdella & Mamelle (1989)	4.5	4.7	9.2	2.04	Children meeting criteria for other forms of 'infantile psychosis' than autism, or a broadened definition of DSM-III
17.	Fombonne & du Mazaubrun (1992)[c]	4.6	6.6	11.2	2.43	Children with mixed developmental disorders
19.	Fombonne et al. (1997)	5.3	10.94	16.3	3.05	Children with mixed developmental disorders

[a]Combined rate divided by autism rate.
[b]Computed by the author.
[c]These rates are derived from the complete results of the survey of three birth cohorts of French children (Rumeau-Rouquette et al., 1994).

with a first peak of incidence in the first year of life (Volkmar & Nelson, 1990).

RATES OF OTHER PERVASIVE DEVELOPMENTAL DISORDERS

Several studies have provided useful information on rates of syndromes similar to autism but falling short of strict diagnostic criteria (Table 2.6). As the screening procedures and subsequent diagnostic assessments differed from one study to another (Table 2.2), these groups of disorders are not comparable across studies. In addition, as they were not the group on which the attention was focused, their phenomenological description is often insufficient in the available reports. Different labels have been used to characterize them such as the triad of impairments defined by Wing & Gould (1979) as involving impairments in reciprocal social interaction, communication and imagination. These groups would be overlapping with current diagnostic labels such as atypical autism and PDD-NOS, which does little to clarify their relationship with a narrower definition of autism. Eight of the 19 surveys yielded estimates of the prevalence of these developmental disorders, with six studies showing higher rates for the nonautism disorder than the rates for autism. The ratio of the combined rate of all developmental disorders to the rate of autism varied from 1.44 to 4.33 (Table 2.6) with a mean value of 2.6. In other words, for two children with autism assessed in epidemiological surveys, about three children were found to have severe impairments of a similar nature. This group has been less studied but it is clear from these figures that they are a very substantial group whose treatment needs are likely to be as important as those of children with autism.

Asperger's syndrome is a condition that has received much attention during the last decade. Yet, epidemiological studies of its prevalence and characteristics are sparse, probably due to the fact that it was acknowledged as a separate diagnostic category only recently in both the *International Classification of Diseases* (ICD-10) and DSM-IV. At least four different diagnostic schemes have been proposed to operationalize its definition and no definite consensus has been reached yet about the validity of these competing definitions. Only one epidemiological study has been conducted which investigated its prevalence (Ehlers & Gillberg, 1993). These authors surveyed 1519 children aged 7 to 16 years old from five normal schools on the outskirts of Göteborg (Sweden). A questionnaire was used for screening and the intensive assessment relied on a combination of direct assessment, observation and parent/teacher interviews. The prevalence for definite cases was estimated to be 28.5 per 10 000 (95% CI computed by us: 0.6–56.5) for ICD-10 criteria and 35.7 per 10 000 (95% CI: 4.5–66.9) for the authors' own diagnostic criteria. These estimates are based on a handful of cases and, as suggested by the wide confidence intervals, they are relatively imprecise. Higher rates were computed by the authors when they included possible or suspected cases. Replication of these figures in other samples is clearly needed before some meaningful picture can be drawn.

OTHER CORRELATES

Time trends

Anecdotal reports have suggested that more cases of autism were seen in specialized centres, which suggests that the prevalence is perhaps going up. Observations from clinically referred samples, however, are confounded by many factors such as referral patterns, availability of services and changes in diagnostic practices to name only a few. Therefore, epidemiological studies are crucial to assess secular changes in the incidence of a disorder. As shown before, epidemiological surveys of autism each possess unique design features which could account for most of the between studies variations in rates, and time trends are therefore difficult to gauge from published rates. In addition, as mentioned before, the correlation between prevalence rate and year of publication was nonsignificant. Nevertheless, epidemiological studies can be used to assess time trends in two instances: (1) when repeated surveys using the same methodology have been conducted in the same geographical area at different points in time, and (2) when large studies have produced specific prevalence rates for successive birth cohorts. In the latter case, increased rate among the most recent birth cohorts could be interpreted as indicating a secular increase in the incidence of the disorder. The surveys conducted in Sweden and in France shed some light on this issue. The Göteborg studies provided three prevalence estimates which increased over a short period of time from 4.0 (1980) to 6.6 (1984) and 9.5 (1988), the gradient being even steeper if rates for the urban area alone are considered (4.0, 7.5 and 11.6); however, comparison of these rates is not straightforward as different age groups were included in each survey. For example, the rate in the first survey for the youngest age group (which resembles more closely the children included in the other two surveys) was 5.1 per 10 000. Second, the increase in prevalence in the second survey was explained by improved detection among the mentally retarded and that of the third survey by cases born to immigrant parents. That the majority of the latter group was born abroad suggests that migration into the area could be a key explanation. Taken in conjunction with a progress- ive broadening of the definition of autism over time by the authors (Gill- berg et al., 1991), these findings do not provide solid evidence for an increased prevalence rate.

The French surveys (studies 17 and 19) derived from much larger sample sizes. In the first study (study 17), prevalence estimates were available for the two birth cohorts of children born in 1972 and 1976. The rates were similar (5.1 and 4.9) and not statistically different. Furthermore, in the same investigation, the age specific rate of autism for the birth cohort 1981 was lower (3.1) (Rumeau-Rouquette et al., 1994), most probably reflecting a poorer sensitivity among the youngest age groups. In any case, the findings did not suggest increasing rates in the most recent cohorts. These findings of a stable prevalence rate were independently replicated in two different ways. First, another survey conducted with the same methodology but in different French regions a few years later (study 19) led to a similar (Table 2.4) overall prevalence estimate compared with the first survey. In the latter survey which included birth cohorts from 1976 to 1985, the age specific rates showed no trend towards an increase (Fombonne et al., 1997). Sec- ond, another French survey (study 14) conducted at a different time in a different area with a different methodology also yielded a similar preva- lence estimate of 5.1 for DSM-III defined autism among school aged children. The consistency of estimates from these various surveys and their stability across birth cohorts is impressive. Some weight should be given to these results as they derive from a total target population of 735 343 children and a number of 389 children with autism. The available epi- demiological evidence does not therefore suggest that the prevalence of autism has increased and several reasons could easily account for an artefactual impression of an increase (Fombonne, 1996).

Autism and immigrant status

Some investigators have mentioned the possibility that rates of autism might be higher among immigrants (Wing, 1980; Gillberg, 1987; Gillberg et al., 1991). Five of the 17 children with autism identified in the Camberwell

Table 2.7. *Autism and social class*

1.	Lotter (1967)	Father's occupation significantly higher than control group and population norms; similar trend for parental education
2.	Brask (1970)	No social class difference
3.	Treffert (1970)	Significantly higher educational level (fathers and mothers) and occupational level (fathers) compared with parents of psychiatric controls
4.	Wing et al. (1976)	No difference compared with local census data
5.	Hoshino et al. (1982)	Significantly higher social class and parental education compared with national norms
7.	McCarthy et al. (1984)	*Perhaps* a skew towards higher SES applying only to 'nuclear' autism (as opposed to autism associated with MR or medical disorders), no quantitative assessment
8.	Steinhausen et al. (1986)	No difference compared with census data (slight trend towards upper-middle class preponderance)
14.	Cialdella & Mamelle (1989)	No difference compared with census data
15.	Ritvo et al. (1989)	Educational and occupational levels of parents close to those of the population
16.	Gillberg et al. (1995)	No significant difference with a representative sample of the population
17.	Fombonne & du Mazaubrun (1992)	No difference compared with census data
19.	Fombonne et al. (1997)	No difference compared with census data

MR: mental retardation; SES: socioeconomic status.

study were of Caribbean origin (study 4; Wing, 1980) and the estimated rate was 6.3 per 10 000 for this group compared with 4.4 per 10 000 for the rest of the population (Wing, 1993). The wide confidence intervals associated with rates from this study (Table 2.4) indicate no statistical significance. In addition, this area of London had received a large proportion of immigrants from the Caribbean region in the 1960s and, under circumstances where migration flux in and out of an area is happening, estimation of population rates should be viewed with much caution. Yet, Afro-Caribbean children referred from the same area were recently found to have higher rates of autism than referred controls (Goodman & Richards, 1995); however, the sample was small (total of 18 children) and differential referral patterns to a tertiary centre could not be ruled out. Similarly, the findings from the Göteborg studies paralleled an increased migration flux in the early 1980s in this area (Gillberg, 1987); they too were based on relatively small numbers (19 children from immigrant parents). Taken altogether, the combined results of these two studies (studies 4 and 16) should be interpreted in the specific methodological context of these investigations. Both studies had low numbers of identified cases and both groups of authors have relied upon broadened definitions of autism. Unfortunately, other studies have not systematically reported the proportion of immigrant groups in the areas surveyed (Table 2.1). In two studies where these proportions were low (studies 11 and 12), rates of autism were in the upper range of rates. Conversely, in other populations where immigrants contributed substantially to the denominators (studies 14, 17 and 19), rates were in the rather low band. Finally, it is unclear what common mechanism could explain the putative association between immigrant status and autism as the origins of the immigrant parents (especially in study 16) were very diverse and, in fact, represented all the continents. With this heterogeneity in mind, it is unclear what common biological features might be shared by these immigrant families and what would be a plausible mechanism. The association of immigrant status with autism remains therefore uncertain.

Autism and social class

Twelve of the 19 studies provided information on the social class of the families of autistic children (Table 2.7). Of these, four studies (1, 2, 3 and 5) suggested an association between autism and social class or parental education. The year of data collection for these four investigations was

59

before 1980 (Table 2.1) and all studies conducted thereafter provided no evidence for the association. Thus, the epidemiological results suggest that the earlier findings were due to artefacts in the availability of services and in the case finding methods, as already shown in other samples (Schopler et al., 1979; Wing, 1980).

CONCLUSIONS

This review concludes that the best available estimate of autism is 5.0 per 10 000. This estimate takes into account the fact that rates for the school age period must be closer to the true prevalence rate and also that a small proportion of cases is missed in each survey whose results therefore underestimate the population rate. The methodology of epidemiological surveys is well established and relies on a multistage case finding method. Epidemiological surveys can provide an invaluable starting point for the investigation of developmental disorders in countries where such investigations have not been conducted. Epidemiological samples may be used in various ways, i.e. to estimate the needs for specialized services or to provide a sampling base to select unbiased samples for case control studies. The main features of autism are the consistent associations with mental retardation in about 80% of cases, with a preponderance of males (a male: female ratio of 3.7:1), with some rare and genetically determined medical conditions such as tuberous sclerosis, and no association with social class. All surveys identified a larger group of children whose impairments have commonalities with those of autism. Future research should focus on this group on which basic data are lacking as well as on some more specific variants of autistic spectrum disorders such as Asperger's syndrome. In future epidemiological studies, reliance on current diagnostic methods of interview and observation, which have now become standard in clinical practice and research, should help to enhance comparability between surveys and to allow for more meaningful differentiation within the group of pervasive developmental disorders.

REFERENCES

Aussilloux, C., Collery, F. & Roy, J. (1989). Epidémiologie de l'autisme infantile dans le département de l'Hérault. *Revue Française de Psychiatrie*, 7, 24–8.
Bohman, M., Bohman, I. L., Björck, P. O. & Sjöholm, E. (1983). Childhood psychosis in a northern Swedish county: some preliminary findings from an epidemiological survey. In *Epidemiological Approaches in Child Psychiatry*, ed. M. H. Schmidt & H.

Remschmidt, pp. 164–73. Stuttgart: Georg Thieme.

Brask, B. H. (1970). A prevalence investigation of childhood psychoses. In *Nordic Symposium on the Care of Psychotic Children*. Oslo: Barnepsychiatrist Forening.

Bregman, J. D. & Volkmar, F. R. (1988). Autistic social dysfunction and Down's syndrome. *Journal of the American Academy of Child and Adolescent Psychiatry*, **27**, 440–1.

Bryson, S. E., Clark, B. S. & Smith, I. M. (1988). First report of a Canadian epidemiological study of autistic syndromes. *Journal of Child Psychology and Psychiatry*, **4**, 433–45.

Burd, L., Fisher, W. & Kerbeshan, J. (1987). A prevalence study of pervasive developmental disorders in North Dakota. *Journal of the American Academy of Child and Adolescent Psychiatry*, **26**, 700–3.

Cialdella, P. H. & Mamelle, N. (1989). An epidemiological study of infantile autism in a French department. *Journal of Child Psychology and Psychiatry*, **30**, 165–75.

Deykin, E. Y. & McMahon, B. (1979). The incidence of seizures among children with autistic symptoms. *American Journal of Psychiatry*, **136**, 1310–12.

Dunn, L. M. & Dunn, L. M. (1981). *Peabody Picture Vocabulary Test – Revised*. Circle Pines, Minnesota: American Guidance Service.

Ehlers, S. & Gillberg, C. (1993). The epidemiology of Asperger's syndrome. A total population study. *Journal of Child Psychology and Psychiatry*, **34**, 1327–50.

Fombonne, E. (1996). Is the prevalence of autism increasing? *Journal of Autism and Developmental Disorders*, **6**, 673–6.

Fombonne, E. & du Mazaubrun, C. (1992). Prevalence of infantile autism in four French regions. *Social Psychiatry and Psychiatric Epidemiology*, **27**, 203–10.

Fombonne, E., du Mazaubrun, C., Cans, H. & Grandjean, H. (1997). Autism and associated medical disorders in a large French epidemiological sample. *Journal of the American Academy of Child and Adolescent Psychiatry*, **36**, 1561–9.

Ghaziuddin, M., Tsai, L. & Ghaziuddin, N. (1992). Autism in Down's syndrome: presentation and diagnosis. *Journal of Intellectual Disability Research*, **35**, 449–56.

Gillberg, C. (1984). Infantile autism and other childhood psychoses in a Swedish region: epidemiological aspects. *Journal of Child Psychology and Psychiatry*, **25**, 35–43.

Gillberg, C. (1987). Infantile autism in children of immigrant parents. A population-based study from Göteborg, Sweden. *British Journal of Psychiatry*, **150**, 856–8.

Gillberg, C. & Coleman, M. (1996). Autism and medical disorders: a review of the literature. *Developmental Medicine and Child Neurology*, **38**, 191–202.

Gillberg, C. & Forsell, C. (1984). Childhood psychosis and neurofibromatosis: more than a coincidence. *Journal of Autism and Developmental Disorders*, **13**, 1–8.

Gillberg, C., Gillberg, C. & Ahlsén, G. (1994). Autistic behaviour and attention deficits in tuberous sclerosis: a population-based study. *Developmental Medicine and Child Neurology*, **36**, 50–6.

Gillberg, C., Schaumann, H. & Gillberg, I. C. (1995). Autism in immigrants: children born in Sweden to mothers born in Uganda. *Journal of Intellectual Disability Research*, **39**, 141–4.

Gillberg, C., Steffenburg, S. & Schaumann, H. (1991). Is autism more common now than ten year ago? *British Journal of Psychiatry*, **158**, 403–9.

Goodman, R. & Richards, H. (1995). Child and adolescent psychiatric presentations of second-generation Afro-Caribbeans in Britain. *British Journal of Psychiatry*, **167**, 362–9.

Haga, H. & Miyamoya, Y. (1971). A survey on the actual state of so-called autistic children in Kyoto prefecture. *Japanese Journal of Child Psychiatry*, **12**, 160–7.

Herder, G. A. (1993). Infantile autism among children in the county of Nordland: prevalence and etiology. *Tidsskrift tar den Norske Laegeforening*, **113**, 2247–9.

Hoshino, Y., Yashima, Y., Ishige, K., Tachibana, R., Watanabe, M., Kancki, M.,

Kumashiro, H., Ueno, B., Takahashi, E. & Furukawa H. (1982). The epidemiological study of autism in Fukushima Ken. *Folia Psychiatrica et Neurologica Japonica*, **36**, 115–24.

Howlin, P., Wing, L. & Gould, J. (1995). The recognition of autism in children with Down syndrome. Implications for intervention and some speculations about pathology. *Developmental Medicine and Child Neurology*, **37**, 406–14.

Ishii, T. & Takahashi, O. (1983). The epidemiology of autistic children in Toyota, Japan: prevalence. *Japanese Journal of Child and Adolescent Psychiatry*, **24**, 311–21.

Jastak, S. & Wilkinson, G. S. (1984). *The Wide Range Achievement Test – Revised.* Wilmington, Del. : Jastak.

Krug, D. A., Arick, J. R. & Almond, P. J. (1980). Behavior Checklist for identifying severely handicapped individuals with high levels of autistic behavior. *Journal of Child Psychology and Psychiatry*, **21**, 221–9.

Lotter, V. (1966). Epidemiology of autistic conditions in young children: I. Prevalence. *Social Psychiatry*, **1**, 124–37.

Lotter, V. (1967). Epidemiology of autistic conditions in young children: II. Some characteristics of the parents and children. *Social Psychiatry*, **1**, 163–73.

McCarthy, P., Fitzgerald, M. & Smith, M. A. (1984). Prevalence of childhood autism in Ireland. *Irish Medical Journal*, **77**, 129–30.

Matsuishi, T., Shiotsuki, M., Yoshimura, K., Shoji, H., Imuta, F. & Yamashita, F. (1987). High prevalence of infantile autism in Kurume City, Japan. *Journal of Child Neurology*, **2**, 268–71.

Mouridsen, S. E., Bachmann-Andersen, L., Sörensen, S. A., Rich, B. & Isager, T. (1992). Neurofibromatosis in infantile autism and other types of childhood psychoses. *Acta Paedopsychiatrica*, **55**, 15–18.

Nakai, M. (1971). Epidemiology of autistic children in Gifu-Ken. *Japanese Journal of Child Psychiatry*, **12**, 262–6.

Reynell, J. K. (1978). *Reynell Developmental Language Scales – Revised.* Windsor, UK: NFER-Nelson Publishing Company Ltd.

Ritvo, E. R., Freeman, B. J., Pingree, C., Mason-Brothers, A., Jorde, L., Jenson, W. R., McMahon, W. M., Petersen, P. B., Mo, A. & Ritvo, A. (1989). The UCLA-University of Utah epidemiologic survey of autism: prevalence. *American Journal of Psychiatry*, **146**, 194–9.

Rumeau-Rouquette, C., du Mazaubrun, C., Verrier, A., Mlika, A., Bréart, G., Goujard, J. & Fombonne, E. (1994). *Prévalence des Handicaps: Évolution dans Trois Générations d'Enfants* 1972, 1976, 1981. Paris, Editions INSERM.

Rutter, M. (1970). Autistic children: infancy to adulthood. *Seminars in Psychiatry*, **2**, 435–50.

Rutter, M., Bailey, A., Bolton, P. & Le Couteur, A. (1994). Autism and known medical conditions: myth and substance. *Journal of Child Psychology and Psychiatry*, **35**, 311–22.

Schopler, E., Andrews, C. E. & Strupp, K. (1979). Do autistic children come from upper-middle-class parents? *Journal of Autism and Developmental Disorders*, **9**, 139–51.

Schopler, E., Reichler, R. J. & Renner, B. R. (1986). *The Childhood Autism Rating Scale (CARS) for Diagnostic Screening and Classification of Autism.* New York: Irvington.

Smalley, S. L., Tanguay, P. E., Smith, M. & Gutierrez, G. (1992). Autism and tuberous sclerosis. *Journal of Autism and Developmental Disorders*, **22**, 339–55.

Sparrow, S., Balla, D. & Cicchetti, D. (1984). *Vineland Adaptive Behavior Scales (Survey Form).* American Guidance Service, Circle Pines, Minnesota.

Steffenburg, S. & Gillberg, C. (1986). Autism and autistic-like conditions in Swedish rural and urban areas: a population study. *British Journal of Psychiatry*, **149**, 81–7.

Steinhausen, H. -C., Göbel, D., Breinlinger, M. & Wohlloben, B. (1986). A community survey of infantile autism. *Journal of the American Academy of Child Psychiatry*, **25**, 186–9.

Stutsman, R. (1984). *Merrill-Palmer Scale of Mental Tests*, (reprinted). Los Angeles: Western Psychological Services.

Sugiyama, T. & Abe, T. (1989). The prevalence of autism in Nagoya, Japan: a total population study. *Journal of Autism and Developmental Disorders*, **19**, 87–96.

Tanoue, Y., Oda, S., Asano, F. & Kawashima, K. (1988). Epidemiology of infantile autism in Southern Ibaraki, Japan: differences in prevalence in birth cohorts. *Journal of Autism and Developmental Disorders*, **18**, 155–66.

Treffert, D. A. (1970). Epidemiology of infantile autism. *Archives of General Psychiatry*, **22**, 431–8.

Volkmar, F. R. & Nelson, D. S. (1990). Seizure disorders in autism. *Journal of the American Academy of Child and Adolescent Psychiatry*, **1**, 127–9.

Wechsler, D. (1974). *Wechsler Intelligence Scale for Children – Revised*. Windsor: NFER Publishing Co.

Wignyosumarto, S., Mukhlas, M. & Shirataki, S. (1992). Epidemiological and clinical study of autistic children in Yogyakarta, Indonesia. *Kobe Journal of Medical Sciences*, **38**, 1–19.

Wing, L. (1980). Childhood autism and social class: a question of selection? *British Journal of Psychiatry,,* **137**, 410–7.

Wing, L. (1993). The definition and prevalence of autism: a review of the literature. *Adolescent Psychiatry*, **2**, 61–74.

Wing, L. & Gould, J. (1979). Severe impairments of social interactions and associated abnormalities in children: epidemiology and classification. *Journal of Autism and Developmental Disorders*, **9**, 11–29.

Wing, L., Yeates, S. R., Brierly, L. M. & Gould, J. (1976). The prevalence of early childhood autism: comparison of administrative and epidemiological studies. *Psychological Medicine*, **6**, 89–100.

Zahner, G. E. P. & Pauls, D. L. (1987). Epidemiological surveys of infantile autism. In *Handbook of Autism and Pervasive and Developmental Disorders*, ed. D. J. Cohen, A. M. Donnellan & R. Paul, pp. 199–207. New York: John Wiley.

3

Psychological factors in autism

Margot Prior and Sally Ozonoff

INTRODUCTION

Reviewing psychological factors in autism presents a major challenge, given the vast amount of research that has accumulated over the past 50 years. In that time we have moved from largely speculative notions of what underlies the puzzling set of symptoms that autistic children present to us (Kanner, 1943) to a comprehensive knowledge of their strengths and weaknesses in a broad range of psychological domains. The key to the puzzle of autism, however, continues to alternately approach and recede from our grasp, much as it has done for several decades. Fortunately, our understanding of psychological factors has developed alongside increasingly productive approaches to the education and treatment of autistic children so that theory and practice can build on each other. This review of psychological aspects of autism is divided into sections covering the major domains of perception, cognition, affect, language and social behaviour.

One important issue that needs to be kept in mind concerns the powerful and pervasive influence of level of functioning on the symptoms, behaviours and capabilities of autistic children. Low and high functioning autistic children are both the same in their core deficits, and very different in their adaptive level, and this makes some of our conclusions rather qualified. While the central social and communicative deficits may be common, there are clear differences in levels and profiles of abilities across the spectrum of autistic conditions and many differences between low and high functioning children.

This is seen perhaps most vividly in considering children with Asperger's syndrome. These children share key symptom criteria for autism but they are generally at the upper end of the spectrum in terms of their cognitive and language capacities and they are frequently less socially isolated as well. So far, the data indicate that the similarities between autism and Asperger's syndrome may well outweigh the differences and hence it is debatable whether they require separate diagnostic categories on the basis of current research data. This is currently a very active research area which focuses on putative differentiating features of autism and Asperger's syndrome or, alternatively, which seeks evidence for the conceptualization of autism/Asperger's syndrome as more validly described via a 'spectrum of severity' heuristic (Gillberg & Gillberg, 1989; Szatmari et al., 1989, 1995; Ozonoff et al., 1991b).

SENSORIMOTOR AND PERCEPTUAL DEVELOPMENT

Many early studies of autistic children investigated their sensory and perceptual abilities. As this disorder is of very early onset, it seems reasonable to suggest that perceptual development at its most basic level may be disturbed in some way. Overall, both earlier and recent studies converge in the conclusion that basic sensory and perceptual abilities are not fundamentally abnormal. Nevertheless, autistic children are well known for their deviant response patterns to various kinds of sensory stimuli, and both under and over responsiveness are seen not only to differing degrees within the autistic population but even within the one child. Disturbed perception of auditory stimulation has been particularly noted (Prior, 1979).

Many low functioning children show sensory anomalies similar to those seen in sensorily handicapped children, such as peculiar and perseverative gazing at lights or moving fans; running water or sand through their hands repetitively; peering closely and persistently at objects; and flicking fingers in front of the eyes.

An interesting study of young low functioning autistic children based on home movies reported by Losche (1990) suggested that sensory motor development was normal at least during the infancy period, but that with increasing age autistic children showed increasing delays and even regressions in their development, with aimless and stereotyped behaviour being particularly a feature.

Testing young autistic children using Piagetian scales of sensorimotor development indicates that they develop normal object permanence but show notable deficits in vocal and gestural imitation (Sigman & Ungerer,

1984a). These deficits appear to diminish with age and with verbal skill development (Morgan et al., 1989). Autistic children often develop adequate rote learning ability (figurative schemas of representation according to Piagetian theory), at least commensurate with their mental age level (Green et al., 1995), but do not develop operative representation or the ability to form and manipulate symbolic material, and to develop conceptual structures. Hence for most children there is a low ceiling on their sensorimotor and cognitive development.

The acquisition of imitation and language skills is associated with more sophisticated levels of Piagetian type skills such as means-end reasoning (Abrahamsen & Mitchell, 1990). Lack of imitation skills is a notable feature of autism and is a distinguishing diagnostic characteristic. Deficiencies are apparent from the first year of life (Prior et al., 1975) when the normally expected simple imitative games do not appear. Difficulties in using gestures, in imitating communicative and social behaviours are persistent and pervasive (Wing, 1976, 1981), except perhaps in the very highest functioning children. Ohta (1987), Sigman & Ungerer (1984a) and Hertzig et al. (1989) have all reported autism specific imitation deficits in comparative studies covering motor, vocal, sensorimotor, symbolic and affective behaviours across a range of ages. While early conceptualizations of these deficits stressed the apparent absence of the desire to imitate, more recent research has questioned whether the deficits are due to conceptual and symbolic impairments, or perhaps to more basic problems with organizing, coordinating and integrating body movements. Smith & Bryson (1994) in reviewing imitation and action in autism have suggested that difficulties with motor imitation are characteristic of children with other developmental disorders, especially those involving language impairments; hence at least some of the difficulties may be nonspecific. The relations are complex as the impairments seem to be present even when other areas of cognitive and language functioning are relatively high, and some groups with similar levels of language impairment and mental retardation such as Down's syndrome children nevertheless show good imitation skills (Prior, 1977).

The other line of argument which is salient is that autistic children have representational deficits, and hence imitation and action deficits may be the product of lack of social cognitive abilities which are necessary for the understanding of why and how imitation works in the social and communicative domain. The 'chicken and egg' problem here is one which requires prospective studies of very young autistic children in which stages of development of various skills and the sequence of their emergence can be minutely tracked.

Most researchers would agree with Shapiro & Hertzig (1991) that it is 'integrative deficits' which are central to any sensory and perceptual dysfunction, i.e. the autistic child is unable to coordinate and integrate varying kinds of sensory input and to form a coherent functional picture of the world. This applies across all modalities and may be fundamental to all of the other deficits.

Temple Grandin, an autistic adult, in reflecting on her early life has described her experience as 'sensory jumbling' (Grandin, 1995: 150) an expression which seems to describe well the problems for autistic children.

MOTOR DEVELOPMENT

Evidence that autistic children show neurodevelopmental and motor abnormalities has slowly gathered over the years. Early descriptions of these children suggested that they were graceful and skilful and had few signs of motor impairment. This was part of the puzzle. Systematic studies of motor performance including those of DeMyer et al. (1972) and Jones & Prior (1985) uncovered clear signs of delayed or abnormal motor and sensorimotor development. Wing (1976) had also reported clumsiness and difficulties in planning and executing organized motor programmes such as riding a tricycle or managing more than one motor task at a time. Problems in producing gesture, either by imitation or spontaneously, may underlie the well-known failure of autistic children to use gesture to communicate as do normal children. Motor dyspraxias and neurodevelopmental signs such as choreiform movements, balance problems, gait abnormalities, (Damasio & Maurer, 1978) and impaired body imitation abilities are now believed characteristic of autism (Damasio & Maurer, 1978; Manjiviona & Prior, 1995).

Moreover, motor milestones are reported to be slow in a substantial proportion of cases (DeMyer et al., 1981), although it is not clear whether neurologically handicapped autistic children are different from those without measurable signs on these indices. The increasing proportion of children in research studies who have evidence of central nervous system (CNS) dysfunction along with their autism, may be influencing the trend away from earlier Kannerian type beliefs where there was emphasis on the apparent normality of motor development in children with this diagnosis. Recent studies, using standardized tests of motor impairment and including Asperger's syndrome and higher functioning autistic children as subjects (Ghaziuddin et al., 1994; Manjiviona & Prior, 1995), have shown that both groups show signs of neuromotor clumsiness across a range of gross and fine, and upper and lower body, motor performance. These findings are of particular interest given the belief that clumsiness is a marked feature of Asperger's syndrome rather than autism, and that it might be a diagnostically differentiating sign. It appears that this belief is highly questionable. Investigations of observed gait and locomotion abnormalities in autistic children have provided evidence for theories of cerebellar dysfunction (Hallet et al., 1993).

THE ROLE OF ATTENTION

Many investigations have documented attentional abnormalities in individuals with autism. Early studies, for example, suggested that arousal modulating systems were dysfunctional, leading to fluctuations between states of over- and under arousal (Hutt et al., 1964; Ornitz & Ritvo, 1968). Later work, using cortical event related potentials, confirmed that orienting and processing of novel stimuli by autistic persons is reduced (Courchesne et al., 1985; Dawson et al., 1986). Many individuals with autism appear to have 'over focused' attention, responding to only a subset of environmental cues during learning situations (Lovaas et al., 1979). Consistent with overly focused attention is a deficit in shifting attention. Individuals with autism, even those who are high functioning, with IQs in the normal range, appear to have difficulty moving their attention from one spatial location to another (Casey et al., 1993; Wainwright-Sharp & Bryson, 1993; Courchesne et al., 1994).

This pattern of attentional dysfunction distinguishes children with autism from those with attention deficit hyperactivity disorder (ADHD), another childhood condition involving attention problems. While children with ADHD have little difficulty moving attention (Swanson et al., 1991), they demonstrate severe impairment in sustaining attention and controlling impulses (Douglas & Peters, 1979). In contrast, a number of studies have suggested that the ability to sustain attention is a relatively spared function in autism (Garretson et al., 1990; Buchsbaum et al., 1992; Casey et al., 1993).

Overall then, autistic children show clearly deviant attention to their environment. They can be oblivious, avoidant and selectively or over focused. They may selectively avoid attending to socially relevant stimuli, probably because they cannot comprehend their meaning. They have difficulty controlling arousal aspects of attention; they show impairments in the ability to shift attention, to select salient rather than irrelevant or arbitrary attributes of stimuli to be processed, and they are easily distracted by irrelevant stimuli (Burack, 1994). More work comparing autistic children with other clinical groups is needed in this area of functioning because attention deficits are such a ubiquitous phenomenon in a range of psychiatric disorders. As a majority of autistic children are unable to participate in the common experimental tasks used to assess attention there is a great challenge in finding ways to objectively assess their problems.

Abnormal attentional processes in autism are highly likely to be associated with difficulties in understanding the meaning of environmental stimuli, leading to poor choices of what to attend to in the absence of clear directives, and strong tendencies to over focus in order to try to achieve some measure of control over an overwhelming input. This in turn restricts adaptive learning and perpetuates the difficulties. In more able autistic individuals, learning of concrete rules and strategies to apply to tasks seems to facilitate attentional and behavioural control. It is much more rare for it to lead to the development of spontaneous and flexible attentional strategies which can be applied to new problems.

MOTIVATION

In the early years of the study of autism the question of whether autistic children 'could' or 'would' (i.e. were able versus willing) engage with others, and with the kinds of tasks set for them, was a salient preoccupation for researchers and carers alike. As a result of the belief that autistic children were actually intelligent beings 'locked up' in their autistic aloneness, it was thought that they had at least normal abilities; the challenge was to motivate them to demonstrate their capacities. The major evidence for this was in the occasional case showing high levels of ability in a self-chosen area.

The curiosity and information gathering which is so central to the behaviour of normal young children is almost universally absent to a remarkable degree. These children also lack the 'wh' questions which characterize the language of normally developing young children.

Finding ways to motivate autistic children to do intelligence tests was important in underpinning our attempts to explore other key factors, and also as a possible explanation for their behaviour.

Little attention has been paid in the recent literature, however, to this issue as it was more clearly recognized during the 1970s and 1980s that autism involved severe cognitive deficits (Rutter, 1983) and that 'can't' rather than 'won't' was the answer to the question. Skills in persuading autistic children, especially the higher functioning ones, to comply with our experiments and assessments for example, have improved dramatically, allowing greater confidence that the performance we observe is a reliable and valid estimate of their capacities. This remains somewhat idiosyncratic; many children are relatively inaccessible, and many are mostly motivated by preoccupations and by ensuring security and routine, so that one never feels totally certain that there may not be some ability which could be elicited if one could get past the barrier. Researchers who have devised ways of enhancing motivation via the use of rewards of both concrete and social kinds have shown that it is possible to increase learning potential at least in some areas and some of the time (Koegel & Koegel, 1995). With low functioning children and adolescents whose behavioural repertoires are severely limited and deviant, motivating them to learn more adaptive behaviour remains a substantial challenge.

GENERAL INTELLECTUAL FUNCTION

The majority of children with autism function intellectually in the mentally handicapped range (e.g. IQ of less than 70). DeMyer et al. (1974), in an early study, found that close to half their sample functioned in the severe–profound range of mental retardation (IQ of less than 35); one-quarter demonstrated abilities in the moderately handicapped range (IQ 35–50); a fifth functioned in the mildly retarded range (IQ 50–70); and only 6% obtained IQ scores in the nonretarded range (IQ more than 70). The low representation of higher functioning cases in this sample is likely a reflection of the era (the early 1970s) in which there was not nearly as great a recognition of mild forms of autism as there is today. A more recent study found that 23% of a preschool aged autistic sample demonstrated IQ scores in the moderately mentally handicapped range of functioning, 48% in the mild range and 29% in the nonretarded range (Lord & Schopler, 1988); children functioning in the severe and profound ranges were not included in this study (Chapter 2).

While the results of these two investigations are not completely convergent, they are consistent, along with many others (Freeman et al., 1985; Ritvo et al., 1989), in finding that the majority of autistic individuals are mentally handicapped. Approximately one-quarter of people with autism, however, function in the intellectually normal range and do not demonstrate comorbid mental retardation. In general, girls with autism obtain lower scores on intellectual tests and represent a smaller proportion of high functioning cases than boys (Konstantareas et al., 1989; Lord & Schopler, 1985).

Children with autism demonstrate a wide scatter of skills on cognitive testing. In general, they have difficulty with tasks that involve language, imitation, abstract or conceptual reasoning, and executive function skills such as sequencing, organization, planning and flexibility (Green et al., 1995; Lincoln et al., 1995; Ozonoff, 1995a). They are detail oriented, but have difficulty 'seeing the big picture', and can be quite literal in their thinking. Learning, in general, is characterized by difficulty in seeing relations between pieces of information, identifying central patterns or themes, distinguishing relevant from irrelevant information, and deriving meaning (Frith, 1989). Such difficulties are apparent across the autistic continuum and are present in even very high functioning individuals (Grandin, 1995).

Conversely, individuals with autism tend to perform well on tasks that are visual in nature, tasks that have concrete materials to manipulate and tasks in which the stimulus materials themselves suggest what is required (DeMyer et al., 1974; Schopler et al., 1995). Strengths in visual–spatial processing, eye–hand coordination, attention to detail and rote memory abilities have been found in a number of different studies (Green et al., 1995; Lincoln et al., 1995).

This general pattern of strengths and weaknesses leads to a characteristic profile on intellectual testing. On standard intelligence tests such as the Wechsler scales (e.g. WPPSI-R, WISC-III, WAIS-R), most studies report higher performance than verbal IQ (for a review see Lincoln et al., 1995). Intersubtest variability is the norm. Reflecting the strengths in visual–spatial processing and rote memory often seen in autism, scores on the Block Design, Object Assembly, and Digit Span subtests are often the highest in a profile (Shah & Frith, 1983, 1993; Happe, 1994a; Freeman et al., 1985; Asarnow et al., 1987; Lincoln et al., 1988). In contrast, scores on the Comprehension subtest are typically the lowest in a Wechsler Verbal Scale Profile (Lockyer & Rutter, 1970; Freeman et al., 1985; Asarnow et al., 1987; Lincoln et al., 1988), reflecting deficits in conceptual reasoning, social judgement and perhaps the ability to reason about others' minds (Happe, 1994a,b). Scores on the Picture Arrangement and Coding subtests are often the lowest on the performance scale profile (Freeman et al., 1985; Lincoln et al., 1988), probably associated with the sequential and analytical difficulties

71

of autism. These patterns appear to be independent of IQ level and severity of autistic symptomatology (Fein et al., 1985; Freeman et al., 1985; Lincoln et al., 1988).

Consistent patterns are obtained on other intelligence tests as well. For example, on the Kaufman Assessment Battery for Children, high scores are obtained on both the Triangles subtest, a measure analogous to the Wechsler Block Design task, and Number Recall, similar to Digit Span (Allen et al., 1991). Similarly, profile patterns on the Stanford–Binet Intelligence Scales demonstrate highest performance on the Pattern Analysis subtest, a measure of visual–spatial function, and lowest performance on the Absurdities subtest, a measure of verbal conceptual reasoning and social judgement (Carpentieri & Morgan, 1994; Harris et al., 1990). Similar discrepancies between visuospatial function and verbal, practical reasoning have been found on the Griffiths Mental Development Scale (Sandberg et al., 1993). Testing with a nonverbal measure of intellectual function, such as the Leiter International Performance Scale (Arthur, 1949), again elicits better performance on the more concrete, visual items than those that require some degree of abstract reasoning (Maltz, 1981).

Very little research has been carried out on variations in cognitive performance as a function of pervasive developmental disorder (PDD) subtype, with no studies yet having examined issues of subtest variability or cognitive strengths and weaknesses in children with Rett's or disintegrative syndrome. There has been some suggestion that the cognitive profile of individuals with Asperger's syndrome may differ from that of autism. In his initial description of the syndrome, Asperger (1944) stated that the children he was studying were extremely clumsy and demonstrated delays in both gross and fine motor development. Motor deficits have been shown to correlate with poor visuospatial skills (Henderson et al., 1994), stimulating recent exploration of visual–spatial functions in individuals with Asperger's syndrome. One recent study found that verbal IQ was significantly higher than Performance IQ in a sample with Asperger's syndrome (Klin et al., 1995), a pattern opposite the typical findings in autism. Additionally, subjects with Asperger's syndrome in this study showed deficits on tests of fine and gross motor ability, visual–motor integration, visuospatial perception, visual memory and nonverbal concept formation. Conversely, high functioning autistic subjects of similar overall IQ performed well on these tests, but demonstrated deficits on measures of auditory perception, verbal memory, articulation, vocabulary and verbal output (Klin et al., 1995). This suggests that the strengths and weaknesses of autism and Asperger's syndrome may be different, with the former group performing well on visuospatial tasks and poorly on language tasks, and the opposite pattern being indicative of the Asperger group. If so, this might suggest that different patterns of underlying brain damage are responsible for the two PDD subtypes, with left hemisphere dysfunction predominating in the autistic group and right hemisphere damage characterizing the Asperger group. These conclusions must remain tentative, however, as DSM-IV criteria were not used when defining the groups in the Klin et al. study (1995) and there are contrary results from other research teams (Ghaziuddin et al., 1994; Majiviona & Prior, 1995; Szatmari et al., 1995).

A number of studies have suggested that IQ scores are relatively stable across time and development in individuals with autism. Correlations of IQ scores in preschool and school age are generally statistically significant and similar to values seen in nonhandicapped children (Lord & Schopler, 1988). Scores are more stable and predictive the older the age at initial assessment (Lord & Schopler, 1989). Scores can and do change, however, with a proportion of children changing IQ grouping levels as they age (e.g. from moderately to mildly retarded, etc.) (Lord & Schopler, 1989; Freeman et al., 1991). Thus, narrow categorization of intellectual level based on early IQ scores may not be appropriate.

ACADEMIC FUNCTIONING

The performance profile seen on measures of education and academic function is similar to that obtained on intellectual tests. Academic skills requiring primarily rote, mechanical or procedural abilities are generally intact, while those relying upon more abstract, conceptual or interpretive abilities are typically deficient. For example, in the reading domain, Minshew et al. (1994) found that high functioning autistic individuals performed as well as or better than normal controls matched on age and IQ on tests of single word oral reading, non word reading and spelling. These measures all require phonological decoding skills and thus indicate preserved or even advanced knowledge of grapheme–phoneme correspondence rules in autism. In contrast, autistic subjects in the study performed less well than controls on two measures of reading comprehension.

This pattern, in its most extreme form, is called hyperlexia. This term is used to describe individuals with word recognition skills that are significantly better than predicted by intellectual or educational level. Excellent decoding skills are typically accompanied by relatively poor comprehension abilities (Silberberg & Silberberg, 1967). Hyperlexia has been documented in individuals with autism by a number of researchers (Burd et al., 1987; Welsh et al., 1987; Tirosh & Canby, 1993).

The pattern is quite different from that typically obtained by reading disabled individuals (Vellutino, 1979; Pennington, 1991). In two studies directly comparing the reading profiles of autistic and dyslexic individuals, dyslexic subjects demonstrated deficits on phonological processing measures but strengths in comprehension and interpretation, while autistic subjects displayed the opposite pattern (Frith & Snowling, 1983; Rumsey & Hamburger, 1990). Thus, the profile of reading strengths and weaknesses seen in autism is not simply a reflection of general learning disability, but takes on a highly characteristic pattern.

There has been less empirical work examining mathematical and other academic abilities in autistic individuals. Rumsey & Hamburger (1990) found that high functioning adult males with autism performed as well as matched normal controls and better than dyslexic individuals on a test of arithmetical calculation. Similarly, Minshew et al (1994) found that high functioning autistic individuals performed as well as controls on math computation tasks. Interestingly, in this study autistic individuals showed no deficits in applied aspects of mathematics, thus failing to demonstrate the same discrepancy between mechanical and conceptual abilities apparent in the reading realm. This finding requires independent replication by other research teams, but may suggest that mathematics is a relatively spared academic ability in high functioning cases of autism.

Investigators have also examined age differences in performance on academic tests. Goldstein et al (1994) compared autistic children with autistic adolescents/adults of similar IQ level. They found that both age groups performed better on measures of phonological decoding and mathematics than on measures of reading comprehension and abstract, complex reasoning. In comparison with matched normal controls, some interesting differences as a function of age emerged, however. Younger autistic subjects performed as well as controls on most tests, but older autistic individuals performed significantly less well than matched controls on many of the same measures. These findings may reflect the kinds of skills emphasized in the educational system across the course of development. School work in the early years emphasizes mastery of rote, mechanical procedures, such as letter–sound correspondences and multiplication tables. Later educational curricula, on the other hand, highlight comprehension, conceptualization and analysis skills. Therefore, as Goldstein et al. (1994) suggest, high functioning autistic individuals may perform as well

as peers until grade levels in which abstract, interpretive skills are emphasized, at which point they fall behind.

Predictors of school achievement have also been studied in autistic
samples. Venter et al. (1992) found that performance on academic tests in
adolescence was significantly predicted by early nonverbal IQ and functional speech before age 5 years, while the severity of repetitive, stereotyped
behaviours in preschool was negatively correlated with later academic
achievement.

These studies suggest that high functioning autistic individuals perform
capably in a number of academic domains, at least relative to others of
similar intellectual and mental age level. Deficits are not universal and tend
to cluster in areas requiring conceptual and abstract reasoning. This mirrors the characteristic profile obtained on measures of intellectual function.

'IDIOT SAVANT' OR SPLINTER ABILITIES

Early studies in the field highlighted cases of autism where there were 'islets
of ability' or splinter skills, in a background of general intellectual disability. This was likened to examples of 'idiot savant' abilities which had been
in the literature related to mental retardation for some time. Rimland
(1978) suggested that these cases should be called 'autistic savants'. He
reported that about 10% of autistic individuals showed some high level
special ability or in some cases more than one savant ability. The particular
association between savant abilities and autism is demonstrated by the fact
that the estimate of such cases in the mentally retarded population is about
one in 2000 (Hill 1977, cited in Pring et al., 1995). Their special talents are
notable for the fact that they are of little help in other cognitive and social
areas of their lives.

The kinds of talents described include mathematics, especially 'lightning
calculation'; music, art, mechanical ability, calendrical calculation, memory, geographical knowledge (maps, routes, etc.), as well as multiple skills.
The most common in this list according to Rimland's (1978) study are
musical, memory, artistic, mathematical, geographical and pseudoverbal
(remembering, spelling and pronouncing, but not understanding words)
abilities. Most of these cases showed their gifts by the age of 4 years, and
had reached their peak by 10 years according to parental reports. The
autistic savants are usually functioning in the intellectually disabled range
and are unable to describe or explain their abilities (but for counter
examples on this last point, see Pring et al., 1995). Rimland, in seeking

theoretical and biological explanations for this phenomenon, stressed the ability of these cases to concentrate intensely on their interests, to fixate on details and their abnormal memory processes.

The research group of Hermelin and O'Connor in Britain has provided sophisticated analyses of some autistic savant talents using experimental methods to try to identify the processes involved and their relations to facets of intelligence. They report that preoccupations, or obsessions and repetitive behavioural tendencies are closely associated with idiot savant abilities (Hermelin & O'Connor, 1991). Their experiments indicate that autistic savants do follow simple rules to help them in recall and to calculate dates, for example; furthermore, they are able to abstract, a capacity which is usually extremely limited in the general autistic population (O'Connor, 1989).

A study of calendrical calculators (O'Connor & Hermelin, 1984: 806) suggested that their exceptional ability was not based just on rote memory for dates and days, but involved 'rule-governed calculations and strategies', and that speed of access was influenced by the distance of the date to be recalled from the present.

In seeking explanations for exceptional artistic ability, Pring et al. (1995) emphasize the fact that a substantial proportion of autistic cases show notable superiority with block design tasks by comparison with other subtests of intelligence, which suggests that they have a special ability to segment a holistic stimulus into its component parts. This, they argue, can be especially significant in drawing and painting and is an ability which appears to be independent of general intelligence in artistically talented people. A parallel argument can be made with regard to musical ability and the facility with pitch discrimination (subcomponents of music) within a musical 'gestalt'. Such dissociations may also be important, in for example, geographical abilities, where individuals can remember with absolute fidelity the details of particular streets, places, maps and routes no matter how unusual or obscure they might be. Hermelin's group have linked such abilities to Frith's (1989) 'central coherence' theory in which the core deficit in autism is seen as a failure to derive coherence (meaningful wholes) from the information they may apprehend, leaving them prone to 'modular' (noncoherent) abilities.

Although there is minimal substantive evidence on outcome for autistic savants. Rimland (1978) claims that many of those who 'recover' to some extent from their autism, lose their exceptional abilities. It is also worth noting here that one of the cardinal features of Asperger's syndrome and autistic individuals is their intense preoccupation with special interests.

Although this does not inevitably reach the status of a savant ability, such children are extraordinarily knowledgeable (and pedantic) about their favourite topics (such as computers, trains, timetables, sport, astronomy, anatomy, geography, etc.) albeit in a nonfunctional way. Asperger and autistic children are rarely able to reflect upon and describe how they have acquired this knowledge and it helps little in their everyday adjustment.

MEMORY

The memory of autistic individuals has been extensively studied. Some investigators have suggested that autism is a primary disorder of memory, likening it to an amnesic syndrome (Boucher & Warrington, 1976; Hetzler & Griffin, 1981; DeLong, 1992; Bachevalier, 1994). This theory was first put forth by Boucher & Warrington (1976), who outlined the behavioural similarities between autistic children and animals with hippocampal and other medial temporal lesions. The amnesic analogy has received some support from anatomical data, in that a number of studies have documented temporal and limbic malformations in autism (Hauser et al., 1975; Bauman & Kemper, 1985, 1988; Hoon & Reiss, 1992; White & Rosenbloom, 1992).

In addition to behavioural and anatomical similarities, it has also been proposed that the pattern of functioning in memory tests is similar in autistic and amnesic patients (Boucher & Warrington, 1976; DeLong, 1992; Bachevalier, 1994). Amnesic subjects typically demonstrate three patterns that have been hypothesized to also exist in autistic individuals: (1) intact short term and rote memory abilities, (2) reduced primacy but normal recency effects, and (3) better performance under cued than free recall conditions. A number of experimental investigations have been carried out to explore the validity of this analogy and are reviewed below.

Rote memory

Kanner (1943) was the first to note the good rote memories of children with autism. In the opening paragraphs of his seminal paper describing the syndrome of autism, Kanner commented upon the extraordinary memories of the children he was studying, particularly their ability to recite long lists of items or facts. Many have suggested that the echolalic tendencies of autistic individuals indicate an above average auditory rote memory

(Hermelin & O'Connor, 1970; Hermelin & Frith, 1971). Early experimental studies confirmed the observations that short term and rote memorial processes were largely intact in autistic individuals. In a series of studies, Hermelin & Frith (1971) demonstrated that the short term auditory memory of children with autism was as good as that of normal and mentally handicapped individuals of similar mental age. Autistic subjects were as able to repeat back strings of words as the other groups, although there were some qualitative differences in how they did this (see below). Prior & Chen (1976) demonstrated that once autistic, retarded and normal subjects matched on mental age were equated for pre-existing list learning and acquisition differences, the three groups were equally capable of recalling both single items and lists in a visual memory task. They concluded that differences in performance on memory tasks between autistic and nonautistic samples may be a function of learning and acquisition deficiencies, rather than primary memory difficulties.

The rote memory of people with autism appears to diverge from that of amnesic individuals in the ability to learn paired associate lists, however. Boucher & Warrington (1976) found that autistic children were able to learn lists of word pairs as easily as normal children and better than retarded controls of higher verbal ability. Similar results on a paired associate learning task have been reported more recently by Minshew & Goldstein (1993) in high functioning autistic adolescents and adults. This is in contrast to amnesics, who typically demonstrate extraordinary difficulty on this type of learning task (Boucher & Warrington, 1976), thus weakening the strongest version of the autistic-amnesic analogy.

Primary versus recency effects

O'Connor & Hermelin (1967) were the first to note that primacy effects in list learning tended to be weaker than recency effects in autistic children; these results were replicated by Boucher (1981). This pattern is also characteristic of amnesic adults (Baddeley & Warrington, 1970). Hermelin & Frith (1971) attempted, unsuccessfully, to attenuate strong recency effects by composing sentences in which the beginning part of the word string was made up of meaningful sentence fragments, while the latter part was composed of random verbal material. Their autistic group continued to demonstrate strong recency and weak primacy effects even under these conditions. As recency effects rely more purely on rote auditory mechanisms, while recall of the first part of a list requires further processing and encoding of the material (Craik & Lockhart, 1972), less developed primacy effects in autism may be secondary to organizational and encoding impairments rather than to memory deficits per se, an issue to which we return below.

Free versus cued recall

Another point of similarity between autism and amnesia cited by Boucher & Warrington (1976) is the finding that cued recall is significantly better than free recall for both groups. This finding has been replicated recently by Tager-Flusberg (1991). Others, however, have found mild impairments relative to controls in both free and cued recall conditions, suggesting a general recall inefficiency in autism that is not specific to the method of testing retention (Minshew & Goldstein, 1993).

Other patterns: the role of organization and meaning

It has been suggested that autistic individuals encounter difficulty remembering material that requires further encoding, organization or use of meaning to facilitate recall (DeLong, 1992; Minshew & Goldstein, 1993). In a pioneering series of experiments, Hermelin, O'Connor and colleagues found that the advantage in remembering meaningful over random material typically seen in normally developing individuals is not apparent in autism, i.e. individuals with autism do not appear to use the syntactic and semantic cues that aid others in recalling material. For example, two studies demonstrated that autistic children were just as capable of recalling random verbal material (e.g. unconnected words) as they were of remembering meaningful sentences (Hermelin & O'Connor, 1967; Hermelin & Frith, 1971). In contrast, matched mentally handicapped children demonstrated a significant advantage in remembering words in the context of a meaningful sentence. Similarly, early studies demonstrated that autistic children did not semantically cluster or 'chunk' related items when recalling word lists (O'Connor & Hermelin, 1967; Hermelin & Frith, 1971).

Later experiments clarified, however, that autistic children are not incapable of using semantic cues in recall, just less efficient in doing so. Fyffe & Prior (1978) failed to replicate earlier results, finding that autistic children recalled sentences significantly better than random word lists. Relative to controls, however, recall of sentences was deficient, while recall of random material was adequate. Thus, while the autistic group did appear to make use of meaning in recall, their advantage was not as great as in the mentally handicapped or normally developing control groups. Tager-Flusberg (1991) replicated this pattern, finding that recall of related and unrelated word lists was equivalent within the autistic group; however, their memory for meaningful material was less efficient than that of controls. Thus, the ability of autistic individuals to utilize meaning, structure and semantic cues in recall appears to be poorer than that of matched controls, but by no means absent.

In a recent study utilizing visual rather than verbal stimuli, however, autistic individuals were found to be significantly impaired in the recall of random material but adequate relative to controls in remembering meaningful stimuli (Ameli et al., 1988). This may indicate that inefficient use of meaning to facilitate recall is relatively specific to the verbal domain, reflecting the general language difficulties of autism, rather than being a universal memorial deficit of the disorder. Thus, similarities between autism and amnesia may exist only under selective experimental conditions, such as when verbal material must be processed.

Deficits in working memory have also been found in autism. Working memory is defined as the ability to maintain information in an activated, online state to guide cognitive processing (Baddeley, 1986). More so than other memory operations, working memory serves a dynamic function and has been referred to as a 'computational workspace' (Baddeley, 1986). Typical working memory tasks require subjects to simultaneously hold information online, process it and store results for later recall, thus requiring a significant amount of organization and processing of the material to be remembered. A recent study of working memory in autistic individuals, using sentence and counting span measures (Bennetto et al., 1996), found that subjects with autism were significantly impaired relative to controls on working memory tasks, but not on measures of short and long term recognition memory, cued recall or new learning ability.

The evidence reviewed here suggests that autism is not a primary disorder of memory. Rather, difficulty appears to occur at the stage of encoding and organizing material. It is the overlay or additional requirement of higher order processing that makes certain memory tasks difficult for autistic individuals. As summarized by DeLong (1992), the deficit does not appear to be an acquisition, storage or retention impairment, but an interaction with the kind of information being processed and the operations being performed on the information. As with intellectual and academic functions, memory deficits appear to be selective, rather than widespread and all-encompassing. Concrete, rote and mechanical processes are spared; once abstraction, organization and use of meaning are required, however, performance declines.

SOCIAL DEVELOPMENT AND BEHAVIOUR

Impairments in perceiving and processing social and emotional cues in people and in the environment from the beginning of life seem to be at the heart of the disorder (Rutter, 1983). On the basis of a large epidemiological study of children with autism and developmental disorders, Wing & Gould (1979) proposed that the deficits of autistic children were encompassed by a 'triad of impairments' in imagination, communication and socialization. This conceptualization is immediately appealing because it captures the core features across all levels of functioning and it provides direction for exploring why these features might cohere and provide clues about the basis of the autistic disorder. In the remainder of the chapter, social behaviour, communicative/language capacities and theoretical approaches to bringing together research in these domains are the focus.

Social impairments are apparent very early in life in the majority of cases. As infants, autistic individuals are reported as not cuddly but rather stiff and resistant to contact, or else passive and floppy. They do not mould their bodies in anticipation of being picked up. Some appear placid and undemanding of human attention and are described as exceptionally 'good' babies; others are difficult to manage, their needs cannot be identified and satisfied, and they are impossible to comfort (Prior et al., 1975).

Their self-isolation and lack of communication is sometimes interpreted as a sign of deafness even though they may show an unpredictable or idiosyncratic reaction to particular sounds. Earlier researchers (e.g. De-Myer, 1976) suggested that severely handicapped young children do not discriminate between people, but more recent research (e.g. Walters et al., 1990; Dissananayake & Crossley, 1996) has shown that autistic children do show responsiveness and attachment to familiar carers, at least at a level consistent with their mental age. In fact, a number of studies during the last decade have reported evidence of attachment to carers in young autistic children which is not too dissimilar from that seen in nonautistic groups (Sigman et al., 1986; Rogers et al., 1991). This has represented a small breakthrough in understanding, since for decades it has been so widely believed that a central and causal mechanism in autism was a lack of bonding and attachment. This work suggests that their nonresponsiveness is not always 'pervasive'. Attachment behaviour can be seen across the spectrum in various forms but may be more likely to be observable in higher functioning children.

Nevertheless, it is true that autistic children seek help and comfort less often than do normal and intellectually disabled children; they show less mutual eye contact, less attention to people and events, and show more avoidant behaviour. Contact is most frequently 'on their terms' (Wing, 1976).

Aloofness, indifference, passivity, distractibility, noncompliance, along with lack of cooperation and engagement in the activities of others, are characteristic of these children although they may vary on a continuum from almost totally withdrawn to occasional or 'active but odd' contact (Wing & Gould, 1979), based entirely on their own interests and needs. The severity of their social deficits is related to IQ and language capacities, with the lowest functioning children the most difficult to engage.

A number of researchers have examined 'joint attention' and social behaviour in autistic children in both laboratory and naturalistic settings. Joint attention refers to the child's propensity, normally present from around 12 months of age, to show by pointing, bringing or otherwise indicating an object or event which they wish to share with a partner. It also encompasses eye contact with the partner related to the interest of the object, so called referential looking. It is a key component of normal social development and one which is notably absent in most autistic children. This deficit is believed to offer a key to the understanding of their deviance in social development because of its significance in the normal developmental pathway to social and communicative competence. Mundy & Sigman (1989a) have summarized a number of studies confirming the near universality of joint attention deficits in young autistic children, and drawing on this work in developing a theory which incorporates the cognitive and affective impairments central to autism (on this topic see debate among Baron-Cohen, 1989a; Harris, 1989; Mundy & Sigman, 1989a,b).

Joint attention behaviour can be increased when adult carers provide structure and modelling for such interaction although it is rarely spontaneously shown (Kasari et al., 1993). Baron-Cohen (1989b) in a study of protodeclarative versus protoimperative pointing has also shown that deficits in pointing to objects of interest are in the shared interest aspect (protodeclarative), rather than representing an inability to indicate the presence of an object (protoimperative pointing).

Although a lack of joint attention behaviours is evident even when controlling for IQ (Mundy et al., 1990), like other deficit behaviours, they

82

are less marked in higher functioning children. Joint attention skills are also associated with the development of language skills (Mundy et al., 1987), with correlations around 0.5 and 0.6 being reported by Mundy et al. (1990) in a longitudinal study of 4–5 year olds, based on observations of social and play interactions in the laboratory and assessment with the Reynell Developmental Language Scales. Mundy & Sigman (1989a: 174) assert that 'a disturbance of nonverbal joint attention behaviours is a fundamental characteristic of young autistic children' and that this 'may be regarded as an important manifestation of early aspects of autistic developmental process'. They consider whether social skill deficits are better explained via a model which emphasizes cognitive impairments (Baron-Cohen, 1988) or one which emphasizes deficits in the development of affect in interaction with carers (Kanner, 1943; Hobson, 1989). They argue that problems in gestural joint attention skills reflect deficits in affective processes as well as social/cognitive factors.

While there is little disagreement that joint attention deficits are one of the keys to autism and that they are related to the expression of other core social impairments, the nature of their role remains the subject of debate (Baron-Cohen, 1989a; Mundy & Sigman, 1989a,b; Harris, 1989).

Longitudinal studies which can map the timing and emergence of joint attention skills within the context of cognitive and affective development in other domains will be helpful in understanding this issue. Moreover, future studies assessing the effects of training in joint attention and related reciprocal social behaviours may not only provide adaptive avenues for treating autistic children but may answer some questions concerning the temporal and causal role of these impairments in the development of the disorder.

While rarely demonstrating joint interest and reciprocal activities, some children will enlist partners for repetitive games, preoccupations or obsessions such as verbal routines which may not vary, and do not take into account the other person's independent or contributory role.

Some will make pseudosocial approaches to complete strangers which are inappropriate and deviant. For example, older children have been known to try to stroke the hair or the breasts of complete strangers.

The hallmark of the condition, at every age and stage, and every level of functioning, is lack of reciprocal social interaction. Even high functioning individuals with Asperger's syndrome who are actively seeking to make contact with others suffer from lack of insight into the thoughts, feelings, plans and wishes of others. Try as they might, they cannot master the skills necessary for true reciprocity of social communication. Empathy remains a mystery even to those who appear to have made a good adjustment (Wing, 1981; Sigman et al., 1992).

Apart from the absence of appropriate social skills there is also the presence of much unacceptable deviant and socially embarrassing behaviour. These behaviours include stereotypies such as rocking, head banging, self-stimulatory and self-injurious behaviour such as hand biting and head punching, screaming and temper tantrums often in highly public places such as supermarkets; aggressive and hyperactive behaviour; purloining desired objects or those which are part of an obsession (for example taking certain flowers or leaves from people's gardens); and socially embarrassing eating, toileting and sometimes verbal behaviours. There are some famous examples in the literature of even high functioning individuals making comments which might be true but which would rarely be uttered by a nonhandicapped person. Few of these kinds of deviant behaviours are distinctive to autism by comparison with the 'absent' behaviours which are more discriminative of an autism diagnosis. They contribute to the fact that the majority of these children are extraordinarily difficult to manage and to socialize. It is these kinds of behaviours which are likely to have some children excluded from normal educational and social environments and make it more likely that they will be kept in special, segregated and more restrictive settings.

Comparative studies of autistic and other handicapped as well as normal groups using standardized tests such as the Vineland Adaptive Behaviour Scales show their severe handicaps in social and communicative domains, with scores well below expectation taking into account their mental age levels. Dysfunctional social behaviours found in a study of this genre by Rodrigue et al. (1991) were pervasive, especially in the use of play and leisure times, in interpersonal relating and in coping skills. Their autistic subjects also showed behaviours not apparent in normal children at any age. Naturalistic observational studies of social behaviour (Buitelaar et al., 1991) confirm deficits in reciprocal social and communicative skills across varying levels of severity of autism.

Peer interaction is significantly impaired and most commonly almost completely absent, even in children who relate reasonably well to adults. Attempts to train peer interaction skills have had limited success and there are persistent and seemingly intransigent difficulties in spontaneous initiation of interactions (Walters et al., 1990). One important aspect of Asperger's syndrome individuals which indicates some difference from autism is the finding that they often would like to interact with peers but are handicapped by their lack of skills in doing so (Eisenmajer et al., 1996).

They are also often conscious of and can describe their difficulties. Higher functioning autistic and Asperger's syndrome individuals sometimes do have a particular 'friend', usually a child with similar social problems or obsessive interests.

EMOTION PERCEPTION

Experimental research on the emotion perception abilities of autistic individuals was originally stimulated by Hobson's account of early affective development (Hobson, 1986a, 1989). Hobson highlighted the inborn capacity of normal infants and children to recognize the salience of social and affective cues, make 'emotional touch' with others and affectively experience close personal relationships. He hypothesized that this inborn mechanism does not develop properly in autistic children, accounting for many of their aberrant social behaviours. In addition, his theory predicts that children with autism should have particular difficulty with experimental tasks that require recognition of emotional states in other people.

Using a crossmodal paradigm in which subjects had to match affective and nonaffective auditory and visual stimuli, Hobson (1986a,b) found that the autistic group committed significantly more errors than controls matched on nonverbal IQ when matching affective material, but performed as well as controls on nonaffective tasks. Weeks & Hobson (1987) demonstrated that autistic children preferred to sort faces by nonemotional attributes, such as hairstyles and accessories, than by emotional expressions. When required to sort faces by emotion, performance was significantly impaired relative to controls.

Other researchers, using different but related paradigms, have replicated the finding that autistic individuals are selectively impaired on affective tasks, relative both to performance of comparison subjects matched on nonverbal IQ and to their own performance on nonaffective control tasks (MacDonald et al., 1989; Bormann-Kirschkel et al., 1995). Young children with autism pay little attention to the emotional displays of others, tending to ignore them or engage in alternate activities, relative to both normally developing and mentally retarded controls (Sigman et al., 1992). Finally, two studies have found that autistic individuals are impaired in recognizing the meanings of emotion related nouns and adjectives, relative to concrete, nonemotional terms (Hobson & Lee, 1989; Van Lancker et al, 1991).

Two methodological issues have been raised concerning these studies, however, by both Hobson himself (1991) and others (Braverman et al.,

1989; Ozonoff et al., 1990). First, in many studies the affective and nonaffective comparison tasks were not of equal difficulty, with the latter typically being easier for all groups. Thus, the finding that group differences exist on emotion recognition tasks, but not on nonaffective control tasks, does not necessarily indicate a specific deficit in emotion perception. Second, and even more importantly, the role of verbal ability in emotion perception was not adequately controlled in early studies. If some verbal mediation is required to process affective information, then failure to match on verbal ability may account for group differences, rather than a primary deficit in emotion perception being responsible. Most studies reviewed above matched control samples on nonverbal IQ alone.

Both of these issues were addressed in three subsequent investigations by Hobson et al. (1988a,b, 1989a), who found that when autistic individuals were matched with control subjects on the basis of verbal ability, group differences were no longer apparent on emotion sorting, matching and naming tasks. This finding has been replicated by several research teams (Braverman et al., 1989; Davies et al., 1994; Ozonoff et al., 1990; Prior et al., 1990; Serra et al., 1995), each of whom found that group differences on emotion perception tasks were dependent on the nature of the control group used, i.e. group differences evident when controls were matched on nonverbal ability disappeared when matching was instead on the basis of verbal mental age or IQ. Language ability and verbal IQ can account for large amounts of variance in emotion perception scores, with intercorrelations in the 0.60–0.70 range (Fein et al., 1992). Capps et al. (1992) found deficits in recognizing only more complex emotions, such as pride and embarrassment. Since these emotions require some social referencing and social comparison, it has been suggested that deficits on such tasks may be more reflective of theory of mind difficulties than emotion perception impairments (Baron-Cohen, 1991a).

These results suggest that there are a number of moderating variables that account for variance in emotion perception abilities in autism. Group differences between autistic and control samples may be secondary to linguistic, cognitive, pragmatic or theory of mind deficits of autism, rather than reflecting a specific emotion processing impairment. Finally, research has demonstrated that emotion perception deficits are not specific to the autistic population, having also been documented in individuals with mental retardation (Hobson et al., 1989b), learning disabilities (Holder & Kirkpatrick, 1991) and schizophrenia (Novic et al., 1984; Walker et al., 1984).

LANGUAGE

The majority of autistic children do not develop communicative language. A number of these mute children may use grunting, pointing or instrumental touching or pulling to communicate needs, and a minority may have a few words used for similar purposes. Use of gesture to communicate is notably restricted. It is rare for an autistic child to gain language if he/she has not done so by the age of about 6 years. Prognosis for children with language before 2 years of age appears to be enhanced (Rogers & DiLalla, 1990) and for nonspeaking children is universally poor.

Even for speaking children, however, the communicative functions of language are impaired or limited in significant ways. The intention to communicate may be said to underlie both language and social behaviour and it is this which often appears abnormal in autistic children. An alternative view for which there is some support is that many of these children wish to communicate but do not know how to do so effectively, i.e. this is a fundamental biologically based, cognitive impairment. Recent proposals about the centrality of the lack of a theory of mind in autism which are discussed below, provide a way of bringing the elements of the social/cognitive/language picture together in a way that makes sense.

The kinds of abnormalities noted over the years in autistic children's language have included concreteness, literalness, pronomial reversal, deviant or monotonous prosodic features, metaphorical language, inability to initiate or sustain a conversation, ritualistic and inflexible language, and insensitivity to the listener's response to a conversation (Tager-Flusberg, 1981, 1982). These deficits, however, exist on a continuum across the population of autistic children, and there are marked individual differences (Wetherby, 1986).

The language abnormalities appear to be present early in life as noted in a lack of (or abnormal) babbling, lack of the normal preference for attending to human speech (Klin, 1991), signs of incomprehension of the language environment, delay in first words, and in developing phrase speech; regressions after initial speech development; failure to imitate sounds and speech, echolalia, both immediate and delayed; and in some cases, repeating of rhymes or jingles with no apparent communicative function, often as the only form of speech.

Perhaps the most universal language deficit in autism is that associated with pragmatics, i.e. language used to communicate socially (Tager-Flusberg & Anderson, 1991). This transcends the individual differences in levels of speech competence, as it is seen in every autistic person to some degree. Even very high functioning cases have difficulty adapting their discourse to the listener's response, in perceiving what the listener might be wanting or thinking, and in imagining where to go next in the conversation. Some of such individuals are able to articulate that they experience this problem, they wish to overcome it, but are unable to adapt their conversation and thinking no matter how well motivated (see the collection of personal accounts in Schopler & Mesibov, 1992). They also have difficulty understanding and responding to complex questions.

Tager-Flusberg and colleagues, in a series of studies (e.g. Tager-Flusberg, 1989; Tager-Flusberg et al., 1990) have explored the acquisition of language in autistic children over time and compared them with normal and Down's syndrome children. While autistic children are similar to matched comparison groups in the early stages of their language development, especially with their mothers and in familiar settings, as they grow older they become increasingly divergent. They become more prone to use routines, recoding and simple responses, rather than developing more sophisticated discourse as do normal children, and they appear unaware that conversation provides an opportunity for giving new knowledge or for sharing experience. Their vocabularies can also be limited or stereotyped (Tager-Flusberg, 1981), and prosody is frequently deviant, even in high functioning cases.

A naturalistic observational study of communication in the school setting and including autistic children across a wide range of cognitive abilities (Stone & Caro-Martinez, 1990), showed that the most common form of communication was instrumental, in the form of 'motoric acts', i.e. touching another person to gain their attention or to obtain a desired end. The most common recipient was the teacher, although speaking children were also likely to target communication to peers or observers. The speaking group also used more gestures, made comments and gave information, even though overall any spontaneous communication was rare.

Volden & Lord (1991) have analysed the indiosyncratic language and neologisms sometimes reported as a feature of autism, and compared their utterances with those of mentally retarded and normal children matched on chronological age. Most of their high functioning autistic sample produced unusual words, phrases or neologisms, and these were also seen, albeit to a lesser extent, in mentally handicapped children. The autistic children more often used peculiar forms of speech which were neither semantically nor phonologically similar to the appropriate English word, by comparison with control groups. Volden and Lord see these linguistic idiosyncrasies as part of a broader language impairment in autism which is not simply a function of developmental delay.

Most recent work confirms that autistic children are consistent with their mental age level in the mechanics or formal aspects of language such as order of acquisition of speech sounds, in measures of syntax and language content, and length and complexity of utterances (Green et al., 1995); it is the semantic and pragmatic, or socially relevant aspects which they cannot master. Abstract words, i.e. those with no concrete referents, are rarely understood or used; hence 'thinking', 'feeling' 'wanting', kinds of messages in normal social communicative behaviour leave all but the highest functioning cases at a loss.

Comprehension can be impaired and there is a lack of focus on the meaning aspects of language. Their problems have been linked to a language disorder known as 'semantic-pragmatic disorder' (Bishop, 1989), described as 'a set of behaviours that are loosely associated, which shade into autism at one extreme and normality at the other' (Brook & Bowler, 1992: 62). Primary characteristics of this communication disorder encompass the use of language which may be fluent and complex but which is inappropriate or out of tune with the social context. Comprehension is also impaired. The semantic pragmatic language impairments which are shared with high functioning autistic (and with Asperger's syndrome) cases include comprehension deficits, literal interpretations of messages, perseveration, deficits in turn taking and problems with maintaining conversational topics. The two diagnostic groups also share deficits in symbolic play and joint referencing behaviour. Comparisons of social impairments between autism and semantic pragmatic language disorder underline the heterogeneity and variation in levels especially within the latter group. But as Bishop (1989) has noted, autistic children can have other kinds of language disorders, and children with semantic-pragmatic disorder are often not autistic and their communication difficulties are less extensive than those common in autism.

Attempts to train autistic children in the use of speech and in sign language have identified serious limitations in that even when children learned words or signs, they were limited in their ability to use such skills to generate spontaneous 'new' utterances and tended to remain at a relatively parrot like level (Harris, 1975). At least with higher functioning children, however, there has been documented success in improving communication and language competence especially through intensive home based training programmes based on behavioural principles (Lovaas, 1987; Howlin, 1989), although there are always limitations to the level of success achieved.

Severely autistic children remain relatively resistant to improvement despite the best efforts of parents and teachers.

THEORY OF MIND

The last part of this chapter provides a brief discussion of recent theorizing about key underlying deficits in autism including 'Theory of Mind' and executive functioning, two aspects of the disorder which have been linked heuristically at behavioural and neuropsychological levels. The theory of mind hypothesis represents an attempt to bring together what is known about the social, cognitive and communication problems of autistic children across the developmental period, with the aim of providing a coherent, integrated and comprehensive explanation of the psychological characteristics of the disorder (Frith, 1989). Beginning with the experimental studies of Baron-Cohen, Frith and colleagues in Britain (for a summary, see Happe & Frith, 1995), this hypothesis has had considerable influence over autism research in most domains, and in most countries, in recent years. A number of their studies have demonstrated that autistic children have difficulty understanding false belief, ignorance and second order belief (beliefs about beliefs) in other people; in the concept of pretence, and of emotional reactions based on beliefs (Baron-Cohen, 1991a, b).

In essence, the theory of mind explanation of such deficits in autism argues that autistic children are unable to perceive and comprehend the thoughts and feelings of others, i.e. that other people have 'minds'. They suffer from 'mind blindness' (Happe & Frith, 1995). They do not apprehend the fact that individuals have beliefs, thoughts, feelings, plans and intentions, i.e. mental states which influence their actions; nor are they able to comprehend that the thoughts, feelings and actions of other people need to be taken into account in social transactions as guides to reciprocal behaviours. Their behaviour reflects the absence of such knowledge. Their difficulties in understanding pretence, states of ignorance, states of knowledge and emotions which are based on beliefs means that they are unable to provide 'mentalistic' explanations for behaviour, and they cannot predict other's behaviour (Tager-Flusberg & Sullivan, 1994). Their spontaneous language rarely includes terms or comments which refer to mental states such as belief, although they may refer to less mentalistic concepts such as desire, emotion and perception (Tager-Flusberg, 1992). More sophisticated apperception involving mind reading such as cheating, lying, deceiving and understanding jokes are a mystery to them by this theory (but see Leekam & Prior, 1994 for evidence regarding lying and joking).

A variety of experimental tasks and procedures has been used to assess mentalizing ability in autistic children, usually involving comparisons with other groups of similar levels of language and cognitive capacities. Probably the most common tasks are enacted scenarios involving dolls or people whose knowledge or belief states must be intuited, so that predictions about their behaviour can be accurately made. For example, children may be asked what another person would think if they were presented with a box of Smarties (correct answer = there are Smarties in there). While another character either real or puppet like is demonstrably absent, the child is shown that there are really pencils in the box. They are then asked what the absent character believes are the contents of the box. Normal children above the age of 4 years will correctly answer 'Smarties'. Autistic children are more likely to answer 'pencils', thus demonstrating an inability to imagine what the other character will believe on the basis of access to information. Many other creative ways of assessing this ability at varying levels of sophistication and abstraction have been reported in the literature (Baron-Cohen, 1991b; Bowler, 1992; Happe, 1994c; Leekam & Prior, 1994), and naturalistic studies have also illustrated the mentalizing deficits in autism.

Leslie (1987) has conceptualized the core psychological impairments as a 'metarepresentational deficit', i.e. the ability to think about thoughts (one's own and other peoples'). Without such abilities, it is argued, it is no wonder that the autistic individual cannot 'read minds', a capacity which is necessary to explain and predict the behaviour of others in the social world. This makes life confusing and frightening, leading to withdrawal and avoidance.

The earliest signs of this key deficit can be observed in the lack of joint attention skills, communicative gestures and sharing of objects of interest and information with others (Baron-Cohen, 1991b). These behaviours are seen as developmental precursors to mentalizing ability. There is ongoing debate, however, concerning the direction of relations between these impairments, i.e. what is precursor to what? Given that higher functioning autistic children, particularly those with good verbal skills, are notably less handicapped in theory of mind abilities, perhaps higher levels of social and communicative capacities allow development of mentalizing ability. It has also been noted that mentalizing deficits may not always be absent, although they are inevitably delayed in their appearance for those children who do have this capacity (Baron-Cohen, 1989c).

Klin et al. (1992) have claimed that the social impairments characteristic of autism emerge in the earliest developmental stages, before the emergence of precursors to theory of mind capacities, an argument which was also put in 1989 by Mundy & Sigman. It is also possible as Leekam (1993) and others have suggested, that communicative ability and mental state knowledge develop independently, albeit in parallel, rather than being causally related.

Not all autistic children lack a theory of mind, hence claims to have discovered the 'core' and universal explanation for autism are weakened. Findings that children diagnosed with Asperger's syndrome as well as a substantial proportion of more verbally capable autistic cases are often able to solve the theory of mind tasks conventionally used in this genre of research (Eisenmajor & Prior, 1991; Ozonoff et al., 1991b; Bowler, 1992), have lead the proponents of the theory to suggest that such cases may 'hack out' or 'compute' solutions, using compensatory cognitive mechanisms which, however, do not constitute evidence for a 'true' theory of mind (Happe & Frith, 1995). Whether this is true remains a question for exploration, but in any case, however successful the theory might be in explaining the social, language and imaginative impairments of autistic children, it may not satisfactorily encompass other key deficits such as the lack of spontaneous activity and language, the repetitive and ritualistic behaviours including obsessions and preoccupations, islets of ability, lack of generalization skills, resistance to learning, and stereotypic behaviour.

Nevertheless, if one considers that these latter behaviours are characteristic of developmental delays and abnormalities in a general sense, whereas the triad of social, communicative and imaginative impairments are autism specific, the theory has considerable explanatory power (for a discussion of current theoretical debate, see Klin et al., 1992; Happe, 1994c). Even for those children who do acquire some elements of theory of mind, albeit often later in development by comparison with normal children, this remains limited and inflexible, and rarely develops into the complex reflexive capacities involved in thinking about the thinking or shared knowledge of others, i.e. those behaviours that serve as guideposts to normal social interaction.

While 'Theory of Mind' has made a major contribution in bringing together much of what is known about autistic behaviours, there are some findings which challenge the boundaries, if not the essence of this theory. Not every autistic child lacks a theory of mind; many Asperger's syndrome or high functioning autistic individuals are able to demonstrate theory of mind, at least in experimental studies (Bowler, 1992), and with some kinds of tasks (Happe, 1994b), despite the fact that their core social and communicative deficiencies are clearly apparent, especially when subtlety and flexibility in social encounters are called for. There is great variability in theory of mind abilities across samples of children with autistic spectrum disorders. Furthermore, this capacity is clearly associated with language ability (Eisenmajer & Prior, 1991; Ozonoff et al., 1991b; Tager-Flusberg, 1993; Tager-Flusberg & Sullivan, 1994). Other linguistically handicapped children, including deaf individuals (Peterson & Siegal, 1995) may show theory of mind handicaps, but not the other social and pragmatic impairments, so it is not necessarily distinctive of autism. Moreover, it is possible that 'mentalizing' problems are simply one aspect of a more pervasive collection of cognitive impairments and in that sense the theory does not have comprehensibility.

In addition, there is the unresolved difficulty of knowing how such a relatively 'modular' deficit could be connected to any biologically based impairment with aetiological significance for autism, a disorder which has such broad and devastating consequences for the majority of cases.

Although explanations in terms of an autism specific metarepresentational deficit have been a primary focus, there is a variety of alternative interpretations for the responses of autistic children on theory of mind tasks. Harris (1989) and Ozonoff et al. (1994) have suggested that executive function deficits may have considerable explanatory power for autism related impairments. Bowler (1992) also makes reference to problem solving based on slow and cumbersome routes which handicap everyday social interaction but which may allow solutions to be generated for theory of mind experimental tasks.

Many researchers believe that there are multiple cognitive deficits in autism and that they cannot all be encompassed in this theory. It has been however a very fruitful one in generating a research agenda which may take us a little closer to identifying the nature, the timing of emergence and the consequences of various facets of the social cognitive deficits, and their relations to other parts of the puzzle of autism. Finding any kind of biological substrate for such a range of psychological impairments remains a great challenge. Recent research has drawn connections between the kinds of behaviours adduced to indicate theory of mind deficits and those which are believed to indicate problems with executive functions. In the final section some of this recent experimental and theoretical work is reviewed.

EXECUTIVE FUNCTION

Investigation of executive function ability has been an active area of research with autistic individuals since Rumsey's pioneering empirical work in 1985. Executive function skills are those goal directed, future oriented cognitive abilities thought to be mediated by the frontal cortex (Duncan, 1986), including planning, inhibition, flexibility, organization and self-monitoring. Studies documenting deficits in this realm predate Rumsey's work by 40 years, however. Several early investigations described impairments that appear to overlap with what is now called 'executive function', although they were not characterized as such in the original citations. This began with the cognitive studies of Frith (1972), and Hermelin & O'Connor (1970: 126), who, in summarizing the deficits underlying poor performance on several experiments, stated that their autistic subjects 'had a tendency to persist in a once given response rather than select an alternative one'. Boucher (1977) further examined this phenomenon in a maze learning task in which two alternate, but equally correct, routes were available to complete a maze. While ability matched normal controls frequently alternated their maze solutions between the correct choices, autistic children were more likely to stick with one solution strategy, using it over and over again. When a novel solution was presented to subjects on later trials, those in the autistic group were less likely than those in the control group to try the new maze route.

Evidence of executive dysfunction was present in each of these early studies, although none used the same experimental paradigms as present day investigations or described their results using the same terminology. In recent years, autistic individuals of all ages and functioning levels have been tested on measures presumed to require the executive system. Rumsey (1985) studied verbal, high functioning adult men with residual state autism. As have many studies since, the Wisconsin Card Sorting Test (WCST) was used to investigate executive function abilities. Relative to a normal control sample matched on age, deficits were found on most WCST variables, including number of categories completed, total errors, perseverative responses and perseverative errors. In following investigations, Rumsey & Hamburger (1988, 1990) found that autistic individuals sorted significantly fewer WCST categories than age matched controls; this pattern was not a general consequence of learning or developmental disorders, as WCST impairment was found only in the autistic group and was not apparent in a comparison sample with severe dyslexia.

Prior & Hoffmann (1990: 588) administered a simplified version of the

WCST to children with autism and matched controls. Despite such simplifications and the provision of task structure, the autistic group committed significantly more errors and perseverative responses than controls. They also performed significantly less well than controls on the Milner Maze Test, demonstrating deficits in planning and difficulty in learning from mistakes. The autistic group 'perseverated with maladaptive strategies, made the same mistakes repeatedly, and seemed unable to conceive of a strategy to overcome their difficulties'.

The WCST was also administered to individuals with high functioning autism by Szatmari et al. (1990). This study was particularly interesting because 80% of the control group met criteria for ADHD or conduct disorder, two childhood conditions also hypothesized to involve executive dysfunction (Chelune, et al., 1986; Lueger & Gill, 1990). Despite this conservative choice of control group, autistic subjects still made significantly more perseverative errors and completed fewer categories on the WCST than the comparison sample. Ozonoff et al. (1991a) reported similar results and, in addition, found that the autistic group committed significantly fewer failures to maintain set than the control group, a variable logically and conceptually opposite to that of perseveration. An added executive function measure, the Tower of Hanoi, was best able to discriminate between the autistic and learning disabled groups and predict group membership. Performance on this test classified 80% of the subjects in each group correctly, while other neuropsychological variables (e.g. theory of mind, memory, emotion perception and spatial abilities) predicted group membership at no better than chance levels. The classification power of this executive function measure was unexpected, as one-quarter of the control sample met criteria for ADHD. Ozonoff & McEvoy (1994) demonstrated that deficits on the Tower of Hanoi and WCST were stable over a 2 year period, with a tendency for executive function abilities to decline relative to controls over time.

Two investigations have failed to find deficits on the WCST in autistic individuals (Schneider & Asarnow, 1987; Minshew et al., 1992), although experimental design factors may account for the Schneider and Asarnow findings. Minshew et al. (1992) found no group differences in perseverative or nonperseverative WCST errors relative to matched normal controls, but did, however, document evidence of executive dysfunction on a different executive function measure, the Goldstein-Scheerer Object Sorting Test, in which autistic subjects were less able to shift set than controls.

The only investigation to examine executive functions in preschool age autistic children was conducted by McEvoy et al. (1993). They used several developmentally simple measures of prefrontal function that were first developed for use with nonhuman primates and human infants (Diamond & Goldman-Rakic, 1986). In the spatial reversal task, an object is hidden in one of two identical wells outside of the subject's vision. The site of hiding remains the same until the subject successfully locates the object on four consecutive trials, after which the site of hiding is changed to the other well. Thus, successful search behaviour requires flexibility and set shifting. Autistic children made significantly more perseverative errors than children with either the mental or chronological age matched groups. No group differences were evident on three other executive function measures, although this appeared secondary to significant floor and ceiling effects that made these tasks less developmentally appropriate for the sample.

A recent research trend has been the use of computerized experimental paradigms designed to examine specific aspects of executive function and more precisely identify the nature of the executive function impairments underlying autism. Hughes et al. (1994) developed a computerized set shifting task suitable for use with both low and high functioning individuals with autism. Significant group differences were found, with the autistic sample engaging in highly perseverative and inflexible strategies. A number of internal controls were built into the task, eliminating several other executive function deficits (e.g. inhibition, rule reversal, transfer of learning) as explanations for poor task performance and highlighting the flexibility impairment of the autistic group.

Ozonoff and colleagues, in a series of papers, have suggested that flexibility is a more dysfunctional component of executive function than inhibition. In a computerized Go-NoGo task designed to isolate and separately examine flexibility and inhibition operations in high functioning autistic subjects (Ozonoff et al., 1994), they found that the autistic group was not impaired relative to controls when inhibiting responses, but was very deficient at shifting set. In contrast, matched comparison subjects with Tourette's syndrome experienced no difficulty in either the inhibition or flexibility conditions. Two additional aspects of inhibitory function, the ability to inhibit voluntary motor responses and the ability to inhibit processing of distractor stimuli during a cognitive task, were found to be unimpaired in autistic subjects in a later study (Ozonoff & Strayer, 1997). These results suggest that inhibition may be a spared component of executive function in autism, standing in contrast to the impairments in flexibility found in other studies (Rumsey, 1985; Prior & Hoffmann, 1990; Ozonoff et al., 1991a; Hughes et al., 1994).

It has also been suggested that executive dysfunction may underlie some aspects of the social cognition deficit of autism. In a study designed to examine theory of mind and strategic deception abilities (Russell et al., 1991), autistic subjects were taught to play a game in which they competed with an experimenter for a piece of candy. The candy was placed in one of two boxes with windows that revealed the contents of the box to subjects, but not to the experimenter. The objective of the task was to 'fool' the experimenter into looking for the candy in the empty box. It was explained that the strategy of pointing to the empty box would be successful in winning the candy, whereas pointing to the box that actually contained the chocolate would result in losing it. Even after many trials, the autistic subjects were unable to point to the empty box, despite the consequences of this strategy. Russell et al. (1991) first attributed these results to a perspective taking deficit that caused an inability to engage in deception. In a follow-up study, Hughes & Russell (1993) demonstrated that significant group differences remained even after the element of social deception was removed from the task. Subjects were simply instructed to point to the empty box to get the candy. Even with no opponent present, the autistic subjects persisted in using the inappropriate strategy. On the basis of these results, Hughes & Russell (1993) reattributed the autistic subjects' pattern of performance to a deficit in disengaging from the object and using internal rules to guide behaviour, rather than to a social or perspective taking dysfunction.

Several other studies have highlighted the related and interdependent nature of social/cognitive and executive function skills (Grattan & Eslinger, 1989; Szatmari et al., 1989; Ozonoff et al., 1991a; Berger et al., 1993). It has been suggested that executive function and perspective taking abilities may share a common neural substrate (Ozonoff & McEvoy, 1994; Ozonoff, 1995a), with recent functional neuroimaging research indicating that theory of mind capacities may be subserved by the prefrontal cortex (Baron-Cohen et al., 1994; Fletcher et al., 1995). Alternatively, certain executive function skills, such as flexibility, may be a prerequisite for empathy and other social behaviours. Ozonoff (1995b) recently demonstrated that autistic individuals perform more similarly to controls on computerized versions of the WCST that do not require any verbal or social interaction than on standardly administered versions of the test. These studies suggest that the social cognition and executive function deficits of autism may not be completely separable, independent areas of dysfunction. It is also clear, however, that executive function difficulties cannot completely account for the social disabilities of autism, as nonautistic individuals with severe executive function disorders do not demonstrate the same magnitude or quality of social disturbance as in autism (Bishop, 1993).

While it is likely that executive function deficits in some form or other are a feature of a number of childhood disorders involving social and cognitive impairments, the linking of Theory of Mind and executive functions in both experimental and naturalistic studies seems to have promise for further research development, and for contributing to the understanding of psychological aspects of autism spectrum disorders.

REFERENCES

Abrahamsen, E. P. & Mitchell, J. R. (1990). Communication and sensorimotor functioning in children with autism. *Journal of Autism and Developmental Disorders,* **20,** 75–85.

Allen, M. H., Lincoln, A. J. & Kaufman, A. S. (1991). Sequential and simultaneous processing abilities of high-functioning autistic and language-impaired children. *Journal of Autism and Developmental Disorders,* **21,** 483–502.

Ameli, R., Courchesne, E., Lincoln, A., Kaufman, A. S. & Grillon, C. (1988). Visual memory processes in high-functioning individuals with autism. *Journal of Autism and Developmental Disorders,* **18,** 601–15.

Arthur, G. (1949). The Arthur adaptation of the Leiter International Performance Scale. *Journal of Clinical Psychology,* **5,** 345–9.

Asarnow, R. F., Tanguay, P. E., Bott, L. & Freeman, B. J. (1987). Patterns of intellectual functioning in non-retarded autistic and schizophrenic children. *Journal of Child Psychology and Psychiatry,* **28,** 273–80.

Asperger, H. (1944). 'Autistic psychopathy' in childhood. *Archiv fur Psychiatrie und Nervenkrankheiten,* **117,** 76–136.

Bachevalier, J. (1994). Medial temporal lobe structures and autism: a review of clinical and experimental findings. *Neuropsychologia,* **32,** 627–48.

Baddeley, A. D. (1986). *Working Memory.* Oxford: Clarendon Press.

Baddeley, A. D. & Warrington, E. K. (1970). The distinction between long and short-term memory. *Journal of Verbal Learning and Verbal Behaviour,* **9,** 176–89.

Baron-Cohen, S. (1988). Social and pragmatic deficits in autism: cognitive or affective? *Journal of Autism and Developmental Disorders,* **18,** 379–402.

Baron-Cohen, S. (1989a). Joint-attention deficits in autism: towards a cognitive analysis. *Development and Psychopathology,* **1,** 185–9.

Baron-Cohen, S. (1989b). Perceptual role taking and protodeclarative pointing in autism. *British Journal of Developmental Psychology,* **7,** 113–27.

Baron-Cohen, S. (1989c). The autistic child's theory of mind: a case of specific developmental delay. *Journal of Child Psychology and Psychiatry,* **30,** 285–97.

Baron-Cohen, S. (1991a). Do people with autism understand what causes emotion? *Child Development,* **62,** 385–95.

Baron-Cohen, S. (1991b). The theory of mind deficit in autism: how specific is it? *British Journal of Developmental Psychology,* **9,** 301–14.

Baron-Cohen, S., Ring, H., Moriarty, J., Schmitz, B., Costa, D. & Ell, P. (1994). Recognition of mental state terms: clinical findings in children with autism and a functional neuroimaging study of normal adults. *British Journal of Psychiatry,* **165,** 640–9.

Bauman, M. & Kemper, T. L. (1985). Histoanatomic observations of the brain in early infantile autism. *Neurology,* **35,** 866–74.

Bauman, M. & Kemper, T. L. (1988). Limbic and cerebellar abnormalities: consistent findings in infantile autism. *Journal of Neuropathology and Experimental Neurology*, **47**, 369.

Bennetto, L., Pennington, B. F. & Rogers, S. J. (1996). Impaired and intact memory functions in autism: a working memory model. *Child Development*, **67**, 1816–1835.

Berger, H. J. C., van Spaendonck, K. P. M., Horstink, M. W. I. M., Buytenhuijs, E. L., Lammers, P. W. J. M. & Cools, A. R. (1993). Cognitive shifting as a predictor of progress in social understanding in high-functioning adolescents with autism: a prospective study. *Journal of Autism and Developmental Disorders*, **23**, 341–59.

Bishop, D. V. M. (1989). Autism, Asperger's syndrome and semantic-pragmatic disorder: where are the boundaries? *British Journal of Disorders of Communication*, **24**, 107–21.

Bishop, D. V. M. (1993). Autism, executive functions, and theory of mind: a neuropsychological perspective. *Journal of Child Psychology and Psychiatry*, **34**, 279–93.

Bormann-Kischkel, C., Vilsmeier, M. & Baude, B. (1995). The development of emotional concepts in autism. *Journal of Child Psychology and Psychiatry*, **36**, 1243–59.

Boucher, J. (1977). Alternation and sequencing behaviour and response to novelty in autistic children. *Journal of Child Psychology and Psychiatry*, **18**, 67–72.

Boucher, J. (1981). Immediate free recall in early childhood autism: another point of behavioural similarity with the amnesic syndrome. *British Journal of Psychology*, **72**, 211–15.

Boucher, J. & Warrington, E. K. (1976). Memory deficits in early infantile autism: some similarities to the amnesic syndrome. *British Journal of Psychology*, **67**, 73–87.

Bowler, D. M. (1992). 'Theory of mind' in Asperger's syndrome. *Journal of Child Psychology and Psychiatry*, **33**, 877–93.

Braverman, M., Fein, D., Lucci, D. & Waterhouse, L. (1989). Affect comprehension in children with pervasive developmental disorders. *Journal of Autism and Developmental Disorders*, **19**, 301–16.

Brook, S. L. & Bowler, D. M. (1992). Autism by another name? Semantic and pragmatic impairments in children. *Journal of Autism and Developmental Disorders*, **22**, 61–81.

Buchsbaum, M. S., Siegel, B. V., Wu, J. C., Hazlett, E., Sicotte, N., Haier, R., Tanguay, P., Asarnow, R., Cadorette, T., Donoghue, D., Lagunas-Solar, M., Lott, I., Paek, J. & Sabalesky, D. (1992). Attention performance in autism and regional brain metabolic rate assessed by positron emission tomography. *Journal of Autism and Developmental Disorders*, **22**, 115–25.

Buitelaar, J. K., van Engeland, H., de Kogel, K. H., de Vries, H. & van Hooff, J. A. R. A. M. (1991). Differences in the structure of social behaviour of autistic children and non-autistic retarded controls. *Journal of Child Psychology and Psychiatry*, **32**, 995–1015.

Burack, J. A. (1994). Selective attention deficits in persons with autism: preliminary evidence of an inefficient attentional lens. *Journal of Abnormal Psychology*, **103**, 535–43.

Burd, L., Fisher, W., Knowlton, D. & Kerbeshian, J. (1987). Hyperlexia: a marker for improvement in children with pervasive developmental disorder? *Journal of the American Academy of Child and Adolescent Psychiatry*, **26**, 407–12.

Capps, L., Yirmiya, N. & Sigman, M. (1992). Understanding of simple and complex emotions in nonretarded children with autism. *Journal of Child Psychology and Psychiatry*, **33**, 1169–82.

Carpentieri, S. C. & Morgan, S. B. (1994). A comparison of patterns of cognitive functioning of autistic and nonautistic retarded children on the Stanford-Binet fourth edition. *Journal of Autism and Developmental Disorders*, **24**, 215–23.

Casey, B. J., Gordon, C. T., Mannheim, G. B. & Rumsey, J. M. (1993). Dysfunctional attention in autistic savants. *Journal of Clinical and Experimental Neuropsychology*,

15, 933–46.

Chelune, G. J., Ferguson, W., Koon, R. & Dickey, T. O. (1986). Frontal lobe disinhibition in attention deficit disorder. *Child Psychiatry and Human Development*, 16, 221–34.

Courchesne, E., Lincoln, A. J., Kilman, B. A. & Galambos, R. (1985). Event-related brain potential correlates of the processing of novel visual and auditory information in autism. *Journal of Autism and Developmental Disorders*, 15, 55–75.

Courchesne, E., Townsend, J., Akshoomoff, N. A., Saitoh, O., Yeung-Courchesne, R., Lincoln, A. J., James, H. E., Haas, R. H. Schreibman, L. & Lau, L. (1994). Impairment in shifting attention in autistic and cerebellar patients. *Behavioural Neuroscience*, 108, 848–65.

Craik, F. I. M. & Lockhart, R. S. (1972). Levels of processing: a framework for memory research. *Journal of Verbal Learning and Verbal Behaviour*, 11, 671–84.

Damasio, A. R. & Maurer, R. G. (1978). A neurological model for childhood autism. *Archives of Neurology*, 35, 777–86.

Davies, S., Bishop, D., Manstead, A. S. R. & Tantam, D. (1994). Face perception in children with autism and Asperger's syndrome. *Journal of Child Psychology and Psychiatry*, 35, 1033–57.

Dawson, G., Finley, C., Phillips, S. & Galpert, L. (1986). Hemispheric specialization and the language abilities of autistic children. *Child Development*, 57, 1440–53.

DeLong, G. R. (1992). Autism, amnesia, hippocampus, and learning. *Neuroscience and Biobehavioural Reviews*, 16, 63–70.

DeMyer, M. (1976). Motor, perceptual-motor and intellectual disabilities of autistic children. In *Early Childhood Autism: Clinical, Educational and Social Aspects*, 2nd edn., ed. L. Wing. Oxford: Pergamon Press.

DeMyer, M. K., Barton, S., Alpern, G. D., Kimberlin, C., Allen, J., Yang, E. & Steele, R. (1974). The measured intelligence of autistic children. *Journal of Autism and Childhood Schizophrenia*, 4, 42–60.

DeMyer, M. K., Barton, S. & Norton, J. A. (1972). A comparison of adaptive, verbal and motor profiles of psychotic and non-psychotic subnormal children. *Journal of Autism and Childhood Schizophrenia*, 2, 359–77.

DeMyer, M. K., Hingtgen, J. N. & Jackson, R. K. (1981). Infantile autism reviewed: a decade of research. *Schizophrenia Bulletin*, 7, 388–451.

Diamond, A. & Goldman-Rakic, P. S. (1986). Comparative development in human infants and infant rhesus monkeys on cognitive functions that depend on prefrontal cortex. *Society of Neuroscience Abstracts*, 12, 742.

Dissanayake, C. & Crossley, S. A. (1996). Proximity and sociable behaviours in autism: evidence for attachment. *Journal of Child Psychology and Psychiatry*, 37, 149–56.

Douglas, V. I. & Peters, K. G. (1979). Toward a clearer definition of the attentional deficit of hyperactive children. In *Attention and Cognitive Development*, ed. G. A. Hale & M. Lewis, pp. 173–247. New York: Plenum Press.

Duncan, J. (1986). Disorganization of behaviour after frontal lobe damage. *Cognitive Neuropsychology*, 3, 271–90.

Eales, M. J. (1993). Pragmatic impairments in adults with childhood diagnoses of autism or developmental receptive language disorder. *Journal of Autism and Developmental Disorders*, 23, 593–617.

Eisenmajer, R. & Prior, M. (1991). Cognitive linguistic correlates of 'theory of mind' ability in autistic children. *Journal of Autism and Developmental Disorders*, 9, 351–64.

Eisenmajer, R., Prior, M., Leekam, S., Wing, L., Gould, J. & Ong, B. (1996). A comparison of clinical symptoms in individuals diagnosed with autism and Asperger Syndrome. *Journal of the American Academy of Child and Adolescent Psychiatry*, 35, 1523–31.

Fein, D., Lucci, D., Braverman, M. & Waterhouse, L. (1992). Comprehension of affect in context in children with pervasive developmental disorders. *Journal of Child Psychology and Psychiatry*, **33**, 1157–67.

Fein, D., Waterhouse, L., Lucci, D. & Snyder, D. (1985). Cognitive subtypes in developmentally disabled children: a pilot study. *Journal of Autism and Developmental Disorders*, **15**, 77–95.

Fletcher, P. C., Happe, F., Frith, U., Baker, S. C., Dolan, R. J. & Frackowiak, R. (1995). Other minds in the brain: a functional imaging study of theory of mind in story comprehension. *Cognition*, **57**, 2.

Freeman, B. J., Lucas, J. C., Forness, S. R. & Ritvo, E. R. (1985). Cognitive processing of high-functioning autistic children: Comparing the K-ABC and the WISC-R. *Journal of Psychoeducational Assessment*, **4**, 357–62.

Freeman, B. J., Rahbar, B., Ritvo, E. R., Bice, T. L., Yokota, A. & Ritvo, R. (1991). The stability of cognitive and behavioural parameters in autism: a twelve-year prospective study. *Journal of the American Academy of Child and Adolescent Psychiatry*, **30**, 479–82.

Freeman, B. J., Ritvo, E. R., Needleman, R. & Yokota, A. (1985). The stability of cognitive and linguistic parameters in autism: a five-year prospective study. *Journal of the American Academy of Child Psychiatry*, **24**, 459–64.

Frith, U. (1972). Cognitive mechanisms in autism: experiments with color and tone sequence production. *Journal of Autism and Child Schizophrenia*, **2**, 160–73.

Frith, U. (1989). *Autism: Explaining the Enigma*. Oxford: Basil Blackwell.

Frith, U. & Snowling, M. (1983). Reading for meaning and reading for sound in autistic and dyslexic children. *British Journal of Developmental Psychology*, **1**, 329–42.

Fyffe, C. & Prior, M. (1978). Evidence for language recoding in autistic, retarded, and normal children: a re-examination. *British Journal of Psychology*, **69**, 393–402.

Garretson, H. B., Fein, D. & Waterhouse, L. (1990). Sustained attention in children with autism. *Journal of Autism and Developmental Disorders*, **20**, 101–14.

Ghaziuddin, M., Butler, E., Tsai, L. & Ghaziuddin, N. (1994). Is clumsiness a marker for Asperger's syndrome? *Journal of Intellectual Disability Research*, **38**, 519–27.

Gillberg, I. C. & Gillberg, C. (1989). Asperger syndrome: some epidemiological considerations. A Research note. *Journal of Child Psychology and Psychiatry*, **30**, 631–8.

Goldstein, G., Minshew, N. J. & Siegel, D. J. (1994). Age differences in academic achievement in high-functioning autistic individuals. *Journal of Clinical and Experimental Neuropsychology*, **16**, 671–80.

Grandin, T. (1995). How people with autism think. In *Learning and Cognition in Autism*, ed. E. Schopler & G. B. Mesibov, pp. 137–156. New York: Plenum Press.

Grattan, L. M. & Eslinger, P. J. (1989). Higher cognition and social behaviour: changes in cognitive flexibility and empathy after cerebral lesions. *Neuropsychology*, **3**, 175–85.

Green, L., Fein, D., Joy, S. & Waterhouse, L. (1995). Cognitive functioning in autism: an overview. In *Learning and Cognition in Autism*, ed. E. Schopler & G. B. Mesibov, pp. 13–31. New York: Plenum Press.

Hallett, M., Lebiedowska, M. K., Thomas, S. L., Stanhope, S. J. et al. (1993). Locomotion of autistic adults. *Archives of Neurology*, **50**, 1304–8.

Happe, F. G. E. (1994a). Wechsler IQ profile and theory of mind in autism. *Journal of Child Psychology and Psychiatry*, **35**, 1461–71.

Happe, F. G. E. (1994b). Annotation: current psychological theories of autism: the 'Theory of Mind' account and rival theories. *Journal of Child Psychology and Psychiatry and Allied Disciplines*, **35**, 215–29.

Happe, F. G. E. (1994c). An advanced test of theory of mind: understanding of handicapped, and normal children and adults. *Journal of Autism and Developmental Disorders*, **24**, 129–54.

Happe, F. & Frith, U. (1995). Theory of mind in autism. In *Learning and Cognition in Autism*, ed. E. Schopler & G. B. Mesibov, pp. 177–97. New York: Plenum Press.

Harris, P. L. (1989). The autistic child's impaired conception of mental states. *Development and Psychopathology*, **1**, 191–5.

Harris, S. L. (1975). Teaching language to non-verbal children– with emphasis on problems of generalization. *Psychological Bulletin*, **82**, 565–80.

Harris, S. L., Handleman, J. S. & Burton, J. L. (1990). The Stanford-Binet profiles of young children with autism. *Special Services in the Schools*, **6**, 135–43.

Hauser, S. L., DeLong, G. R. & Rosman, N. P. (1975). Pneumographic findings in the infantile autism syndrome: a correlation with temperal lobe disease. *Brain*, **98**, 667–88.

Henderson, E. S., Barnett, A. & Henderson, L. (1994). Visuospatial difficulties and clumsiness: on the interpretation of conjoined deficits. *Journal of Child Psychology and Psychiatry*, **35**, 961–9.

Hermelin, B. & O'Connor, N. (1967). Remembering of words by psychotic and subnormal children. *British Journal of Psychology*, **58**, 213–18.

Hermelin, B. & O'Connor, N. (1970). *Psychological Experiments with Autistic Children*. New York: Pergamon.

Hermelin, B. & O'Connor, N. (1991). Talents and preoccupations in idiot-savants. *Psychological Medicine*, **21**, 959–64.

Hermelin, B. & Frith, U. (1971). Psychological studies of childhood autism: can autistic children make sense of what they see and hear? *Journal of Special Education*, **5**, 107–17.

Hertzig, M. E., Snow, M. E. & Sherman, M. (1989). Affect and cognition in autism. *Journal of the American Academy of Child and Adolescent Psychiatry*, **28**, 195–9.

Hetzler, B. E. & Griffin, J. L. (1981). Infantile autism and the temporal lobe of the brain. *Journal of Autism and Developmental Disorders*, **11**, 317–30.

Hill, A. L. (1977). Idiot savants: rate of incidence. *Perceptual and Motor Skills*, **44**, 161–2.

Hobson, R. P. (1986a). The autistic child's appraisal of expressions of emotion. *Journal of Child Psychology and Psychiatry*, **27**, 321–42.

Hobson, R. P. (1986b). The autistic child's appraisal of expressions of emotion: a further study. *Journal of Child Psychology and Psychiatry*, **27**, 671–80.

Hobson, R. P. (1989). Beyond cognition: a theory of autism. In *Autism: Nature, Diagnosis and Treatment*, ed. G. Dawson, pp. 22–48. New York: Guilford.

Hobson, R. P. (1991). Methodological issues for experiments on autistic individuals' perception and understanding of emotion. *Journal of Child Psychology and Psychiatry*, **32**, 1135–58.

Hobson, R. P. & Lee, A. (1989). Emotion-related and abstract concepts in autistic people: evidence from the British Picture Vocabulary Scale. *Journal of Autism and Developmental Disorders*, **19**, 601–23.

Hobson, R. P., Ouston, J. & Lee, A. (1988a). Emotion recognition in autism: Coordinating faces and voices. *Psychological Medicine*, **18**, 911–23.

Hobson, R. P., Ouston, J. & Lee, A. (1988b). What's in a face? The case of autism. *British Journal of Psychology*, **79**, 411–53.

Hobson, R. P., Ouston, J. & Lee, A. (1989a). Naming emotion in faces and voices: abilities and disabilities in autism and mental retardation. *British Journal of Developmental Psychology*, **7**, 237–50.

Hobson, R. P., Ouston, J. & Lee, A. (1989b). Recognition of emotion by mentally retarded adolescents and young adults. *American Journal on Mental Retardation*, **93**, 434–43.

Holder, H. B. & Kirkpatrick, S. W. (1991). Interpretation of emotion from facial expressions in children with and without learning disabilities. *Journal of Learning Disabilities*, **24**, 170–7.

Hoon, A. H. & Reiss, A. L. (1992). The mesial temporal lobe and autism: case report and review. *Developmental Medicine and Child Neurology*, **34**, 278–9.

Howlin, P. (1989). Changing approaches to communication training with autistic children. Special issue: *Autism. British Journal of Disorders of Communication*, **24**, 151–68.

Hughes, C. & Russell, J. (1993). Autistic children's difficulty with mental disengagement from an object: its implications for theories of autism. *Developmental Psychology*, **29**, 498–510.

Hughes, C., Russell, J. & Robbins, T. W. (1994). Evidence for executive dysfunction in autism. *Neuropsychologia*, **32**, 477–92.

Hutt, S. J., Hutt, C., Lee, D. & Ounsted, C. (1964). Arousal and childhood autism. *Nature*, **204**, 908–9.

Jones, V. & Prior, M. (1985). Motor imitation abilities and neurological signs in autistic children. *Journal of Autism and Developmental Disorders*, **15**, 37–46.

Kanner, L. (1943). Autistic disturbances of affective content. *Nervous Child*, **2**, 217–50.

Kasari, C., Sigman, M. & Yirmiya, N. (1993). Focused and social attention of autistic children in interactions with familiar and unfamiliar adults: a comparison of autistic, mentally retarded, and normal children. *Development and Psychopathology*, **5**, 403–14.

Klin, A. (1991). Young autistic children's listening preferences in regard to speech: a possible characterization of the symptom of social withdrawal. *Journal of Autism and Developmental Disorders*, **21**, 29–42.

Klin, A., Volkmar, F. R. & Sparrow, S. S. (1992). Autistic social dysfunction: some limitations of the theory of mind hypothesis. *Journal of Child Psychology and Psychiatry*, **33**, 861–76.

Klin, A., Volkmar, F. R., Sparrow, S. S., Cicchetti, D. V. & Rourke, B. P. (1995). Validity and neuropsychological characterization of Asperger's syndrome: convergence with nonverbal learning disabilities syndrome. *Journal of Child Psychology and Psychiatry*, **36**, 1127–40.

Koegel, L. K. & Koegel, R. L. (1995). Motivating communication in children with autism. In *Learning and Cognition in Autism*, ed. E. Schopler & G. B. Mesibov, pp. 73–87. New York: Plenum Press.

Konstantareas, M. M., Homatidis, S. & Busch, J. (1989). Cognitive, communication, and social differences between autistic boys and girls. *Journal of Applied Developmental Psychology*, **10**, 411–24.

Leekam, S. R. (1993). Children's understanding of mind. In *The Child as Psychologist*, ed. M. Bennett, UK: Harvester Wheatsheaf.

Leekam, S. R. & Prior, M. (1994). Can autistic children distinguish lies from jokes? A second look at second-order belief attribution. *Journal of Child Psychology and Psychiatry*, **35**, 901–15.

Leslie, A. M. (1987). Pretence and representation: the origins of 'Theory of Mind'. *Psychological Review*, **94**, 412–26.

Leslie, A. M. (1992). Pretence, autism, and the theory-of-mind module. *Current Directions in Psychological Science*, **1**, 18–21.

Lincoln. A. J., Allen, M. H. & Kilman, A. (1995). The assessment and interpretation of intellectual abilities in people with autism. In *Learning and Cognition in Autism*, ed. E. Schopler & G. B. Mesibov, pp. 89–117. New York: Plenum Press.

Lincoln, A. J., Courchesne, E., Kilman, B. A., Elmasian, R. & Allen, M. (1988). A study of intellectual abilities in high-functioning people with autism. *Journal of Autism and Developmental Disorders*, **18**, 505–24.

Lockyer, L. & Rutter, M. (1970). A five- to fifteen-year follow-up study of infantile psychosis: patterns of cognitive ability. *British Journal of Social and Clinical Psychology*, **9**, 152–63.

Lord, C. & Schopler, E. (1985). Differences in sex ratios in autism as a function of measured intelligence. *Journal of Autism and Developmental Disorders*, **15**, 185–93.

Lord, C. & Schopler, E. (1988). Intellectual and developmental assessment of autistic children from preschool to schoolage: clinical implications of two follow-up studies. In *Diagnosis and Assessment in Autism*, ed. E. Schopler & G. B. Mesibov, pp. 167–81. New York: Plenum Press.

Lord, C. & Schopler, E. (1989). The role of age at assessment, developmental level, and test in the stability of intelligence scores in young autistic children. *Journal of Autism and Developmental Disorders*, **19**, 483–99.

Losche, G. (1990). Sensorimotor and action development in autistic children from infancy to early adulthood. *Journal of Child Psychology and Psychiatry*, **31**, 749–61.

Lovaas, O. I. (1987). Behavioural treatment and normal educational and intellectual functioning in young autistic children. *Journal of Consulting and Clinical Psychology*, **55**, 3–9.

Lovaas, O. I., Koegel, R. L. & Schreibman, L. (1979). Stimulus overselectivity in autism: a review of research. *Psychological Bulletin*, **86**, 1236–54.

Lueger, R. J. & Gill, K. J. (1990). Frontal lobe cognitive dysfunction in conduct disorder adolescents. *Journal of Clinical Psychology*, **46**, 696–706.

MacDonald, H., Rutter, M., Howlin, P., Rios, P., LeCouteur, A., Evered, C. & Folstein, S. (1989). Recognition and expression of emotional cues by autistic and normal adults. *Journal of Child Psychology and Psychiatry*, **30**, 865–77.

McEvoy, R. E., Rogers, S. J. & Pennington, B. F. (1993). Executive function and social communication deficits in young autistic children. *Journal of Child Psychology and Psychiatry*, **34**, 563–78.

McManus, I. C., Murray, B., Doyle, K. & Baron-Cohen, S. (1992). Handedness in childhood autism shows a dissociation of skill and preference. *Cortex*, **28**, 373–81.

Maltz, A. (1981). Comparison of cognitive deficits among autistic and retarded children on the Arthur adaptation of the Leiter International Performance Scales. *Journal of Autism and Developmental Disorders*, **11**, 413–26.

Manjiviona, J. & Prior, M. (1995). Comparison of Asperger syndrome and high-functioning artistic children on a test of motor impairment. *Journal of Autism and Developmental Disorders*, **25**, 23–39.

Minshew, N. J. & Goldstein, G. (1993). Is autism an amnesic disorder? Evidence from the California Verbal Learning Test. *Neuropsychology*, **7**, 209–16.

Minshew, N. J., Goldstein, G., Muenz, L. R. & Payton, L. R. (1992). Neuropsychological functioning in nonmentally retarded autistic individuals. *Journal of Clinical and Experimental Neuropsychology*, **14**, 749–61.

Minshew, N. J., Goldstein, G., Taylor, H. G. & Siegel, D. J. (1994). Academic achievement in high-functioning autistic individuals. *Journal of Clinical and Experimental Neuropsychology*, **16**, 261–70.

Morgan, S. B., Cutrer, P. S., Coplin, J. W. & Rodrigue, J. R. (1989). Do autistic children differ from retarded and normal children in Piagetian sensorimotor functioning? *Journal of Child Psychology and Psychiatry*, **30**, 857–64.

Mundy, P. & Sigman, M. (1989a). The theoretical implications of joint-attention deficits in autism. *Development and Psychopathology*, **1**, 173–84.

Mundy, P. & Sigman, M. (1989b). Second thoughts on the nature of autism. *Development and Psychopathology*, **1**, 213–18.

Mundy, P., Sigman, M. & Kasari, C. (1990). A longitudinal study of joint attention and language development in autistic children. *Journal of Autism and Developmental Disorders*, **20**, 115–28.

Mundy, P., Sigman, M., Ungerer, J. & Sherman, T. (1987). Play and nonverbal communication correlates to language development in autistic children. *Journal of Autism and Developmental Disorders*, **17**, 349–63.

Novic, J., Luchins, D. J. & Perline, R. (1984). Facial affect recognition in schizophrenia: is there a differential deficit. *British Journal of Psychiatry*, **144**, 533–7.

O'Connor, N. (1989). The performance of the 'idiot-savant': implicit and explicit. *British Journal of Disorders of Communication*, **24**, 1–20.

O'Connor, N. & Hermelin, B. (1967). Auditory and visual memory in autistic and normal children. *Journal of Mental Deficiency Research*, **11**, 126–31.

O'Connor, N. & Hermelin, B. (1984). Idiot savant calendrical calculators: Maths or memory? *Psychological Medicine*, **14**, 801–6.

Ohta, M. (1987). Cognitive disorders of infantile autism: a study employing the WISC, spatial relationships, conceptualization and gesture imitations. *Journal of Autism and Developmental Disorders*, **17**, 45–62.

Ornitz, E. M. & Ritvo, E. R. (1968). Perceptual inconstancy in early infantile autism. *Archives of General Psychiatry*, **18**, 76–98.

Ozonoff, S. (1995a). Executive functions in autism. In *Learning and Cognition in Autism*, ed. E. Schopler & G. B. Mesibov, pp. 199–219. New York: Plenum Press.

Ozonoff, S. (1995b). Reliability and validity of the Wisconsin Card Sorting Test in studies of autism. *Neuropsychology*, **9**, 491–500.

Ozonoff, S. & McEvoy, R. E. (1994). A longitudinal study of executive function and theory of mind development in autism. *Development and Psychopathology*, **6**, 415–31.

Ozonoff, S., Pennington, B. F., & Rogers, S. J. (1990). Are there emotion perception deficits in young autistic children? *Journal of Child Psychology and Psychiatry*, **31**, 343–61.

Ozonoff, S., Pennington, B. F. & Rogers, S. J. (1991a). Executive function deficits in high-functioning autistic individuals: Relationship to theory of mind. *Journal of Child Psychology and Psychiatry*, **32**, 1081–105.

Ozonoff, S., Rogers, S. J. & Pennington, B. F. (1991b). Asperger's syndrome: evidence of an empirical distinction from high-functioning autism. *Journal of Child Psychology and Psychiatry*, **32**, 1107–22.

Ozonoff, S. & Strayer, D. L. (1997). Inhibitory function in nonretarded children with autism. *Journal of Autism and Developmental Disorders*, **27**, 59–77.

Ozonoff, S., Strayer, D. L., McMahon, W. M. & Filloux, F. (1994). Executive function abilities in autism: an information processing approach. *Journal of Child Psychology and Psychiatry*, **35**, 1015–31.

Pennington, B. F. (1991). *Diagnosing Learning Disorders: a Neuropsychological Framework*. New York: Guilford Press.

Peterson, C. C. & Siegal, M. (1995). Deafness, conversation and theory of mind. *Journal of Child Psychology and Psychiatry*, **36**, 459–74.

Pring, L., Hermelin, B. & Heavey, L. (1995). Savants, segments, art and autism. *Journal of Child Psychology and Psychiatry*, **36**, 1065–76.

Prior, M. R. (1977). Psycholinguistic disabilities of autistic and retarded children. *Journal of Mental Deficiency Research*, **21**, 37–45.

Prior, M. R. (1979). Cognitive abilities and disabilities in infantile autism: a review. *Journal of Abnormal Child Psychology*, **7**, 357–80.

Prior, M. R. & Chen, C. S. (1976). Short-term and serial memory in autistic, retarded, and normal children. *Journal of Autism and Childhood Schizophrenia*, **6**, 121–31.

Prior, M. R., Dahlstrom, B. & Squires, T. (1990). Autistic children's knowledge of thinking and feeling states in other people. *Journal of Child Psychology and Psychiatry*, **31**, 587–602.

Prior, M. R. & Hoffmann, W. (1990). Neuropsychological testing of autistic children through an exploration with frontal lobe tests. *Journal of Autism and Developmental Disorders*, **20**, 581–90.

Prior, M., Perry, D. & Gajzago, C. (1975). Kanner's syndrome or early-onset psychosis: a taxonomic analysis of 142 cases. *Journal of Autism and Childhood Schizophrenia*, **5**, 71–80.

Rimland, B. (1978). Inside the mind of the autistic savant. *Psychology Today*, August, 69–80.

Ritvo, E. R., Freeman, B. J., Pingree, C., Mason-Brothers, A., Jorde, L., Jenson, W. R., McMahon, W. M., Petersen, P. B., Mo, A. & Ritvo, A. (1989). The UCLA-University of Utah epidemiologic survey of autism: prevalence. *American Journal of Psychiatry*, **146**, 194–9.

Rodrigue, J. R., Morgan, S. B. & Geffken, G. R. (1991). A comparative evaluation of adaptive behaviour in children and adolescents with autism, Down's syndrome, and normal development. *Journal of Autism and Developmental Disorders*, **21**, 187–96.

Rogers, S. J., & DiLalla, D. L. L. (1990). Age of symptom onset in young children with pervasive developmental disorders. *Journal of the American Academy of Child and Adolescent Psychiatry*, **29**, 863–72.

Rogers, S. J., Ozonoff, S. & Maslin-Cole, C. (1991). A comparative study of attachment behaviour in young children with autism or other psychiatric disorders. *Journal of the American Academy of Child and Adolescent Psychiatry*, **30**, 483–8.

Rumsey, J. M. (1985). Conceptual problem-solving in highly verbal, nonretarded autistic men. *Journal of Autism and Developmental Disorders*, **15**, 23–36.

Rumsey, J. M. & Hamburger, S. D. (1988). Neuropsychological findings in high-functioning autistic men with infantile autism, residual state. *Journal of Clinical and Experimental Neuropsychology*, **10**, 201–21.

Rumsey, J. M. & Hamburger, S. D. (1990). Neuropsychological divergence of high-level autism and severe dyslexia. *Journal of Autism and Developmental Disorders*, **20**, 155–68.

Russell, J., Mauthner, N., Sharpe, S. & Tidswell, T. (1991). The 'windows task' as a measure of strategic deception in preschoolers and autistic subjects. *British Journal of Developmental Psychology*, **9**, 331–49.

Rutter, M. (1983). Cognitive deficits in the pathogenesis of autism. *Journal of Child Psychology and Psychiatry*, **24**, 513–32.

Sandberg, A. D., Nyden, A., Gillberg, C. & Hjelmquist, E. (1993). The cognitive profile in infantile autism: a study of 70 children and adolescents using the Griffiths mental development scale. *British Journal of Psychology*, **84**, 365–73.

Schneider, S. G. & Asarnow, R. F. (1987). A comparison of cognitive-neuropsychological impairments of nonretarded autistic and schizophrenic children. *Journal of Abnormal Child Psychology*, **15**, 29–46.

Schopler, E. & Mesibov, G. B. (1992). High Functioning Individuals with Autism. New York: Plenum Press.

Schopler, E., Mesibov, G. B. & Hearsey, K. (1995). Structured teaching in the TEACCH system. In *Learning and Cognition in Autism*, ed. E. Schopler & G. B. Mesibov, pp. 243–68. New York: Plenum Press.

Serra, M., Minderaa, R. B., van Geert, P. L. C., Jackson, A. E., Althaus, M. & Til, R. (1995). Emotional role-taking abilities of children with a pervasive developmental disorder not otherwise specified. *Journal of Child Psychology and Psychiatry*, **36**, 475–90.

Shah, A. & Frith, U. (1983). An islet of ability in autistic children: a research note. *Journal of Child Psychology and Psychiatry*, **24**, 613–20.

Shah, A. & Frith, U. (1993). Why do autistic individuals show superior performance on the block design task? *Journal of Child Psychology and Psychiatry*, **34**, 1351–64.

Shapiro, T. & Hertzig, M. E. (1991). Social deviance in autism: a central integrative failure as a model for social non engagement. *Psychiatric Clinics of North America*, **14**,

19–32.

Sigman, M. D., Kasari, C., Kwon, J. & Yirmiya, N. (1992). Responses to the negative emotions of others by autistic, mentally retarded, and normal children. *Child Development*, **63**, 796–807.

Sigman, M., Mundy, P., Sherman, T. & Ungerer, J. (1986). Social interactions of autistic, mentally retarded and normal children and their caregivers. *Journal of Child Psychology and Psychiatry*, **27**, 647–56.

Sigman, M. & Ungerer, J. (1984a). Cognitive and language skills in autistic, mentally retarded and normal children. *Developmental Psychology*, **20**, 293–302.

Sigman, M. & Ungerer, J. A. (1984b). Attachment behaviours in autistic children. *Journal of Autism and Developmental Disorders*, **14**, 231–44.

Silberberg, N. & Silberberg, M. (1967). Hyperlexia: specific word recognition skills in young children. *Exceptional Children*, **34**, 41–2.

Smith, I. M. & Bryson, S. E. (1994). Imitation and action in autism: a critical review. *Psychological Bulletin*, **116**, 259–73.

Stone, W. L. & Caro-Martinez, L. M. (1990). Naturalistic observations of spontaneous communication in autistic children. *Journal of Autism and Developmental Disorders*, **20**, 437–53.

Swanson, J. M., Posner, M., Potkin, S., Bonforte, S., Youpa, D., Fiore, C., Cantwell, D. & Crinella, F. (1991). Activating tasks for the study of visual-spatial attention in ADHD children: a cognitive anatomic approach. *Journal of Child Neurology*, **6**, (Suppl.), S119–S127.

Szatmari, P., Archer, L., Fisman, S., Streiner, D. L. & Wilson, F. (1995). Asperger's syndrome and autism: differences in behaviour, cognition, and adaptive functioning. *Journal of the American Academy of Child and Adolescent Psychiatry*, **34**, 1662–71.

Szatmari, P., Bartolucci, G., Bremner, R., Bond, S. & Rich, S. (1989). A follow-up study of high-functioning autistic children. *Journal of Autism and Developmental Disorders*, **19**, 213–25.

Szatmari, P., Tuff, L., Finlayson, M. A. J. & Bartolucci, G. (1990). Asperger's syndrome and autism: neurocognitive aspects. *Journal of the American Academy of Child and Adolescent Psychiatry*, **29**, 130–6.

Tager-Flusberg, H. (1981). On the nature of linguistic functioning in early infantile autism. *Journal of Autism and Developmental Disorders*, **11**, 45–56.

Tager-Flusberg, H. (1982). Pragmatic development and its implications for social interaction in autistic children. In *Proceedings of the 1981 International Conference on Autism*, ed. D. Park, pp. 103–7. Washington, DC: NSAC.

Tager-Flusberg, H. (1989). A psycholinguistic perspective on language development in the autistic child. In *Autism: Nature, Diagnosis and Treatment*, ed. G. Dawson, pp. 92–115. New York: Guilford Press.

Tager-Flusberg, H. (1991). Semantic processing in the free recall of autistic children: further evidence for a cognitive deficit. *British Journal of Developmental Psychology*, **9**, 417–30.

Tager-Flusberg, H. (1992). Autistic children's talk about theory of mind. *Child Development*, **63**, 161–72.

Tager-Flusberg, H. (1993). What language reveals about the understanding of minds in children with autism. In *Understanding Other Minds: Perspectives from Autism*, ed. S. Baron-Cohen, H. Tager-Flusberg & D. J. Cohen, pp. 138–57. Oxford: Oxford University Press.

Tager-Flusberg, H. & Anderson, M. (1991). The development of contingent discourse ability in autistic children. *Journal of Child Psychology and Psychiatry*, **32**, 1123–34.

Tager-Flusberg, H., Calkins, S., Nolin, T., Baumberger, T., Anderson, M. & Chadwick-Dias, A. (1990). A longitudinal study of language acquisition in autistic and Down's syndrome children. *Journal of Autism and Developmental Disorders*, **20**, 1–21.

Tager-Flusberg, H. & Sullivan, K. (1994). Predicting and explaining behaviour: a comparison of autistic, mentally retarded and normal children. *Journal of Child Psychology and Psychiatry*, **35**, 1059–75.

Tirosh, E. & Canby, J. (1993). Autism with hyperlexia: a distinct syndrome? *American Journal on Mental Retardation*, **98**, 84–92.

Tubbs, V. K. (1966). Types of linguistic disability in psychotic children. *Journal of Mental Deficiency Research*, **10**, 230–40.

Van Lancker, D., Cornelius, C. & Needleman, R. (1991). Comprehension of verbal terms for emotions in normal, autistic and schizophrenic children. *Developmental Neuropsychology*, **7**, 1–18.

Vellutino, F. R. (1979). *Dyslexia: Theory and Research*. Cambridge, MA: MIT Press.

Venter, A., Lord, C. & Schopler, E. (1992). A follow-up study of high-functioning autistic children. *Journal of Child Psychology and Psychiatry*, **33**, 489–507.

Volden, J. & Lord, C. (1991). Neologisms and idiosyncratic language in autistic speakers. *Journal of Autism and Developmental Disorders*, **21**, 109–30.

Wainwright-Sharp, J. A. & Bryson, S. E. (1993). Visual orienting deficits in high-functioning people with autism. *Journal of Autism and Developmental Disorders*, **23**, 1–13.

Walker, E., McGuire, M. & Bettes, B. (1984). Recognition and identification of facial stimuli by schizophrenics and patients with affective disorders. *British Journal of Clinical Psychology*, **23**, 37–44.

Walters, A. S., Barrett, R. P. & Feinstein, C. (1990). Social relatedness and autism: current research, issues, directions. *Research in Developmental Disabilities*, **11**, 303–26.

Weeks, S. J. & Hobson, R. P. (1987). The salience of facial expression for autistic children. *Journal of Child Psychology and Psychiatry*, **28**, 137–52.

Welsh, M. C., Pennington, B. F. & Rogers, S. J. (1987). Word recognition and comprehension skills in hyperlexic children. *Brain and Language*, **32**, 76–96.

Wetherby, A. M. (1986). Ontogeny of communicative functions in autism. *Journal of Autism and Developmental Disorders*, **16**, 295–316.

White, C. P. & Rosenbloom, L. (1992). Temporal lobe structures and autism. *Developmental Medicine and Child Neurology*, **34**, 556–9.

Wing, L. (1976). *Early Childhood Autism: Clinical, Educational and Social Aspects*, 2nd edn. Oxford: Pergamon Press.

Wing, L. (1981). Asperger's syndrome: a clinical account. *Psychological Medicine*, **11**, 115–29.

Wing, L. & Gould, J. (1979). Severe impairments of social interaction and associated abnormalities in children: epidemiology and classification. *Journal of Autism and Developmental Disorders*, **9**, 11–29.

4

Genetic epidemiology of autism and other pervasive developmental disorders

Peter Szatmari and Marshall B. Jones

INTRODUCTION

Over twenty years ago Hanson & Gottesman (1976) published a review article entitled 'The genetics, if any, of infantile autism and childhood schizophrenia'. As the title suggests, the two authors found little evidence of a genetic role in the aetiology of autism. 'No strong evidence exists', they wrote, 'implicating genetics in the development of childhood psychoses that begin before the age of 5'. The viewpoint expressed in this article was not idiosyncratic and was generally held to be true at the time. Currently, the general viewpoint regarding autism has reversed itself completely. Autism today is thought to be one of the most heritable of all psychiatric conditions, more so than bipolar disorder or schizophrenia, and much more so than alcoholism or antisocial behaviour. The issue today is not whether autism has a genetic basis but what that basis is, the specific genes involved and how they act.

Several developments were responsible for this reversal. The most influential was a series of twin studies, the first of which appeared a year after the Hanson and Gottesman review. Folstein & Rutter (1977) attempted 'to obtain information on all school age autistic twin pairs (same sex twins at least one of whom was autistic) in Great Britain'. This attempt was implemented in a variety of ways, including a list of autistic twin pairs collected over the years by the late Dr M. Carter, a search of the records of all children known to the National Society for Autistic Children, and a request for cases published in the Society's newsletter. These efforts resulted in 11 monozygotic and ten dizygotic pairs. Four of the monozygotic pairs were concordant for autism, which yielded a proband wise concordance rate of 53%. None of the dizygotic pairs was concordant for autism which, of course, yielded a proband wise concordance rate of 0%.

The next twin study (Ritvo et al., 1985a) obtained subjects primarily through an advertisement placed in the newsletter of the National Society for Autistic Children, USA. Unfortunately, this same advertisement also solicited children who came from multiplex sibships, i.e. sibships with more than one affected child. This combined solicitation of both twin and multiplex families could reasonably be expected to skew the twin results toward concordant pairs. Those results were 22 concordant out of 23 monozygotic pairs for a proband wise concordance rate of 98% and four concordant out of 17 dizygotic pairs for a proband wise concordance rate of 38%.

In 1988 Smalley, Asarnow and Spence summarized twin studies of autism to that time. These studies were the Folstein-Rutter and Ritvo studies plus 11 monozygotic and nine dizygotic pairs from single-case studies. They also corrected all of the results for a well-known ascertainment effect, namely that when searches are made for autistic twins, concordant pairs are roughly twice as likely to be located as discordant pairs. Correcting for this effect, Smalley and associates found an overall concordance rate of 64% for the monozygotes and 9% for the dizygotes.

The third study (Steffenburg et al., 1989) was carried out in Denmark, Finland, Iceland, Norway and Sweden. In Denmark and Sweden, cases were obtained primarily through the twin registers maintained in those two countries. In the remaining three countries (none of which maintained national twin registers) cases were obtained through the National Autistic Societies or through specialists who were contacted and asked if they knew of any autistic twins. These efforts succeeded in locating 11 monozygotic pairs plus a triplet, all three of whom were concordant for autism, and ten dizygotic pairs. Ten of the monozygotic pairs were concordant for autism which, together with the concordant triplet, yielded a proband wise concordance rate of 96% (23 of 24). None of the dizygotic pairs was concordant so that in this case, as in the Folstein–Rutter study, the concordance rate for dizygotic pairs was 0%.

Quite recently, Bailey et al. (1995) have reported an extension of the early Folstein–Rutter study. The extension includes 23 monozygotic pairs plus one triplet. Thirteen of the 23 pairs are concordant and all three members of the triplet are autistic, which yields a concordance rate of 73% (29 of 39). The extension also includes 20 dizygotic pairs, none of whom is concordant.

In the same years that these twin studies were being conducted, the analysis of twin data was also developing. For decades concordance rates from twin studies had been made to yield heritability estimates by means of formulas originally advanced by Holzinger (1929). The Holzinger estimates, however, were arbitrary and bore no demonstrable relation to genetic theory. Concordance rates could, however, be related to genetic theory if it were assumed that a person became affected when an underlying, continuous and normally distributed liability exceeded a threshold value. Falconer (1965), who introduced this formulation, also assumed that the underlying liability constituted a final common path for all determinants of the disorder, environmental as well as genetic. Subsequent papers by Edwards (1969) and Smith (1970, 1974) advanced Falconer's approach.

Estimating heritability by reference to an underlying liability continuum brings into play a consideration that was ignored in the Holzinger estimates, i.e. population risk. In the Falconer approach the same concordance rates for monozygotic and dizygotic twins may give rise to very different heritability estimates, depending on population risk. In general, the rarer a condition is the higher the heritability estimate will be for the same concordance rates. Autism is a rare condition. The population risk is generally estimated at between 4 and 10 cases per 10 000. Hence, taking population risk into account tends to reinforce the impression one gets from the raw concordance rates that autism is highly heritable. Using the Falconer approach, heritability estimates for autism based on the summary by Smalley et al. (1988), the North European study by Steffenburg and associates, or the recent extension of the Folstein-Rutter study are all in excess of 90%.

Hanson & Gottesman (1976) based their conclusion that autism was probably not genetic on the result, culled from the literature then available, that 'very few siblings of early onset cases are affected'. By 'early onset cases' the two authors meant 'cases where the proband's disorder begins before the age of 5'. For this group of probands they quoted a 1.8% rate of 'schizophrenia or schizophrenic like childhood psychosis in siblings'. Given that 'schizophrenia or schizophrenic like', while it might include autism, could also include psychotic or retarded children who were not specifically autistic, the figure of 1.8% should probably be regarded as an upper bound. Even if the true risk to siblings was considerably less than 1.8%, say 1.0%, it would still be 25 times greater than the population risk and, in the next two decades, estimates of sibling risk would increase steadily.

In their review of the literature, Smalley et al. (1988) summarized six

111

'recent studies' of sibling risk, all published after the Hanson & Gottesman paper and all focused on autism specifically. Their estimate of the sibling risk of autism, based on all six studies was 2.7%, a substantial increase over the estimate made by Hanson and Gottesman.

About the same time as the Smalley et al. review, Jones & Szatmari (1988) pointed out that autistic children tended to be born late in their sibships. In this respect autistic children were similar to children with Down's syndrome or cerebral palsy. They suggested that the explanation was also similar. The parents of children with burdensome conditions that become apparent at birth or in early childhood were less likely to have more children than other parents. They abbreviated their family because the burden of the child they already had was great and they feared, in addition, the probability of having another such child. If every autistic child was the last in his or her sibship, then no sibship could have more than one affected child and the risk to siblings would be zero. The conclusion, however, that autism was not genetic would plainly not be warranted. If the tendency not to have any more children after the birth of an affected child was complete, a condition could be completely determined genetically and the risk to siblings could still be zero.

In the presence of stoppage rules, as the tendency not to have more children is called, the segregation ratio has to be estimated by the recurrence risk, i.e. the risk to children born after the first affected child. This, in turn, requires a population with large families and little tendency to be deterred by the birth of handicapped children. The Mormon population in Utah is such a population. In an apparently complete survey of autism in this population Ritvo et al. (1989) reported a sibling risk of 4.5% and a recurrence risk of 8.6%. The sibling risk is somewhat higher than has been reported in most other studies, so perhaps the recurrence risk may somewhat overestimate the true segregation ratio. Even so, using the recurrence risk (and thereby avoiding an underestimate due to stoppage rules) yields an estimate of the segregation ratio that is twice that given by Smalley et al. (1988) and very much larger than the estimate made by Hanson and Gottesman.

As a result of these twin and family studies, six reviews (Folstein & Rutter, 1977; Reiss et al., 1986; Pauls, 1987; Smalley et al., 1988; Silliman et al., 1989; Rutter et al., 1990) have all concluded that a genetic aetiology is plausible for autism. Although individually many of the older studies suffered from convenience sampling, poorly standardized diagnostic procedures, nonblind assessments of relatives, etc. the consistency of results across studies is impressive.

This chapter reviews more recent data on the role, rather than the existence or extent, of genetic factors in autism/pervasive developmental disorder (PDD), focusing specifically on findings and issues not covered in previous reviews. This involves consideration of issues that are commonly seen in other complex disorders, such as variable expressivity, pleiotropy and genetic heterogeneity. The chapter concludes with a discussion of a genetic model for autism/PDD and several unresolved issues that must be addressed before further progress is possible.

VARIABLE EXPRESSIVITY AND PLEIOTROPY

Variable expressivity refers to the phenomenon whereby the genes for a disorder also confer susceptibility to milder or incomplete manifestations of the same disorder, even some that may fall below the threshold for a diagnosis. Variable expressivity is often seen in dominant Mendelian disorders such as tuberous sclerosis and neurofibromatosis, and in complex genetic disorders due to a dynamic mutation such as the fragile X syndrome and Huntington's disease.

Several studies taken as a whole indicate that the genes for autism also confer susceptibility to milder or incomplete manifestations of autism. For example, the cotwins of monozygotic autistic probands can have atypical autism or Asperger's syndrome (Folstein & Rutter, 1977; Bailey et al., 1995), and the risk of Asperger's syndrome and atypical autism in the nontwin siblings of autistic probands is roughly 3% (Bolton et al., 1994). Thus, the overall risk of both autism and other PDDs to siblings of PDD probands is 5–6% (Szatmari et al., 1993) even without taking account of stoppage. The risk, relative to the general population, cannot be calculated in this case because systematic data on the population prevalence of the other forms of PDD are not available.

Another type of impairment that has recently been reported to occur in first degree relatives is a 'lesser variant' of PDD characterized by similar impairments in reciprocal social interaction, communication and interests but not enough to merit a diagnosis of any form of PDD, even Asperger's syndrome. For example, Piven et al. (1994) report that parents of autistic children were more often rated as aloof, untactful and unresponsive on a standardized personality interview than parents of Down's syndrome controls. Similarly, Bolton et al. (1994) found that roughly 20% of siblings of autistic probands had social or communication impairments or a restricted pattern of interests compared with 3% of siblings of Down controls

($P < 0.001$). Similar findings have been reported by Landa et al. (1992) and Narayan et al. (1990) using other measures. In these studies the ratings of social impairment were not conducted blind to proband status and the control group of parents of children with Down's syndrome (in the Piven et al. and Landa et al. studies) were ascertained from a parent support group. Such parents might be expected to have better social skills than parents who do not belong to such organizations and this makes the comparison difficult to interpret.

Two controlled studies have looked at the prevalence of milder social impairments in collateral second and third degree relatives of PDD probands. This is a useful design as second and third degree relatives share genes with an autistic child but do not generally live with him/her. Thus, if elevated rates of a condition are found in extended relatives this can be taken as reasonable evidence that the elevated risk in siblings and parents is due to genetic factors, not shared environmental factors. Pickles et al. (1995) reported that the lesser variant was found in 6% of male second and third degree relatives of autistic probands compared with 3% in similar relatives of children with Down's syndrome. The finding of similar rates in second and third degree relatives is inconsistent with a purely genetic model but may have to do with the precision of measurement and low numbers. Szatmari et al. (unpublished results) have also investigated rates of this same lesser variant in extended relatives. Families with two or more children affected with PDD were compared with families with a single affected male or female child and families that had either adopted a PDD child or were step parents to a PDD child. The use of such a group controls for familiarity with PDD among informants and allows for similar sampling procedures in proband and control families. It has been shown, for example, that familiarity with a disease can change rates of other conditions as reported by family history (Gibbons et al., 1993; Chapman et al., 1994). Even with this design, Szatmari et al. (unpublished results) found that rates of the lesser variant were more common among biological relatives of PDD probands than among nonbiological relatives, indicating that informant bias is not a major issue.

Based on their twin study, Folstein & Rutter (1977) originally postulated that what is inherited in autism is not so much the disorder itself but rather more broadly based cognitive impairments, particularly in language. While several early family history studies have supported this finding (August et al., 1981; Minton et al., 1982; Baird & August, 1985), more recent studies using direct testing of parents and siblings have failed to confirm this result (Freeman et al. 1989; Gillberg et al. 1992; Szatmari et al., 1993). Previous studies often failed to exclude siblings affected with PDD and so the cognitive impairments reported may have been a part of the sibling's PDD instead of being due to a pure learning disorder. It appears as if cognitive impairments are part of the autism phenotype only if associated with social-communication problems as well.

If it is true that variable expressivity exists (but is limited to other forms of PDD and the lesser variant), the next question is whether genetic or environmental factors account for these variations in severity. The best design to answer this question is to see whether concordant monozygous twins are more alike in severity than concordant dyzygous twins. This would demonstrate that genetic factors account for variations in severity rather than environmental factors which can be either shared or non-shared. The one twin study with concordant dyzygous twins did not address this issue (Ritvo et al. 1985a). An alternative design is to see whether the variation among affected (nontwin) siblings is less than the variation seen between affected PDD children from different families. The comparison of variation between and within families is estimated using an intraclass correlation coefficient (similar to a Pearson correlation). Spiker et al. (1994) found very low correlations between affected siblings on IQ and autistic symptoms using a sample of 37 multiple incidence families with autism. In contrast, Szatmari et al. (1996) found an Intraclass Correlation Coefficient (ICC) of 0.62 for a measure of nonverbal IQ and for socialization scores in a sample of 23 multiple incidence families with PDD children. Lower but still significant correlations were also observed for autistic symptoms (J.E. MacLean et al., unpublished results). Possible reasons for these discrepant findings are that the Szatmari et al. (1996) and MacLean et al. (unpublished results) studies employed a sample of PDD children (allowing for more variation between families) and a single measure of nonverbal IQ for all children (eliminating an extraneous source of variation within families). The Spiker et al. (1994) study used children with strictly defined autism, reducing variation within families, and a variety of different IQ measures, adding variation between families. Thus, the results from the former studies indicate that familial, presumably genetic, factors account for the variation in severity seen between PDD children. Such high correlations in clinical features are also seen in disorders caused by dynamic mutations because the number of trinucleotide repeats will vary between families but will be similar within a family (Snell et al., 1993). These findings also have implications for heterogeneity (see below).

Another active area of investigation is whether the genes for autism/PDD confer susceptibility to qualitatively different disorders such as affective disorders or substance abuse. For example, if the genes involved in serotonin transmission are involved in the aetiology of autism (Young et al. 1982), these genes may confer susceptibility to other psychiatric disorders that are also associated with serotonin transmission.

Several studies have reported that parents and siblings of autistic probands have increased rates of affective and anxiety disorders. Two studies have used control groups and direct interviews of first degree relatives. For example, Piven et al. (1991) measured rates of psychiatric disorders using the Schedule of Affective Disorders and Schizophrenia Lifetime version (SADS-L) in parents of autistic children compared with parents of children with Down's syndrome. Elevated rates of anxiety disorders were found (23.5% versus 2.9%). Smalley et al. (1995) conducted semi-structured psychiatric interviews on the parents and siblings of probands with autism and controls with other neurological disorders. They reported that rates of major depression (32.3% versus 11.1%), social phobia (20.2 versus 2.4%) and substance abuse (22.1% versus 0%) were significantly higher in relatives of the autistic children compared with controls.

The key issue is whether this association is due to genetic or environmental mechanisms. It is possible, for example, that the stress of raising a profoundly handicapped child may, by itself, give rise to these disorders. Indeed, a number of studies have reported that parenting stress generated by the child's handicap correlates with the presence of depression in the mothers (Holroyd & McArthur, 1976; Bristol & Schopler, 1983; Peterson, 1984; Wolf et al., 1989). However, Smalley et al. (1995) reported that the majority (64%) of parents of autistic probands had the onset of their mood disorder prior to the birth of the child with autism, compared with 20% of the parents of controls, which suggests that the affective disorder is not due to stress; however, this result needs to be replicated with a larger sample.

The most informative design to resolve this issue is to use twin or adoption studies. None of the twin studies has reported rates of psychiatric disorders in discordant cotwins and there are no adoption studies in autism. Another informative design involves estimating the risk of psychiatric disorders in collateral relatives who do not live with a handicapped child. If these conditions have a genetic relation to autism, second and third degree relatives should also show an increased risk compared with population base rates. In a family history study, Szatmari et al. (1995) did not find that rates of psychiatric symptoms were increased in extended relatives of PDD probands compared with controls. This suggests that the increased rate in parents reported in other studies may be, at least in part, a function of family stress; however, that study reported on rates of symptoms not disorders and used family history not direct interview.

Conclusion

It seems that there is now some agreement that autism is a strongly genetic disorder and that the genes for autism also confer susceptibility to other forms of PDD such as Asperger's syndrome, atypical autism and perhaps to milder forms of social impairment that fall below a threshold for a diagnosis of PDD (the lesser variant). It also seems clear that the genes for autism do not confer susceptibility to learning disabilities or mental retardation unaccompanied by PDD like social impairment. The evidence is not clear whether there is an increased risk for other psychiatric disorders such as affective disorders and social phobia. Further replication of these latter findings is needed as well as twin and adoption studies to determine whether the observed familial aggregation is due to environmental or genetic factors.

AETIOLOGICAL AND GENETIC HETEROGENEITY IN AUTISM/PDD

There are several different meanings of the term 'heterogeneity' in the context of genetic disorders. Aetiological heterogeneity refers to the possibility that a disorder might be caused by both genetic and environmental aetiologies. Genetic heterogeneity, on the other hand, refers to the possibility that autism/PDD might be caused either by several mutations at a single genetic locus (intralocus heterogeneity) or by several genes at different loci (interlocus heterogeneity).

There is, in fact, considerable evidence that PDD is both aetiologically and genetically heterogeneous. For example, autism occasionally occurs with certain viral diseases such as congenital rubella and cytomegalovirus (Garrow et al., 1984). Autism can also occur in association with several different genetic diseases, i.e. tuberous sclerosis, neurofibromatosis, phenylketonuria (PKU), the fragile X syndrome, etc. (Ritvo et al., 1989). Such cases with known disease associations probably only account for 10% of the cases of PDD (Ritvo et al., 1990). Furthermore, the mechanism of the comorbidity in these situations is unclear; is the autism a nonspecific sequelae of the mental retardation or is it the direct result of disruption in certain key brain regions?

Another important question is whether genetic heterogeneity exists among the idiopathic cases of autism/PDD. There are several ways in which genetic heterogeneity can be detected (Khoury et al., 1993). If different mutations are associated with different clinical features, heterogeneity can be detected by seeing if certain clinical features run true within families. The Spiker et al. (1994) data referred to earlier, reported that individual autistic behaviours as assessed by the Autism Diagnostic Interview (ADI) showed little or no correlation among affected siblings from the same family. However, Szatmari et al. (1996) and MacLean et al. (unpublished results) found that IQ, severity of impairment and summary measures of autistic behaviours do appear to run true within families. For example, 66% of probands with IQ below 50 also had affected siblings with IQ below 50, and 80% of probands with IQ above 70 had affected siblings with similar levels of IQ. Thus, variations in severity, but not necessarily specific autistic behaviours, could be due to genetic heterogeneity; high and a low functioning PDD probands could arise from separate genetic mechanisms.

Another way of detecting heterogeneity in complex genetic disorders is to see whether there are differences in recurrence risk to relatives associated with certain clinical features of probands. This way of testing for genetic heterogeneity has proved very successful in mapping genes for other complex genetic diseases such as Alzheimer's disease, breast cancer and diabetes. Ritvo reported a higher risk of autism to siblings of female autistic probands compared with male probands (14% versus 7%); however, power was too low to test this hypothesis with an acceptable type II error. Bolton et al. (1994) reported that the risk of the lesser variant in siblings was higher in lower functioning probands compared with those who were higher functioning (18.6% versus 2.8%). There was, however, no difference in risk for the lesser variant by the sex of the proband.

Conclusion

It is clear that autism can occur as a result of both rare viral aetiologies and several single gene disorders. Among the idiopathic cases of autism, however, the picture is much less clear. There is some tentative evidence which suggests that severity of impairment appears to run true within families. In multiple incidence families, affected siblings tend to show similar levels of functioning. In addition, lower functioning probands may carry a higher risk of the lesser variant to siblings than higher functioning ones and females with autism may carry a higher risk of autism to their siblings. As females with autism tend to be more severely impaired than males, these findings may be converging and suggest that genetic heterogeneity may be signalled by the level of impairment or sex of the proband. Clearly, however, more studies are needed to confirm this suggestion and to determine whether sex and level of impairment are true markers of heterogeneity.

POSSIBLE GENETIC MODELS

Both the low risk to sibs and the anomalous sex ratio (approximately four males to every female) are incompatible with any simple Mendelian or single gene inheritance (i.e. autosomal recessive, dominant or X-linked). These would predict a recurrence risk of at least 25% to sibs, and either an equal sex ratio for autosomal transmission, or an overwhelming number of males compared with females for X-linked recessive transmission. The remaining possible modes of inheritance belong to the spectrum of complex genetic models including complex monogenic (single locus, two allele, with reduced, sex specific, penetrance values for homozygotes and heterozygotes) and multilocus models (Reich et al., 1972; Kidd, 1981; Risch, 1990). The evidence for each of these models is now reviewed in turn.

Complex monogenic models

Evidence for and against the existence of a single major gene determining the liability to develop autism/PDD comes from segregation analysis, linkage studies and studies of candidate genes.

SEGREGATION ANALYSIS

In an early segregation analysis using nuclear families, Ritvo et al. (1985b) reported that the data were most consistent with an autosomal recessive mode of transmission. The ability to discriminate among genetic models using segregation analysis, however, is severely limited by sample size and heterogeneity. Furthermore, the ascertainment scheme used in the study was rather complicated and it is unclear whether any correction for this is possible.

LINKAGE STUDIES

In an early study, Spence et al. (1985) were unable to find significant linkage between autism and 30 standard phenotypic markers. More recently, Ciaranello and colleagues at Stanford have used parametric forms of linkage analysis and exclusion mapping to detect major genes. In a linkage study, the mode of transmission associated with the highest significant lod score would be the correct one and would indicate the presence of a major gene. Testing different modes of transmission and assuming homogeneity, major portions of chromosomes 6, 7, 9, 12, 13, 15 and the X chromosome have been excluded with markers placed 10–15 cM apart (Hallmayer et al., 1993). In a more recent analysis using multipoint sib pair methods, this group could not exclude an X-linked gene of small effect based on a lod score of 1.24 (Hallmayer et al., 1996). This promising finding obviously needs to be replicated with a larger sample and more informative markers in that region.

A potential problem with exclusion mapping in complex genetic disorders is the criterion for exclusion of a region (i.e. a lod score of -2). Clerget-Darpoux (1993) has suggested that this exclusion criterion may be overly conservative if the mode of transmission is mispecified and homogeneity is assumed. Thus promising regions of the genome may be prematurely excluded by this approach.

CANDIDATE GENES – THE X CHROMOSOME

A major locus on the X chromosome has long been an attractive hypotheses for autism in view of the preponderance of affected males and the reported association between autism/PDD and the fragile X syndrome (Szatmari & Jones, 1991). Holden et al. (1996) have conducted extensive DNA analyses of the FMR-1 gene on the X chromosome and the FRAX E and F sites distal to FMR-1 in children from families with two affected male siblings. They did not find any triplet repeat expansions at these sites and the affected children inherited the exact number of CGG repeats from their mothers.

Although the FMR-1, FRAX E and FRAX F genes have been ruled out, it is still possible that another locus on the X chromosome is involved. If such a locus existed, the sex ratio in autism would be familial, i.e. the sex ratio among affected children following the birth of a first affected male would be higher than when the first affected child were female. This would be true even if the genetic basis of autism were polygenic or epistatic. It would also be true even if the locus was present in only a subset of families, thus reducing the proportion of males observed with a major X-linked locus. In a recent report, Jones et al. (1996) found no tendency for the sex ratio among subsequently affected children to be contingent on the sex of the first affected. The size of the sample was, however, too small to exclude the possibility of a small effect. The conclusion, therefore, was the same as the one reached by Hallmayer et al. (1996), namely that if the X chromosome plays any role in the causation of autism, that role is probably a small one.

OTHER CANDIDATE GENES AND ASSOCIATION STUDIES

Candidate genes are genes that a priori, might be involved in the aetiology of autism (for example genes that control serotonin metabolism). In association studies, the frequencies of alleles or genotypes at a candidate locus are compared in autistic children and in unrelated controls. Although such studies are able to detect genes that contribute a relatively small proportion of the variance to a disorder, there is quite a bit of controversy on the use of association studies in complex genetic disorders (Crowe, 1993). A positive association may result from several mechanisms; the marker loci may exist in linkage disequilibrium with susceptibility genes, the measured alleles may be the susceptibility genes themselves or else the result is a false positive and reflects population admixture and stratification. Association studies are also notoriously susceptible to false positive results (Hodge, 1995) and these alternatives cannot be resolved using only the association design.

Several association studies have been carried out in autism. For example, Herault et al. (1994) reported negative results for genes coding for tyrosine hydroxylase, insulin and insulin-like growth factor on the tip of the short arm of chromosome 6. However, this group did report a positive association (Herault et al. 1993) using the HRAS marker on the short arm of chromosome 11. A similar result was reported (Herault et al., 1995) using an overlapping sample and flanking markers. Unfortunately, results for the new and old samples were not reported separately so it is difficult to tell whether this was a true replication or an extension of previous findings.

Warren et al. (1995) have reported that children with autism have immunological abnormalities that indicate a possible role for the HLA system in this disorder. They subsequently reported that autistic children had a higher frequency of a certain allele at an HLA locus on chromosome 6 than unaffected controls (Daniels et al., 1995).

As there is a high rate of false positive findings with association studies, these results need to be replicated. Furthermore, if replicated, there needs to be evidence that the result is not due to population stratification. Nevertheless, it is clear from the available data that there is currently no evidence for a single gene of major effect in autism/PDD. Instead, attention has now focused on the possibility of multilocus models, involving several interacting genes of smaller effect.

Multilocus models

Multilocus models are often differentiated into polygenic and oligogenic models. The polygenic model proposes that autism is caused by many genes each of very small effect. In contrast, oligogenic models postulate that autism/PDD is caused by a small number of genes. In both cases, the genes may interact in an additive or multiplicative (epistatic) manner.

In a polygenic model, the liability to develop autism is normally distributed in the general population and determined by the number of 'autism' genes that a child inherits from both parents. To be consistent with the skewed sex ratio, separate thresholds can be postulated for males and females. The main problem with polygenic models is that further work at characterizing autism genes would be fruitless as each gene would only contribute a tiny portion of the variance to the disorder. In a sense, polygenic models represent the 'null hypothesis' for genetic studies.

The polygenic model is consistent with some but not all aspects of the genetic epidemiology of autism. For example, the relatives of female and low IQ probands should be at higher risk of autism/PDD and the lesser variant than relatives of male probands or those with higher IQ. As reviewed above, there are some limited data to support these predictions. Similarly, a complex segregation analyses performed by Jorde et al. (1991) on nuclear families indicated that the mode of transmission of autism within families (particularly the paucity of affected cousins) was most consistent with polygenic transmission. Unfortunately, complex segregation analysis has little power to discriminate among alternative genetic models (Ott, 1990) particularly if the issue of genetic heterogeneity is ignored, as it was in this study.

Another useful way to differentiate polygenic and oligogenic epistatic models that is not affected by heterogeneity is to estimate the relative risk of a disorder in various classes of relatives. Risch (1990) has pointed out that if a disorder is caused by a single gene (and there are no dominance effects), the relative risk should fall by roughly half as one looks at the relative risk in monozygous cotwins, siblings and second and third degree relatives. For example, in a single gene disorder, the relative risk might fall from 32 in monozygotic cotwins to 16 in first degree relatives to 8 and 4 in second and third degree relatives, respectively. In a polygenic-epistatic model (where many genes each of small effect interact multiplicatively), the risk would fall as a function of the square root of the risk in the previous class of relative. For example, if the relative risk is 16 in first degree relatives, the risk should be 4 in second degree relatives; however, if the multiple genes interact in an additive manner, the overall effect will mimic the single gene pattern (Risch, 1990). In an oligogenic model with epistatic effects, the risk falls more rapidly than for a single gene but more slowly than in a polygenic model.

Although there are data on the rates of autism in twins and siblings, they are much more limited for more distant relatives. Pooling the results of three twin studies with systematic sampling, it is possible to estimate that the risk of autism to monozygotic cotwins is roughly 60%. There were no concordant dizygotic twins found in these three studies so the rate of 3% found in nontwin siblings can be used instead. If the prevalence of autism is taken to be 1 per 10000 (Bryson et al., 1988), the relative risk goes from 600 in monozygotic twins to 30 in siblings. Such a large drop is clearly inconsistent with a single gene model where the relative risk should fall to roughly 300. Under a polygenic (epistatic) model, the relative risk in siblings would be 24 (given the data on monozygotic twins), which is much closer to the observed figure. Using family history from a single informant, Pickles et al. (1995) were unable to detect any second and third degree relatives with autism, a finding that is also consistent with polygenic transmission; however, family history from a single informant will underestimate the true risk to extended relatives.

The data are somewhat different if one focuses on the lesser variant. Pickles et al. (1995) reported on rates of this personality characteristic in monozygotic twins, first, second and third degree relatives. The relative risk of this trait (excluding cases with autism) in monozygotic cotwins and siblings is 6.1 and 3.7, respectively. Model fitting using a latent class analysis with the lesser variant was consistent with a three gene model. In contrast, the relative risk for autism in this data set is 846 in monozygotic cotwins and 29.2 in siblings, a decrement entirely consistent with polygenic-epistatic transmission. Although latent class analysis can account to a certain extent for measurement error using family history, remaining error is likely to produce a pattern consistent with multiple genes (P. Szatmari & M.B. Jones, unpublished results). In other words, it is possible that the Pickles result is a conservative one and the true number of genes involved may be less than three. Szatmari et al. (1996) also looked at the relative risk for the lesser variant in second and third degree relatives of PDD probands using multiple informants which would reduce measurement error. In this sample, the pattern of relative risks was also consistent with one or two genes being involved.

INTRAUTERINE EFFECTS

The term 'intrauterine effects' refers to the possibility that the intrauterine environment may play a role in the aetiology of autism in conjunction with genetic susceptibility in the child. These intrauterine effects may result from genetic conditions in the mother that place the developing fetus at risk. The classic example of this is phenylketonuria (PKU). The children of mothers with PKU often have developmental disabilities and congenital anomalies not because the children have PKU but because high levels of maternal phenylalanine cross the placenta and affect the developing brain (Stevenson & Huntley, 1976). There is currently no evidence of an intrauterine effect in autism/PDD. One of the most consistent findings in autism, however, is that affected children have a higher rate of pregnancy and birth complications than their siblings or controls (Piven et al., 1993). These complications could conceivably arise from a genetic condition in the mother that might affect the fetus. In addition, in a family history study, Szatmari et al. (1995) reported that there were four PDD cases identified among the relatives of PDD probands and all four were on the mother's side of the family. This finding, too, is not inconsistent with a genetic intrauterine effect. The joint interaction of genetic susceptibility in the child and a maternal genetic factor that affects the intrauterine environment would look like an epistatic mode of transmission and so is not inconsistent with the relative risk data in relatives presented earlier.

CONCLUSION

In the past 20 years it has become abundantly clear that autism is a genetic disorder. The studies reviewed above, however, indicate that there is no consensus on the mode of transmission of autism/PDD. The genetic epidemiology of the disorder is complicated by variable expressivity, possible pleiotropy and heterogeneity which makes it difficult to decide who is affected in a pedigree and thus to establish firmly the mode of transmission.

It seems clear, however, that the data do not support a single gene model for autism. Therefore, at least two or more genes need to be considered. What is striking about the relative risk data in various classes of relatives is the fact that the pattern of fall in relative risk seems to be different if one focuses on the lesser variant of autism. The decrement in relative risk for autism is consistent with an epistatic polygenic model whereas for the lesser variant the pattern is consistent with a very small number of genes or even a single gene. In other words, the genetic mechanism for the lesser variant may be different from the mechanism for autism. It may be that the lesser variant is caused by a very small number of genes, whereas autism is caused by additional genes or some other mechanism in addition to the genes for the lesser variant. The form of epistasis is unknown and may include gene–gene or gene–environment interactions. This is not dissimilar to the two-hit hypothesis currently considered as the mechanism for many forms of cancer (Knudson, 1971). What is encouraging at this point is that there is no reason to reject an oligogenic model in favour of a purely polygenic-epistatic one. The report by Hallmayer et al. (1996) suggests that possibly at least one of the genes of small effect may be on the X chromosome. The association studies also provide weaker evidence of other possible genes.

Given the high heritability and risk to siblings, there is no logical reason that mapping autism genes cannot be successful. Linkage studies, however, need to be conducted on genetically homogeneous families where the disorder is caused by one (or a few) major genes. Without such evidence, linkage studies represent a high risk strategy at best and require very large sample sizes. It is hoped that with more accurate knowledge about the inheritance of the lesser variant and a greater ability to identify more genetically homogeneous subgroups, the prospects for identifying 'autism genes' are much more favourable now than they were just a few years ago. Once these genes are identified, it is hoped that a clearer understanding of pathogenesis will be possible and that this will lead to more effective interventions in the future.

REFERENCES

August, G., Stewart, M. A. & Tsai, L. (1981). The incidence of cognitive disabilities in siblings of autistic children. *British Journal of Psychiatry*, **138**, 416–22.

Bailey, A., Le Couteur, A., Gottesman, I., Bolton, P., Simonoff, E., Yuzda, E. & Rutter, M. (1995). Autism as a strongly genetic disorder: evidence from a British twin study. *Psychological Medicine*, **25**, 63–77.

Baird, T. D. & August, G. K. (1985). Familial heterogeneity in infantile autism. *Journal of Autism and Developmental Disorders*, **15**, 315–21.

Bolton, P., Macdonald, H., Pickles, A., Rios, P., Goode, S., Crowson, M., Bailey, A. & Rutter, M. (1994). A case-control family history study of autism. *Journal of Child Psychology and Psychiatry*, **35**, 877–900.

Bristol, M. M. & Schopler, E. (1983). Stress and coping in families of autistic adolescents. In *Autism in Adolescents and Adults*, ed. E. Schopler & G. B. Mesibov, pp. 251–78. New York: Plenum Press.

Bryson, S. E., Clark, B. S. & Smith, I. M. (1988). First report of a Canadian epidemiological study of autism syndromes. *Journal of Child Psychology and Psychiatry and Allied Disciplines*, **29**, 433–45.

Chapman, T. F., Mannuzza, S., Klein, D. F. & Fyer, A. J. (1994). Effects of informant mental disorder on psychiatric family history data. *American Journal of Psychiatry*, **151**, 574–9.

Clerget-Darpoux, F. (1993). Beyond the LOD score paradigm. *Psychiatric Genetics*, **3**, 136.

Crowe, R. R. (1993). Candidate genes in psychiatry: an epidemiologic perspective. *American Journal of Medical Genetics (Neuropsychiatric Genetics)*, **48**, 74–7.

Daniels, W. W., Warren, R. P., Odell, J. D., Maciulis, A., Burger, R. A., Warren, W. L. & Torres, A. R. (1995). Increased frequency of the extended or ancestral haplotype B44-SC30-DR4 in autism. *Neuropsychobiology*, **32**, 120–3.

Edwards, J. H. (1969). Familial predisposition in man. *British Medical Bulletin*, **25**, 58–64.

Falconer, D. S. (1965). The inheritance of liability to certain diseases estimated for the incidence among relatives. *Annals of Human Genetics*, **29**, 51–76.

Folstein, S. & Rutter, M. (1977). Infantile autism: a genetic study of 21 twin pairs. *Journal of Child Psychology and Psychiatry*, **18**, 297–321.

Freeman, B. J., Ritvo, E., Mason-Brothers, A., Pingree, C., Yokota, A., Jenson, W. R., McMahon, W. M., Petersen, P. B., Mo, A. & Schroth, P. (1989). Psychometric assessment of first-degree relatives of 62 autistic probands in Utah. *American Journal of Psychiatry*, **146**, 361–4.

Garrow, B., Bartheleng, C., Savage, D., Leddert, I. & Lelord, A. (1984). Comparison of autistic syndromes with and without associated neurological problems. *Journal of Autism and Developmental Disorders*, **14**, 105–11.

Gibbons, L. E., Ponsonby, A. L. & Dwyer, I. A. (1993). Comparison of prospective and retrospective responses on sudden infant death syndrome by case and control mothers. *American Journal of Epidemiology*, **137**, 654–9.

Gillberg, C., Gillberg, I. C. & Steffenburg, S. (1992). Siblings and parents of children with autism: a controlled population-based study. *Developmental Medicine and Child Neurology*, **34**, 389–98.

Hallmayer, J., Herbert, J. M., Spiker, D., Lotspeich, L., McMahon, W. M., Petersen, P. B., Nicholas, P., Pingree, C., Lin, A. A., Cavalli-Sforza, L. L., Risch, N. & Ciranello, R. D. (1996). Autism and the X-chromosome: multipoint sib pair analysis. *Archives of General Psychiatry*, **53**, 985–9.

Hallmayer, J., Kalaydjieva, L., Underhill, P., Spiker, D., Lotspeich, L., Kraemer, H.,

Wong, D., Ciaranello, R. & Cavalli-Sforza, L. L. (1993). A linkage study of familial autism. *Psychiatric Genetics*, **3**, 128.

Hanson, D. R. & Gottesman, I. I. (1976). The genetics, if any, of infantile autism and childhood schizophrenia. *Journal of Autism and Childhood Schizophrenia*, **6**, 209–34.

Herault, J., Perrot, A., Barthelemy, C., Buchler, M., Cherpi, C., Leboyer, M., Savage, D., LeLord, G., Mallet, J. & Muh, J. P. (1993). Possible association of a Harvey-Ras-1 (HRAS-1) marker with autism. *Psychiatry Research*, **46**, 261–7.

Herault, J., Petit, E., Buchler, M., Martineau, J., Cherpi, C., Perrot, A., Sauvage, D., Barthélemy, C., Müh, J. P. & Lelord, G. (1994). Lack of association between three genetic markers of brain growth factors and infantile autism. *Biological Psychiatry*, **35**, 281–3.

Herault, J., Petit, E., Martineau, J., Perrot, A., Lenoir, P., Cherpi, C., Barthélemy, C., Sauvage, D., Mallet, J., Müh, J. P. & Lelord, G. (1995). Autism and genetics: clinical approach and association study with two markers of HRAS gene. *American Journal of Medical Genetics*, **60**, 276–81.

Hodge, S. E. (1995). An oligogenic disease displaying weak marker associations: a summary of contributions to problem 1 of GAW9. *Genetic Epidemiology*, **12**, 545–54.

Holden, J. J. A., Wing, M., Chalifoux, M., Julien-Inalsingh, C., Schutz, C., Robinson, P., Szatmari, P. & White, B. N. (1996). Lack of expansion of triplet repeats in the FMR1, FRAXE and FRAXF loci in male multiplex families with autism and pervasive developmental disorders. *American Journal of Medical Genetics*, **64**, 399–403.

Holroyd, J. & McArthur, D. (1976). Mental retardation and stress on the parents: a contrast between Down's syndrome and childhood autism. *American Journal of Mental Deficiency*, **80**, 431–6.

Holzinger, K. J. (1929). The relative effect of nature and nurture on twin differences. *Journal of Educational Psychology*, **20**, 241–8.

Jones, M. B. & Szatmari, P. (1988). Stoppage rules and genetic studies of autism. *Journal of Autism and Developmental Disorders*, **18**, 31–40.

Jones, M. B., Szatmari, P. & Piven, J. (1996). Non-familiality of the sex ratio in autism. *American Journal of Medical Genetics*, **67**, 499–500.

Jorde, L. B., Hasstedt, S. J. & Ritvo, E. R. (1991). Complex segregation analysis of autism. *American Journal of Human Genetics*, **49**, 932–8.

Khoury, M. J., Beatty, T. H. & Cohen, B. H. (1993) *Fundamentals of Genetic Epidemiology*. New York: Oxford University Press.

Kidd, K. K. (1981). Genetic models for psychiatric disorders. In *Genetic Research Strategies for Psychobiology and Psychiatry*, ed. E. S. Gershon, S. Mathysse, X. O. Breakfield & R. Ciaranello. New York: Boxwood Press.

Knudson, A. G. (1971). Mutation and cancer: statistical study on retinoblastoma. *Proceedings of the National Academy of Science USA*, **68**, 820–3.

Landa, R., Piven, J., Wzorek, M. M., Gayle, J. O., Chase, G. A. & Folstein, S. E. (1992). Social language use in parents of autistic individuals. *Psychological Medicine*, **22**, 245–54.

MacLean, J. E., Szatmari, P., Jones, M. B., Bryson, S. E., Mahoney, W., Bartolucci, G. & Tuff, L. (1996). Familial factors influence the severity of pervasive developmental disorder: evidence for genetic heterogeneity. Manuscript submitted for publication.

Minton, J., Campbell, M., Green, W. L., Jenings, S. & Samet, C. (1982). Cognitive assessment of siblings of autistic children. *Journal of the American Academy of Child Psychiatry*, **21**, 256–61.

Narayan, S., Moyes, B. & Wolff, W. (1990). Family characteristics of autistic children: a further report. *Journal of Autism and Developmental Disorders*, **20**, 523–35.

Ott, J. (1990). Invited editorial: cutting a gordian knot in the linkage analysis of complex human traits. *American Journal of Human Genetics*, **46**, 219–21.

Pauls, D. (1987). The familiality of autism and related disorders: a review of the evidence. In *Handbook of Autism and Pervasive Disorders*, ed. D. J. Cohen & A. N. Donnellan. New York: John Wiley.

Petersen, P. (1984). Effects of moderator variables in reducing stress outcomes in mothers of handicapped children. *Journal of Psychosomatic Medicine*, **28**, 337–44.

Pickles, A., Bolton, P., Macdonald, H., Bailey, A., Le Couteur, A., Sim, H. C. & Rutter, M. (1995). Latent-class analysis of recurrence risks for complex phenotypes with selection and measurement error: a twin and family history study of autism. *American Journal of Human Genetics*, **57**, 717–26.

Piven, J., Chase, G. A., Landa, R., Wzorek, M., Gayle, J., Cloud, D. & Folstein, S. E. (1991). Psychiatric disorders in the parents of autistic individuals. *Journal of the American Academy of Child and Adolescent Psychiatry*, **30**, 471–8.

Piven, J., Simon, J., Chase, G. A., Wzorek, M., Landa, R., Gayle, J. & Folstein, S. (1993). The etiology of autism; pre-, peri- and neonatal factors. *Journal of the American Academy of Child and Adolescent Psychiatry*, **32**, 1256–63.

Piven, J., Wzorek, M., Landa, R., Lainhart, J., Bolton, P., Chase, G. A. & Folstein, S. (1994). Personality characteristics of the parents of autistic individuals. *Psychological Medicine*, **24**, 783–95.

Reich, T., James, J. W. & Morris, C. A. (1972). The use of multiple thresholds in determining the mode of transmission of semi-continuous traits. *Annals of Human Genetics*, **36**, 163–83.

Reiss, A. L., Feinstein, C. & Rosenbaum, K. N. (1986). Autism and genetic disorders. *Schizophrenia Bulletin*, **12**, 724–38.

Risch, N. (1990). Linkage strategies for genetically complex traits. I. Multilocus Models. *American Journal of Human Genetics*, **46**, 222–8.

Ritvo, E. R., Freeman, B. J., Mason-Brothers, A., Mo, A. & Ritvo, A. M. (1985a). Concordance for the syndrome of autism in 40 pairs of afflicted twins. *American Journal of Psychiatry*, **142**, 74–7.

Ritvo, E. R., Jorde, L. B., Mason-Brothers, A., Freeman, B. J., Pingree, C., Jones, M. B., McMahon, W. M., Petersen, P. B., Jenson, W. R. & Mo, A. (1989). The UCLA-University of Utah epidemiologic survey of autism: recurrence risk estimates and genetic counselling. *American Journal of Psychiatry*, **146**, 1032–6.

Ritvo, E. R., Mason-Brothers, A., Freeman, B. J., Pingree, C., Jenson, W. R., McMahon, W. M., Petersen, P. B., Jorde, L. B., Mo, A. & Ritvo, A. (1990). The UCLA-University of Utah epidemiologic survey of autism: the etiologic role of rare diseases. *American Journal of Psychiatry*, **147**, 1614–21.

Ritvo, E. R., Spence, M. A., Freeman, B. J., Mason-Brothers, A., Mo, A. & Marazita, A. L. (1985b). Evidence for autosomal recessive inheritance in forty-six families with multiple incidences of autism. *American Journal of Psychiatry*, **142**, 187–92.

Rutter, M., Bailey, A., Bolton, P. & Le Couteur, A. (1994). Autism and known medical conditions: myth and substance. *Journal of Child Psychology and Psychiatry*, **35**, 311–22.

Rutter, M., Bolton, P., Harrington, R., Le, C. A., MacDonald, H. & Simouoff, E. (1990). Genetic factors in child psychiatric disorders. I. A review of research strategies. *Journal of Child Psychology and Psychiatry and Allied Disciplines*, **31**, 3–37.

Silliman, E. R., Campbell, M. & Mitchell, R. S. (1989). Genetic influences in autism and assessment of metalinguistic performance in siblings of autistic children. In *Autism: Nature, Diagnosis, and Treatment*, ed. G. Dawson. New York: Guilford Press.

Smalley, S. L., Asarnow, R. F. & Spence, A. (1988). Autism and genetics: a decade of research. *Archives of General Psychiatry*, **45**, 953–61.

Smalley, S. L., McCracken, J. & Tanguay, P. (1995). Autism, affective disorders, and social phobia. *American Journal of Medical Genetics*, **60**, 19–26.

Smith, C. (1970). Heritability of liability and concordance in monozygous twins. *Annals of Human Genetics*, **26**, 85–91.

Smith, C. (1974). Concordance in twins: methods and interpretation. *American Journal of Human Genetics*, **26**, 454–66.

Snell, R. G., MacMillan, J. C., Cheadler, J. P., Fenton, I., Lazarus, P., Davies, P., MacDonald, M. E., Gusella, J. F., Harper, P. S. & Shaw, D. J. (1993). Relationship between trinucleotide repeat expansion and phenotypic variation in Huntington's disease. *Nature Genetics*, **4**, 393–7.

Spence, M. A., Ritvo, E. R., Marazita, M. L., Funderburk, S. J., Sparkes, R. S. & Freeman, B. J. (1985). Gene mapping studies with the syndrome of autism. *Behavior Genetics*, **15**, 1–13.

Spiker, D., Lotspeich, L., Kraemer, H. C., Hallmayer, J., McMahon, W., Petersen, P. B., Nicholas, P., Pingree, C., Wiese-Slater, S., Chiotti, C., Wong, D. L., Dimicelli, S., Ritvo, E., Cavalli-Sforza, L. L. & Ciranello, R. D. (1994). Genetics of autism: characteristics of affected and unaffected children from 37 multiplex families. *American Journal of Medical Genetics* (*Neuropsychiatric Genetics*), **54**, 27–35.

Steffenburg, S., Gillberg, C., Hellgren, L., Andersson, I., Gillberg, I., Jacobsson, G. & Bohman, M. (1989). A twin study of autism in Denmark, Finland, Iceland, Norway and Sweden. *Journal of Child Psychology and Psychiatry*, **30**, 405–16.

Stevenson, R. E. & Huntley, C. C. (1967). Congenital malformations in offspring of phenylketonuric mothers. *Pediatrics*, **40**, 33–45.

Szatmari, P. & Jones, M. B. (1991). IQ and the genetics of autism. *Journal of Child Psychology and Psychiatry*, **32**, 897–908.

Szatmari, P., Jones, M. B., Fisman, S., Tuff, L., Bartolucci, G., Mahoney, W. J. & Bryson, S. E. (1995). Parents and collateral relatives of children with pervasive developmental disorders: a family history study. *American Journal of Medical Genetics* (*Neuropsychiatric Genetics*), **60**, 282–9.

Szatmari, P., Jones, M. B., Holden, J. J. A., Bryson, S., Mahoney, W., Tuff, L., MacLean, J., White, B. N., Bartolucci, G., Schutz, C., Robinson, P. & Hoult, L. (1996). High phenotypic correlations among siblings with autism and PDD. *American Journal of Medical Genetics* (*Neuropsychiatric Genetics*), **67**, 354–60.

Szatmari, P., Jones, M. B., Tuff, L., Bartolucci, G., Fisman, S. & Mahoney, W. (1993). Lack of cognitive impairment in first degree relatives of children with pervasive developmental disorders. *Journal of the American Academy of Child and Adolescent Psychiatry*, **32**, 1264–73.

Warren, R. P., Yonk, J., Burger, R. W., Odell, D. & Warren, W. L. (1995). DR-positive T cells in autism: association with decrease plasma levels of the complement C4B protein. *Neuropsychobiology*, **31**, 53–7.

Wolf, L. C., Noh, S., Fisman, S. N. & Speechley, M. (1989). Psychological effects of parenting stress on parents of autistic children. *Journal of Autism and Developmental Disorders*, **19**, 156–66.

Young, J. G., Kavanagh, M. E., Anderson, G. M., Shaywitz, B. A. & Cohen, D. J. (1982). Clinical neurochemistry of autism and associated disorders. *Journal of Autism and Developmental Disorders*, **12**, 147–65.

5

Neurobiology of autism

Fritz Poustka

INTRODUCTION

The neurobiology of autism covers a wide range of neurophysiological, chemical, neuroimaging and morphological research data. Yet there is no available framework of a unifying aetiological concept of autistic disease from which various causes and consequences of psychiatric and physical symptoms and biological markers can be deduced and explained. Thus, the relevance of the obvious organic aetiology to the syndrome pathogenesis of autism and the deviance and deficiency in the development of the affected child remains unclear. Some medical conditions arise during the course of autism, i.e. seizures, whereas others may be present from very early in life and thus possibly more relevant to etiology.

To review the neurobiological basis and associations in autism is difficult for various reasons. For example, too often findings are given regardless of the small number of cases, the varying severity of mental retardation, the lack of reasonable control groups, the lack of replication studies, the contradictory findings of other research in the same area and the use of different classifying schemes and instruments. Examples are given of the last problem by Eaves & Milner (1993), who examined the relation between two popular screening tests used for autism. Correlations between the Childhood Autism Rating Scale (CARS) and the Autism Behaviour Checklist (ABC) ranged from -0.16 to 0.73 with a median of 0.39, with a moderate correlation on the nominal classification produced by the two tests. Diagnostic problems in neurobiological research further complicated the problem in that the most widely used classification systems in child psychiatry differed in their approach until recently. *The Diagnostic and Statistical Manual of Mental Disorders* (DSM-III-R) diagnostic criteria of autism tended to overdiagnose this disorder compared with the *International Classification of Diseases* (ICD-10) (Fombonne, 1992) and DSM-III (Volkmar & Cohen, 1988; Volkmar et al., 1992). Therefore, DSM-III-R guidelines work more like a screening test (Szatmari, 1992). Examples are given by Volkmar et al. (1992), who compare DSM-III, DSM-III-R and the draft research diagnostic criteria of ICD-10 with each other and with clinical diagnosis. DSM-IV and the Research Diagnostic Criteria of ICD-10 have a similar approach, partly as a result of the DSM-IV autism/ pervasive developmental field trial (Volkmar et al., 1994). The data from the field trial supported the ICD-10 approach, due to the better combination of a reasonable balance of sensitivity/specificity, the coverage of the range of syndrome expression and the ease of use for clinical and research purposes. Thus, most of the older research data obviously relied on screening procedures. Nevertheless, if research data were repeated and are neither too anecdotal nor single case reports they could at least serve as an hypothesis generating approach.

This chapter covers the evidence that suggests the importance of neurobiological mechanisms in syndrome pathogenesis in various fields and medical conditions. Variants such as Asperger's syndrome and atypical autism are mentioned when appropriate and of relevance.

NEUROLOGY AND RELATED CONDITIONS

Neurological dysfunction

In approximately 75% of 166 autistic subjects, abnormal signs were present on neurological examination (Bieber-Martig et al., 1996). A whole range of soft and hard signs were present ranging from cerebral squinting, nystagmus and hypotonus to deficits in gross and fine coordination or hemiparesis of various degrees (Lisch et al., 1993). Both soft and hard signs correlated with the level of intelligence (higher scores in more severely retarded subjects), without significant sex differences if intelligence were taken into account. Four per cent had difficulties in the optomotoric area, 5% in their reflexes, 5% had extrapyramidal abnormal signs, 15% had abnormal muscle tone, 60% dysdiadochokinesia and approximately a third had difficulties with gait or postural positioning. Fifteen per cent of autistic probands who developed at least some language showed problems in articulation and coordination of speech. Sensory deficits were present – 4% with vision and 2% with hearing impairment. These figures are probably biased by problems of the subjects' cooperation during the examination. A third of the probands could only be observed during action, and sensory activity could only be checked superficially in about half of the sample. 'Clumsiness' in this study did not differentiate between high functioning autism (HFA), Asperger's syndrome and autism with mental retardation of slight or moderate degree. Similarly, Ghaziuddin et al. (1994b) could not differentiate probands with Asperger's syndrome from those with HFA in regard to clumsiness as measured by tests of coordination.

There are few studies available with carefully controlled investigations of neurological dysfunction. Hallett et al. (1993) studied only five adults with autism. Three showed some irregularity in their gait, suggesting disturbance of the cerebellum. DeLong & Nohria (1994) reported positive neurological findings in half of the 40 probands with autistic spectrum disorder.

Several additional abnormal signs were studied in autistic children, for example as tone postural dysfunctions, dominance patterns, dermoglyphic patterns and perinatal conditions. Kohen-Raz (1991) mentioned that weight distribution and toe synchronizations are stable from 5 years of age onwards. Kohen-Raz et al. (1992) evaluated postural control in children with autism, in those with mental retardation and in normals. Postural patterns in autistic children differed from that in the other groups and also from adults with vestibular disorders; posture was more variable, less stable with more lateral sway, and the children with autism had more so-called stressful postures, putting excessive weight on one foot, toe or heel. Instability of anteroposterior and total body sway in autistic children, with some insensitivities to visual perception of environmental motion, were also described by Gepner et al. (1995).

Interestingly, age of walking was not delayed in 93% of autistic children nor did age of onset of walking correlate with intellectual disability in a larger study of children with different impairments (Kokubun et al., 1995).

Hand dominance pattern of parents and other relatives of autistic children showed no increased incidence of left handedness (Boucher et al., 1990).

Arrieta et al. (1990) found different digital and palmar dermatoglyphic patterns in autistic boys compared with controls and other differences in autistic girls from the Basque Country, postulating a genetic basis for these differences. Wolman et al. (1990) failed to establish discriminant patterns for dermatoglyphic analysis between autistic and various control groups of children.

PRE- AND PERINATAL CONDITIONS

The aim of many studies since the 1960s was to identify factors that were probably relevant for the aetiology of autism. In this context, several studies found significantly increased rates of obstetric complications in pregnancies resulting in the birth of autistic persons compared with different control groups (Lobascher et al., 1970; Knobloch & Pasamanic, 1975; Deykin & MacMahon, 1980). The abnormalities described were manifold and included pre-, peri- and postnatal complications, such as prolonged time of gestation, neonatal cyanosis, umbilical strangulation and, severe neonatal icterus.

The results of these studies were inconsistent and partly contradictory. Nowadays, they are difficult to interpret for two reasons. First, the diagnostic criteria they used differ from the criteria used at present (i.e. DSM-IV, ICD-10 criteria) and second, the studies themselves probably used variable diagnostic criteria (e.g. inclusion of index probands exhibiting severe mental retardation with known aetiology, such as rubella or tuberous sclerosis; inclusion of probands exhibiting early onset child psychosis).

From these observations, the question arose as to the nature and meaning of the increased birth complication rate and to what extent these complications could have an aetiological function in causing autism. Since the late 1970s, research findings have increasingly shown the important role of genetic factors in the aetiology of autism, and these findings led to a change of view regarding the role of birth complications in the aetiology of autism. It is important to mention that, at this time, objective and reliable instruments to register and measure birth complications were available and used for research: the 'optimality concept' (Prechtl, 1980, modified by Gillberg et al., 1983) and the Rochester Obstetric Scale (Sameroff et al., 1982).

The first strong hint of a genetic factor in the causation of autism was given by Folstein & Rutter's (1977) twin study. They found a highly increased concordance rate for autism in monozygotic twins (36%), but not for dizygotic twins (0%) (MZ: $n = 11$; DZ: $n = 10$). Steffenburg et al. (1989) found even higher concordance rates for monozygotic twins (60%) in contrast to dizygotic twins (3%).

Interestingly, Folstein & Rutter (1977) had found an increased rate of birth complications for autistic twins compared with their nonautistic twin siblings. Obviously twin studies can not be generalized to singletons because twinning itself increases the risk of various complications relative to singletons (Myrianthopoulos & Melnick, 1977). The experience of being a twin also influences behaviour (Rutter & Redshaw, 1991). This finding can, along with the earlier research findings, lead to the conclusion that perinatal stress may be involved in the aetiologically relevant role of birth complications in causing autism. However, there are serious arguments and research findings which are contradictory to this thesis. Birth complications are a nonspecific finding, and they can be observed in autistic as well as in nonautistic, healthy children. If birth complications are an aetiologically relevant factor, autism would be expected to occur with increased frequency in populations with an increased risk for birth complications, such as populations with lower socio-economic status or twin births. This seems not to be so (Steffenburg et al., 1989). The complication factors observed in autistic probands are mostly quite mild, and are not usually known to cause severe brain damage or mental retardation (Gillberg & Gillberg, 1983; Tsai & Stewart, 1983; Bryson et al., 1988; Levy et al., 1988). It is not possible to identify one single birth complication factor or a group of factors regularly associated with autism (Gillberg & Gillberg, 1983; Rutter, 1988). An increased rate of birth complications can also be found in children with cerebral palsy and severe mental retardation (Rantakallio & Wendt, 1985; Nelson & Ellenberg, 1986; Miller, 1989), and in children with chromosomal aberrations and genetically determined disorders (Bailey, 1993).

Gillberg & Gillberg (1983) found complications during the course of pregnancy for every autistic proband who later showed birth complications, and their conclusion was that birth complications could just have been the consequence of a prenatal existing abnormality. Perinatal complications such as birth asphyxia are not associated with autism except for those conditions that are correlated with prenatal complications (Goodman, 1990).

Further research strengthened the presumption that autism is likely to be a genetically determined disorder. An important finding was that the autism rate of first degree relatives of autistic persons is 50- to 100-fold higher than the normal incidence of the disorder, while second degree relatives have a normal incidence. One conclusion is that several interactive genes must be responsible for the disorder, and the large difference between the relative risks for autism in monozygotic and dizygotic twins supports an epistatic model (Risch, 1990a; Jorde et al., 1991; Bailey et al., 1995). Furthermore, Bolton et al. (1994) found a correlation between obstetric suboptimality and family loading for autism and the broader phenotype of autism; in addition, severity of autism in the proband is related to degree of genetic risk.

On the basis of these findings, it appears to be quite unlikely that birth complication factors are directly responsible for the aetiology of autism. In contrast, the concept of autism as a strongly genetically determined disorder supports the assumption that autism is a condition that produces an increased probability of pregnancy and birth complications. Future research has to take into account the probable interactive nature of the relationship between autism and birth complications that are likely to influence the phenotype (severity) of the disorder.

EEG abnormalities and seizure disorders in autism

Early research findings reported an increased incidence of electro-encephalograph (EEG) abnormalities and seizure disorders in autistic persons (Ornitz, 1978). The prevalence of EEG abnormalities reported in the literature is high and in most studies more than half of autistic subjects have EEG abnormalities, regardless of the occurrence of seizures (Tsai et al., 1985), and all regions of the cortex, mostly bilateral, are involved (Minshew, 1991).

The incidence of epileptic seizures in autism ranges from about a quarter to 30% by early adulthood (Deykin & MacMahon, 1979; Rutter, 1984; Volkmar & Nelson, 1990). These values are markedly increased compared with the normal population of children and adolescents (0.5%) (Rossi et al., 1995), and are also increased if compared with other psychiatric populations. Some studies report lower rates. Wong (1993) found only 5% of children with autistic conditions to have epilepsy, with the majority having onset of seizures before the age of 1 year.

Volkmar & Nelson (1990) found histories of seizure disorder in 21% of a sample of autistic subjects ($n = 192$). In a retrospective study undertaken by Carod et al. (1995), 47% of autistic children exhibited some kind of epileptic syndrome. In an inverse approach, Steffenburg et al. (1996) found, in a population of school age children exhibiting the combination of mental retardation and active epilepsy, that 27% had an autistic disorder. All these findings demonstrate a strong association between autism and EEG abnormalities in seizure disorders.

Tuchman et al. (1991) reported different frequencies of seizures according to various comorbid deficits. The major risk factor for epilepsy was severe mental deficiency in combination with motor deficits; 41% of autistic children exhibit epilepsy, in particular those with severe language problems, without language motor deficits, and without associated perinatal or medical disorders or positive family history of epilepsy. Seizures occurred in only 6% of autistic subjects. This rate was analogous to that in dysphasic nonautistic children (8%). The higher percentage in autistic girls (24%, 18 of 74) compared with boys (11%, 25 of 228) was in accordance with the associated comorbidity mentioned above. Similar associations were seen in a study by Elia et al. (1995), leading to the conclusion that seizures are not related to autism (or the severity of autism) itself. Aman et al. (1995) reported that 19% of autistic subjects (all ages) had had epilepsy, but only 13% were taking anticonvulsant drugs. Nearly 19% had more than one seizure per month, nearly 40% had a 3-year seizure-free interval, which could be an indication for anticonvulsant drug withdrawal.

The kind of EEG abnormalities and the types of seizures are various and heterogeneous. EEG abnormalities are described as diffuse or focal spikes, slow waves and paroxysmal spike and wave activity with mixed discharge and mostly bilateral location (Minshew, 1991), and mostly focal and multifocal and typical of benign childhood partial epilepsy with centrotemporal spikes (Rossi et al., 1995). In a study undertaken by Dawson et al. (1995), autistic children showed reduced EEG power in the frontal and temporal regions, but not in the parietal region. Differences were more prominent in the left than in the right hemisphere, and subgroups of autistic children displayed distinct patterns of brain activity ('passive' autistic children displayed reduced alpha EEG power in the frontal region compared with children classified as 'active but odd').

Autistic probands exhibit different types of epilepsy, and no particular epileptic syndrome was found to be more frequently correlated to autism (Elia et al., 1995). Autistic individuals had generalized major motor seizures, hypsarrhythmia, absence episodes, and complex partial and myoclonic seizures (Volkmar & Nelson, 1990; Elia et al., 1995; Rossi et al., 1995).

Forty-five per cent of the subjects with autism observed by Rossi et al. (1995) had their first seizures after the age of 10 years. There appears to be two peaks of onset: early childhood and during adolescence (Volkmar & Nelson, 1990). Volkmar and Nelson discuss the possibility that early onset of seizures could reflect a closer relation to pre- and perinatal complications, and later onset a closer relation with other processes.

Autistic females have seizures more frequently than males (Tuchman et al., 1991, 1992; Elia et al., 1995). There is also a higher proportion of probands exhibiting seizures in combination with a lower level of intellectual functioning (Elia et al., 1995), severe mental deficiency, motor deficit and a positive family history of epilepsy (Tuchman et al., 1991, 1992).

Results of these studies suggest that the higher incidence of epilepsy was not related to organic pre-, peri- and postnatal antecedents or cerebral lesions. Similarly, the severity of autism was not correlated with an increased risk of developing seizures. These findings led to the conclusion that genetic factors may be responsible for both autism and epilepsy (Rossi et al., 1995).

NEUROANATOMY AND BRAIN IMAGING STUDIES

Neuroanatomical findings

Few post-mortem studies on autistic brains have been carried out and no such neurochemical investigation is available. Ritvo et al. (1986) reported a decreased number of Purkinje cells in the cerebellum (vermis and hemispheres) in four autistic subjects. Williams et al. (1980) found no consistent abnormalities in four autistic brains, but reported a heavier brain weight in one of two idiopathic autistic cases.

Bailey et al. (1993b) reported a heavier brain weight in three of four brains of handicapped autistic individuals compared with the normal range in the population. An obvious decrease in neuronal density was not evident. Thus, an excess number of neurons was suggested, due to the epidemiological findings that autistic twins and singletons under the age of 16 years had significantly larger head circumference in 42% and 37%, respectively, of the cases, which suggests signs of megencephaly as a contributory factor to autism. This suggestion was confirmed in a study (Piven et al., 1995) using magnetic resonance imaging (MRI). Volumes of total brain, total brain tissue and total lateral ventricle volumes in 22 male autistic individuals were significantly greater than in a control group and after controlling for height and performance IQ (the later was significantly lower in the autistic individuals). Therefore, enlargement of the brain seems to result from both greater cerebral parenchyma brain tissue and greater lateral ventricle volume.

The most comprehensive study of anatomical alterations was carried out by Bauman & Kemper. The brains of six patients have been studied systematically so far (Bauman & Kemper, 1985; Raymond et al., 1989a,b;

Bauman, 1991; Kemper & Bauman, 1992). Of these one was female, three had severe mental retardation, and one was of normal intelligence (a 12-year-old boy). Three were younger subjects, aged 9, 10 and 12 years, the remainder were in their twenties. Four had had seizures and had been treated with anticonvulsant medication.

No brain showed gross morphological abnormalities. Reduced neuronal cell size and increased cell packing density, most significantly in the medial, cortical and central nuclei of the amygdala, were observed in these cases compared with controls. This involved areas of the forebrain (hippocampus, subiculum, entorhinal cortex, amygdala, mammillary body, anterior cingulate cortex and septum bilaterally). Pyramidal neurons (CA1, CA4) of the hippocampus displayed decreased complexity and extent of the dendritic arbors. In the medial septal nucleus cell packing density was increased and neuronal size reduced. In the nucleus of the diagonal band of Broca (NDB) the neurons were found to be unusually large in the younger autistic brains and numbers of neurons were normal. This was not so in older autistic brains, where the number of neurons of the NDB was reduced and their nuclei were small. Moreover, all six brains had abnormalities in the cerebellum and related inferior olive, with a significant decrease of Purkinje cells and various decreases in granule cells throughout the cerebellar hemisphere. Further retrograde cell loss and atrophy was seen in the olivary nucleus of the brainstem. The three older brains displayed adequate numbers of olivary neurons, but these were but small and pale; the three younger brains were significantly enlarged but with the neurons normal in number and appearance. In summary, these neuroanatomical abnormalities were related to the limbic system, the cerebellum and the related inferior olive.

Bauman & Kemper (1994) came to several conclusions from these findings. The four patients who had had seizures and had received anticonvulsants showed no different abnormalities in their brains compared with the other two without seizures or medication. No differences were found between the brain of the only case with normal intelligence and the brains of the others. Abnormalities in the cerebellum and the related olivary nucleus suggest an onset prior to birth. The limbic system could present a developmental maturational shortening involving its circuitry. Dysfunction in these circuits may disrupt the acquisition and understanding of information. In particular, the substrate of representational memory (involving sensory modalities and mediating of facts, experience and events, and the integration and generalization of information) and not habit memory is impaired by the significant abnormalities in the hippocampal complex, amygdala, entorhinal cortex, septum and medial mammillary body. The occurrence of retrograde loss of olivary neurons after cerebellar lesions could be associated with a cerebellar cortical lesion before the 30th week of gestation. Differences between brains of different ages may be due to establishment of postnatal persistence of the prenatal projection to the cerebellar nuclei because of the early lack of an adequate number of Purkinje cells as target cells for the mature inferior olivary projection. The fetal circuit is then unable to be sustained over time. Finally, subsets of phenotypic expression may stem from a similar abnormal anatomical pattern. Nevertheless, the aetiology of these abnormalities remains unclear.

The relation of cerebellar abnormalities to dysfunctions in autism is less clear. There is some evidence that alternative hypotheses of cerebellar functions may be operating. For example, the lateral cerebellum is strongly engaged during the acquisition and discrimination of sensory information and is not activated by the control of movement per se. This was confirmed by MRI of the lateral cerebellar output during passive and active sensory tasks in healthy volunteers (Goa et al., 1996). The strongest sensory discrimination occurred when sensory discrimination was paired with finger movements. Bauman & Kemper (1994) discuss the involvement of the cerebellum for higher functions (Schmamann, 1991) and the possibilities of disturbances of emotions, behaviour and learning due to cerebellar lesions. However, Peterson (1995) in his review concludes that findings on the cerebellum in autism (in neuroimaging studies) could be an epiphenomenon of early pathophysiological impairment during the development of the central nervous system, i.e. a correlate rather than immediate cause (see below).

Findings of brain imaging studies

CEREBELLUM AND MRI STUDIES

Besides the discussion about the cerebellar abnormalities in anatomical autopsy studies, the findings of MRI studies on alterations in cerebellar regions seem to support the evidence that there could be some gross markers for autism. Investigations by the research group of Courchesne et al. (1988) showed hypoplasia of the cerebellar vermian lobules VI and VII in autistic children, adolescents and adults. Hashimoto et al. (1995) reported similar findings. Courchesne et al. (1994a) provided a meta-analysis on vermal area measures of 78 autistic patients from four separate studies.

Results showed the majority (85–92%) to have cerebellar hypoplasia and 8–16% to have hyperplasia. A similar distribution was reported by Courchesne et al. (1994b). They compared 50 autistic patients (aged 2–40 years) with a control group of 43 patients and found that 16% had cerebellar lobules VI and VII with a smaller area than the mean of the control group and six patients (34%) had larger (hyperplastic) areas. Courchesne (1991) and Courchesne et al. (1994c) postulated that these findings are related to an impairment of autistic individuals to shift rapidly their mental focus of attention between auditory and visual stimuli.

These findings could not be replicated by others and remain somewhat inconclusive for various reasons (Peterson, 1995). Schaefer et al. (1996) concluded from their MRI study of the cerebellar vermis in 102 different patients with a variety of neurogenetic abnormalities and in 125 normals, that hypoplasia of the cerebellar vermal lobules VI and VII was a nonspecific anatomical marker in autism. This nonspecifity is underlined in the studies of Reiss et al. (1988, 1991), who found a significantly decreased area of the cerebellar vermis in the fragile X syndrome.

In various samples of different sizes, no or heterogeneous results of cerebellar volume measures were reported (Piven et al., 1990, 1992; Nowell et al., 1990; Ekman et al., 1991; Hashimoto et al. 1992a; Kleiman et al., 1992; Holttum et al., 1992; Ciesielski & Knight, 1994). In the study of Piven et al. (1992), cerebellar lobules VI–VII were found not to be smaller in autistic subjects compared with a control group of age and IQ comparable male volunteers. No differences were found after multivariate analysis adjusting for mid-sagittal brain area (MSBA), age and IQ (MSBA was significantly larger than that for subjects in various control groups). This exemplifies the difficulties in the interpretation of the studies available so far. The source of the often too conflicting results could be related to problems in the selection of control groups and autistic individuals (Holttum et al., 1992), which should take into consideration developmental variation, IQ, age, socio-economic status (SES), maternal age and possible other underlying medical conditions.

OTHER BRAIN ABNORMALITIES IN MRI STUDIES

Earlier findings of an enlarged ventricular system, mainly based on computed tomography studies, are not considered here. Again, results are conflicting; the relation to developmental delay and regression, use of medication, and seizures, and the often poorly controlled relation to a general enlargement of the ventricular system, all increase the difficulties in interpretating of the findings in recent decades (Minshew & Dombrowski, 1994). Piven et al. (1995) observed larger lateral ventricles in autistic probands but also observed greater brain volume (see above).

A significant smaller size of the brain stem (midbrain and medulla oblongata) in high functioning autistic children was observed by Hashimoto et al. (1993) regardless of the Development Quotient (DQ) or IQ of the autistic children (Hashimoto et al., 1992b). The size of the pons did not differ from controls (Hashimoto et al., 1992a) but had been found to be significantly smaller in earlier reports (Hashimoto et al., 1991). Hsu et al. (1991) could not find any difference in the size of midbrain and pons between normal and autistic children. These results show no unique problems in the pathway to and from the cerebellum. Midbrain abnormalities would also suggest some associations with the neurotransmitter system.

Parietal lobes were abnormal in appearance in nine of 21 autistic patients due to cortical volume loss with some extension to superior frontal and occipital loss (Courchesne et al., 1993). As the size of the corpus callosum in the posterior subregions was observed to be reduced in 51 autistic patients of various levels of mental retardation and ages compared with a control group matched for age and sex, Egaas et al. (1995) postulated an involvement of the parietal lobe over projection fibres in autism. Saitoh et al. (1995) found no malformation in the hippocampal region in autistic cases or in the cerebellar vermian lobules VI and VII or the posterior portion of the corpus callosum.

Observations of cortical malformations are seldom reported. Piven et al. (1990) found cerebral cortical malformations in a controlled study of 13 high functioning male autistic cases consisting of polymicrogyria, macrogyria and schizencephaly. They postulated neuronal defects of migration during the first 6 months of gestation. Berthier et al. (1990) described left frontal macrogyria and bilateral opercular polymicrogyria in two cases with Asperger's syndrome. Focal pachygyria was seen in three of 13 autistic children, which also suggests neuronal migration abnormalities (Shifter et al., 1994).

FUNCTIONAL ABNORMALITIES IN THE BRAIN (PET AND SPECT STUDIES)

There are few studies performed to data that relate autism with functional activation or brain perfusion. Again, these reports are preliminary and not consistent, and controlled studies on larger groups of autistic patients are lacking.

Siegel et al. (1995) compared 14 autistic adults with 25 schizophrenic patients and 20 normal controls and correlated glucose metabolic rate (GMR), using the positron emission tomography (PET) scan, in selected regions of the brain in the continuous performance test. In autistic patients negative correlation of the medial frontal cortical GMR with attentional performance was observed, in contrast to the control groups. GMR asymmetry was observed in an earlier study (Siegel et al., 1992). Autistic adult patients had a left more than a right anterior rectal gyrus GMR, as opposed to the normal right less than left asymmetry in the same region. Low GMR in the left posterior putamen and high GMR in the right posterior calcaric cortex in the autistic cases was also reported. Shifter et al. (1994) (see above) also found hypometabolic abnormalities in four of 13 autistic children who also had abnormalities in MRI. This suggests that it would be fruitful to search for subtle abnormalities using MRI techniques after findings of regional metabolic aberration are revealed by PET.

Gillberg et al. (1993) studied the regional cerebral blood flow (rCBF) using ^{99m}Tc SPECT 26 (single photon emission computed tomography) in patients with autism and 31 autistic-like conditions but with no control group. The main finding in the patients without epilepsy was temporal hypofusion, mostly bilateral but most pronounced on the left side. Nine of 16 patients also had hypoperfused prefrontal and frontal areas; this was most pronounced in patients without mental retardation and was often unilateral, but with no special side preference. This study is partly in agreement with George et al. (1992), who studied a small group of four young autistic adults and controls using high resolution brain SPECT. The total brain perfusion and the regional flow were significantly reduced in the right lateral temporal and right, left and midfrontal lobes compared with the controls.

Metabolic maturation delay was seen in the study using SPECT by Zilbovicius et al. (1995) after reporting a negative earlier result (Zilbovicius et al., 1992). Frontal hypoperfusion was found in five autistic children at age 3–4 years, corresponding to a pattern found in much younger normal children. Three years later normalization of perfusion was seen in the same children. Abnormal rCBF (SPECT, ^{99m}Tc) was studied by Mountz et al. (1995) who reported abnormalities predominantly in the temporal and parietal lobes with more left abnormalities than right in six autistic children. Right temporal hypoperfusion in one, diffusely decreased right hemispheric uptake in another, and decreased frontal and occipital uptake in the third patient with Asperger's syndrome (ages 12–16 years) were found by McKelvey et al. (1995). Chiron et al. (1995) also reported a lack of normal hemispheric asymmetry. Eighteen autistic children, aged 4–17 years, were compared with 10 age matched controls. They showed higher left than right rCBF for the total hemispheres, and sensorimotor and language related cortex to be independent of handiness, sex and age, which suggests a left hemispheric dysfunction.

Autistic children with deficits in the theory of mind performed significantly worse than a control group of children on the ability to recognize mental state terms in a word list (Baron-Cohen et al., 1994). Subsequently in a second experiment, increased rCBF in the right orbitofrontal cortex during the mental state recognition task was observed in normal adult volunteers. This suggests that the right orbitofrontal cortex serves as the basis for this ability. A direct observation of a disability on the theory of mind deficits in autistic children relating to this part of the cortex is lacking. Nevertheless, this study shows a direction for testing clinical and psychological conjectures in association with neurobiology if the approach could be implemented in a more direct way.

Only one study is available to date which points in this direction. Clinical deficits in autism and correlating alterations in high energy phosphate and membrane phospholipid metabolism in the dorsal prefrontal brain of 11 high functioning autistic subjects (aged 12–36 years) were reported by Minshew et al. (1993). The control group of normals was carefully matched for age, sex, IQ, race and socioeconomic status (SES). When the energy status of the brain (in vivo ^{31}P nuclear magnetic resonance spectroscopy; MRS) was compared within groups to neuropsychological and language test scores, a number of significant correlations was observed in the autistic group but not in the control group. Selected scores that correlated with alterations in high energy phosphate and membrane phospholipid metabolism were from the Wisconsin Card Sorting Test, Test of Language Competence, semantic language comprehension tests and secondary memory tests (delayed recall scores from the California Verbal Learning Test). Correlations demonstrated a consistent pattern and were parallel with severity of autism. These findings were reported to be consistent with a hypermetabolic energy state and with undersynthesis and enhanced degradation of brain membranes. Further studies involving a greater number of probands are necessary to develop an understanding of the pathophysiology of autism.

Fritz Poustka

NEUROCHEMISTRY

In his review Cook (1990) stated neurochemistry in autism as the most validated in childhood neuropsychiatric disorders; especially, hyperserotonaemia shows a familial pattern and is found consistently in over 25% of children and adolescents with autism. The role of the neurotransmitter serotonin in autism was studied in urine, serum, plasma platelets, cerebrospinal fluid concentrations and with the serotonin precursor tryptophan and tryptophan depletion and also brain imaging studies.

Biochemical research in autism has two possible advantages. One target is to get a basis for a rationale for treatment (as with selective serotonin receptor inhibitors), the other to gain markers for at least gene 'susceptibility' in examining receptor genes or changes in certain gene products such as neurotransmitters and their receptors.

Serotonin

Most of the more recent studies since Schain & Freedman (1961) have shown elevation of blood serotonin in autistic subjects (Anderson et al., 1987; Minderaa et al., 1987; Naffah-Mazzacoratti et al., 1993). Rolf et al. (1993) investigated platelet levels of serotonin and the amino acids aspartic acid, glutamine, glutamic acid and gamma-aminobutyric acid. Serotonin level was increased and the amino acids decreased in autistic subjects compared with a healthy match control group. Piven et al. (1991) suggested an autosomal recessive defect as the reason for the hyperserotonaemia. This could be a negative influence on fetal brain development (Buznikov, 1984). This result raises the importance of familial patterns of serotonaemia. Furthermore, some investigations study correlations between hyperserotonaemia and symptom patterns related to autism.

The whole blood serotonin (5HT), in contrast to the plasma norepinephrine (noradrenaline), was significantly positively correlated between autistic children and their parents and sibs in a replicated study by Leventhal et al. (1990). Twenty-three of 47 family members had at least one additional member with hyperserotonaemia and of these, 10 (of 23 families) had two or more hyperserotonaemic family members with 5HT more than 270 ng/ml. Family members had a heightened chance for hyperserotonaemia if the autistic child also had raised levels of blood 5HT. In the study by Piven et al. (1991), autistic children had highest hyperserotonaemia compared with their sibs. Serotonin levels in platelet rich plasma were higher in autistic subjects who had affected siblings (affected with either autism or PDD) compared with those autistic probands without affected sibs. The latter also had significantly higher serotonin levels compared with normal controls.

Support for the hypothesis of a maturation defect of monoaminergic systems was seen by Martineau et al. (1992a) in an age matched controlled study of 156 autistic children from 2 to 12 years of age, and mentally retarded nonautistic and normal children. Autistic children had high serotonin levels in urine but this was also found in the nonautistic children. In all three groups the serotonin levels decreased with age. Similar results were seen for dopamine and its metabolite and for norepinephrine and epinephrine (adrenaline).

One possibility of an effect of maturation in altering serotonin blood level was excluded by Tordjman et al. (1995). Although levels of testosterone and whole blood serotonin are significantly negatively correlated, no differences were found in the secretion of androgens (testosterone and dehydroepiandrosterone sulphate) between prepubertal and postpubertal autistic and normal subjects.

Two groups investigated serotonin involvement in autism in comparison with other neuropsychiatric disorders and healthy control groups. Singh et al. (1990) studied lymphocyte binding of [^{3}H]serotonin and found no difference between autistic and healthy children. Yuwiler et al. (1992) found no close relation of elevated blood serotonin to inhibition of serotonin binding to human cortical membranes by antibody rich blood fractions for autism (in contrast to multiple sclerosis).

The variation of level of serotonin in autism may be explained by different binding and uptake mechanisms. Cook et al. (1993a) postulated subgroups in regard to increased serotonin (5-HT) uptake and with decreased 5-HT2 binding, respectively. The affinity for [^{3}H]paroxetine binding was higher in the normoserotonaemic group, whereas the density (Bmax) of platelet 5-HT2 receptor binding sites was significantly lower in the hyperserotonaemic group. The two groups consisted of 12 hyperserotonaemic and 12 normoserotonaemic carefully matched relatives of autistic probands. Earlier, Perry et al. (1991) correlated density of platelet 5-HT2 binding sites between autistic boys and their fathers. Norepinephrine seemed to be involved in the heterologous regulation of 5-HT2 receptors in the platelet due to a negative correlation of norepinephrine and Bmax.

Raised blood levels of serotonin seem to correlate with psychopathological symptoms in family members of autistic subjects. The same research group as above (Cook et al., 1993b, 1994) compared parents who had autistic offspring with parents of children with Down's syndrome. Hyperserotonaemic parents of an autistic child scored significantly higher on a depression scale and on an obsessive–compulsive inventory than parents of children with Down's syndrome and both groups of parents had lower depression scores when peripheral levels of serotonin (in the blood) were not raised. Subjects with autism and an affected sibling with autism had higher platelet serotonin levels than subjects without an affected sibling with autism (Piven et al., 1991). The mechanism involved could, among others (e.g. receptor bindings for HT_2), be located in the role of platelet serotonin transport (Cook et al., 1996). Genetic studies on the role of the serotonin transporter (5-HTT) suggested evidence for 5-HTT as a potential genetic susceptibility factor for autism (Klauck et al., 1997), albeit somewhat contradictory to a recent study (Cook et al., 1997).

One investigation (with some limits on possible bias attributable to race) of an association between cognitive (especially verbal expressive) abilities of autistic probands and first degree relatives (Cuccaro et al., 1993) showed a substantial variance of cognitive performance correlated to whole blood serotonin level adjusted for race and familial classification. Cook et al. (1990) also found a negative correlation between vocabulary performance and whole blood serotonin in their study on autistic children, their sibs and parents. This was also true for plasma norepinephrine. Moreover, self-injurious behaviour and decreased pain sensitivity, often reported in autistic probands (Lisch et al., 1993), was not correlated with whole blood serotonin or plasma norepinephrine level.

A significant lower serum tryptophan to large neutral amino acids ratio was observed by D'Eufemia et al. (1995) in autism compared with normal controls. In approximately a third of the 40 autistic children in the study, this ratio was two standard deviations below the mean value of the control group. This would suggest a low brain tryptophan availability. The observation is strongly supported by the effects of tryptophan depletion in adults with autistic disorders (McDougle et al., 1996). Short-term tryptophan depletion exacerbated a number of behaviour variables such as stereotyped movements. Moreover, autistic subjects were more anxious, significantly less calm and happy after short-term tryptophan depletion compared with sham testing. These changes in behaviour occurred parallel to a significantly reduced plasma free and total tryptophan. No significant changes could be detected in social relationships to people, effectual reactions, sensory responses, language, or repetitive thinking and behaviour. The lack of effects on repetitive thinking may be due to the short time of the depletion.

It is not clear whether serotonin has an effect only on the many symptoms often associated with autism (aggression, motoric stereotype symptoms, aggression, impulsivity) but not on the core features of autism (such as poor communication and reciprocal social interaction). Disturbances of serotonergic pathways have been implicated in many neuropsychiatric disorders that include anxiety, depression, schizophrenia, alcoholism, migraine, aggression and suicidal behaviour (Erdmann et al., 1995; Heath & Hen, 1995; Lappalainen et al., 1995). Moreover, it is unclear whether tryptophan depletion affects neuropeptides, second messenger systems, receptor synthesis or the balance with other neurotransmitter systems such as dopamine and norepinephrine, as discussed by McDougle et al. (1996). Rolf et al. (1993) found decreased values of amino acids such as glutamic acid, glutamine, aspartic acid and gamma-aminobutyric acid as well as hyperserotonaemia, and therefore presumed an imbalance between these neurotransmitters.

The difficulties in understanding the extent and kind of the involvement of the serotonin neurotransmitter system, especially in autism, can be underlined by studies on the cerebrospinal fluid (CSF). The central metabolite of serotonin (5-hydroxyindolacetic acid, 5-HIAA) was examined in the CSF of eight autistic subjects. Anderson et al. (1988) did not find any increase compared with the normal population. Narayan et al. (1993) also did not find marked alterations of serotonin metabolite (5HIAA) CSF concentration (or of the dopamine metabolite, homovanillic acid (HVA)).

McBride et al. (1989) found a reduced number of receptor binding sites in the brain of autistic individuals and suggested this could be due to an autoimmune reaction (Todd et al., 1988; Root-Bernstein & Westall, 1990).

Dopamine

Other research groups favour the hypothesis of an involvement of brain catecholamine dysfunction in the development of autism. As with dopamine metabolism, high urinary levels of the metabolite HVA in autistic children were reported by different authors, especially the research group in Tours (Barthelmy et al., 1988; Garreau et al., 1988; Garnier et al., 1986). Narayan et al. (1993) (see above) and others did not find abnormal levels of CSF HVA in autism. In a study to measure melatonin concentration (because of the association with inhibition of calcium dependent dopamine release from amacrine cells), Ritvo et al. (1993) reported preliminary results of daytime melatonin in the urine in ten autistic subjects and family members and a (poorly matched) control group of normals. The autistic subjects and some of their parents and unaffected sibs showed a persistence of melatonin into the daylight hours in contrast to the control group. Nocturnal melatonin production did not differ.

Most of the receptor genes of dopamine could be localized (among them the D_2-receptor locus of Comings et al. (1991)) but none proved to be a primary aetiological agent for the autistic disorder. In 1989 Buckle et al. found a subunit of the GABA (3) receptor on Xq 28, which Cohen brought into relation with autism (Cohen et al, 1991). Derry & Barnard (1991) found a further receptor gene on the short arm of the X chromosome, namely Xp 21.3, the GABA A alpha 3-subunit gene; however, definite links to autistic phenotypes have not been established.

Opioid peptides

Several studies link neuropeptides such as the endogenous opioids to autism (Lensing et al., 1992; Nagamitsu, 1993; Gillberg, 1995). In the study by Nagamitsu, autistic patients showed no significant difference in CSF beta-endorphin concentration from the controls. A higher level was found in Rett's syndrome and infections involving the central nervous system. Therapeutic studies in autism using the opioid antagonist naltrexone are inconclusive. Willemsen-Swinkels et al. (1995) found no, or a worsening, effect of symptoms in autistic adults and no effect on self-injury behaviour of these agents.

Adrenergic function and others

Other studies tried to exclude or include further biochemical agents in autism. An elevation of epinephrine and norepinephrine in blood was found by Launay et al. (1987) and Barthelemy et al. (1988). Possible abnormalities of dopaminergic and noradrenergic neurotransmission were reported by Realmuto et al. (1990). On the contrary, Minderaa et al. (1994) found no marked abnormalities when they investigated plasma levels and urinary excretion of norepinephrine and epinephrine and their central and peripheral metabolites, respectively (MHPG and vanillylmandelic acid, VMA). Thus, basal noradrenergic functioning seems not to play an important role in autism.

Richdale & Prior (1992) studied cortisol circadian rhythm and dexamethasone suppression test effects in autistic children. No clear effects were found other than a tendency towards a cortisol hypersecretion during the day in autistic children. However, these children were integrated into the normal school system and findings may indicate an environmental stress response.

NEUROPHYSIOLOGY

Brainstem auditory evoked responses

Prolonged transmission of information in the brain may be linked with dysfunctions of information processing, and perceptual, particularly auditory, abnormalities in autism. Yet the evidence which is to be found in these neurophysiological studies is not conclusive. Klin (1993), in his review of ten studies published during the last 25 years, reporting inter-peak latencies of auditory brainstem responses (ABR) in autism, criticized the results as being only suggestive of brainstem involvement in autism. The reports showed prolonged brainstem transmission times in five studies, as well as shortening (one study) or no abnormalities (five studies) in central transmission latencies. Moreover, the studies revealed peripheral hearing impairment in some of the autistic individuals. Some investigations showed congruent findings of prolonged transmission times. Thivierge et al. (1990) studied 20 autistic and 13 mentally retarded subjects and found prolonged interpeak latencies in 80% of autistic subjects. Wong & Wong (1991) also found in a controlled study a longer brainstem transmission time that correlated with autistic features rather than with mental retardation, age or gender. Sersen et al. (1990) observed longer latencies for middle and late components compared with probands with Down's syndrome (who displayed shorter absolute and interpeak latencies for early components of the ABR). Unfortunately, an effect due to sedation could not be ruled out.

Event related potentials (ERP)

ERP studies deal with orienting responses to novel information, modulation of attention, maintaining selective attention and the topographic distribution of ERP components. Studies of ERP in autism again are relatively rare and do not support a strong and unique discriminant effect related to autism. Positive (P) and negative (N) event related potential

149

amplitudes are measured in milliseconds after stimulus onset (e.g. P300 or P3) and such amplitudes are derived by substraction methods (e.g. PN as the ERP difference between the target and a different nontarget stimulus; Nd as the ERP difference between the target stimulus and the same stimulus previously presented as a nontarget).

Oades et al. (1990) published event related potential amplitudes, e.g. N1, P3, PN, Nd, that were reduced in autistic subjects compared with normals, but the components affected varied. Kemner et al. (1995) (see below) reviews auditory ERP studies in autism and concluded that the findings were inconsistent with respect to P3 and N1.

In a carefully designed study, Kemner et al. (1995) could not replicate earlier studies of abnormal mismatch negativity (MMN, resulting from the subtraction of potentials to different nontargets) in autistic children. Abnormal lateralization of abnormal MMN could not be found. Unexpected occipital P3 to deviant stimuli was significantly larger in the active than passive condition. This and the one replication that could be observed, namely the smaller A/Pcz/300, led to the suggestions that the auditory occipital task effect is related to understimulation of the occipital lobe by visual stimuli in autistic children. As the autistic subjects differed not only from the normal control group but also from those with ADHD and with dyslexia, the effects were suggested as highly specific for autism. Kemner et al. (1994) also reported differences specific to autistic children on ERPs to visual and somatosensory stimuli. Only the autistic group displayed a task effect on the visual P2N2 (mismatch activity) and larger P3s in response to novel rather than to deviant stimuli, again compared with hyperactive and dyslexic children. Therefore, abnormalities in processing of proximal and distal stimuli were regarded as specific for autism. No abnormal lateralization was observed.

Some more recent studies revealed abnormalities associated with the primary and secondary auditory cortex when the N1 (which is generated in primary and secondary auditory cortex) did not increase with increasing stimuli in children with autism and with receptive developmental language disorder but not in controls (Lincoln et al., 1995). Lincoln et al. (1993) found an abnormally small amplitude of the P3b that was seen as evidence for difficulties in processing auditory information in children with autism. P3b was significantly diminished in size under focused selective attention conditions in autistic subjects compared with normals, which suggests abnormalities in selective attention in autism (Ciesielski et al., 1990). 'Emotional sounds' appeared to be particularly effective in activating the neural substrate of the P3 generator system. Autistic subjects with normal IQ did not differ in this respect from normals (Erwin et al., 1991). P1 auditory ERP abnormalities in high functioning adult autistic individuals were studied by Buchwald et al. (1992), who suggested that the ascending reticular activating system and their thalamic target cells may be dysfunctional in autism.

Correlation of ERP with attempts to identify idiomatic phrases in high functioning adult autistic probands were found by Strandburg et al. (1993) (greatly reduced N400 to idioms). Additionally, autistic subjects produced larger N1 amplitudes in all tasks and larger P3s in the Idiom Recognition Task and the Continuous Performance Task.

Martineau et al. (1992a,c) observed a cognitive deficit in the ability to maintain crossmodal associations in autism preceded by a more elementary perceptive abnormality when studying auditory evoked responses to simple and crossmodal (auditivo-visual) stimuli in a controlled study of autistic, mentally retarded and normal children. This could be related to dysfunctions of attention, intention, association and communication.

Overall, many of these psychophysiological studies describe different aspects of possible links to some key or associated features of autism. At present an integrated approach to understanding the impairment in perceptual and information processing (Oades & Eggers, 1993) on a neurophysiological level is needed in further studies.

OTHER MEDICAL CONDITIONS

Gillberg (1992) listed a number of syndromes and diseases associated with autism in at least two studies (fragile X syndrome, other X chromosomal anomalies, partial trisomy 15, other chromosomal anomalies, tuberous sclerosis, neurofibromatosis, hypomelanosis, Goldenhar syndrome, Rett's syndrome, Moebius' syndrome, PKU, lactic acidosis, hypothyroidism, rubella embryopathy, herpes encephalitis, cytomegalovirus infection, Williams' syndrome and Duchenne muscular dystrophy). The list could be continued. Fernell et al. (1991) found that 23% of a population of children with infantile hydrocephalus scored high on the Autism Behaviour Checklist. These children consisted of the most brain damaged and mentally retarded group.

More anecdotal reports find correlations between autism and exposure in utero to valproic acid (Christianson et al., 1994), fetal alcohol syndrome (Harris et al., 1995), lead exposure beyond the third year of life and re-exposure (Shannon & Graef, 1996) and thalidomide embryopathy (Stromland et al., 1994). Also reported are syndromes such as Marfan like disorder (and Asperger's syndrome; Tantam et al., 1990), Sotos' syndrome (Morrow et al., 1990), Bachman-de Lange syndrome (Bay et al., 1993), Joubert's syndrome (Holroyd et al., 1993) and Noonan's syndrome (Ghaziuddin et al., 1994a).

Chromosomal aberrations have also been associated with autistic symptom. These include: a de novo translocation t(3;12) (p26.3;q23.3) of tuberous sclerosis and autistic behaviour in children (Fahsold et al., 1991); deletion of chromosome 5 (Barber et al., 1994); inv dup(15)(pter–q13) (Schinzel, 1990); 15q12 deletion (Kerbeshian et al., 1990); tetrasomy 15 (Hotopf & Bolton, 1995); duplication of the 15q11-13 region (Bundey et al., 1994); a partial 16p trisomy with autistic disorder and Tourette's syndrome (Hebebrand et al., 1994); deletion of 17(p11.2 p11.2); Asperger's syndrome in a balanced t(17;19)(p13.3;p11) translocation (Anneren et al., 1995); trisomy 17 (Shaffer et al., 1996); 18q-chromosomal abnormality (Seshadri et al., 1992; Ghaziuddin et al., 1993); Y chromosome (Blackman et al., 1991); Xp duplication (Rao, 1994); 46,X,t(X;8)(p22.13;q22.1) duplication (Bolton et al., 1995), revealing a mixed picture of locations.

Autism is relatively rarely seen in children with Down's syndrome. Again in anecdotal case reports an overlap between these two conditions has been observed (Ghaziuddin et al., 1992; Howlin et al., 1995). Bolton et al. (1994) reported a lesser variant of autism in 1.6–3.2% of the siblings of Down's syndrome cases.

Other associations include causes such as left temporal oligodenroglioma (Hoon & Reiss, 1992), herpes encephalitis at age 31 years (Gillberg, 1991), congenital hypothyroidism (Gillberg et al., 1992), a relationship with Tourette's syndrome (Comings & Comings, 1991; Sverd, 1991), mutation in adenylsuccinate lyase (Stone et al., 1992), PKU (Miladi et al., 1992), gangliosides (Lekman et al., 1995), high levels of glial fibril acidic protein (Rosengren et al., 1992; Ahlsen et al., 1993), and congenital blindness in children (Goodman & Minne, 1995). Some earlier reported abnormalities in autism lost their strength of association or could not be replicated. For example, congenital rubella and autism was noted by Chess (1977) but has not been replicated over time. Chess argued that neither visual nor hearing impairments nor severity of mental retardation was of importance for the autistic symptoms. F Poustka et al. (unpublished results) could not find any case with abnormalities after screening for mucopolisaccharides, oligosaccharides, HPLC-purine and purimidin in 110 autistic subjects within a broad range of IQ levels from severe mental retardation to normal IQ.

Links to autoimmune disorders, C4 deficiency and autism were proposed by Warren et al. (1991, 1994, 1995) and antibodies to myelin basic protein have also been reported (Singh et al., 1993). Daniels et al. (1995) suggested that one or more genes of the major histocompatibility complex are involved in the development of some cases of autism. Alpha interferonaemia, which contributes to allergies and autimmune phenomena, was increased in autistic children in a very preliminary study (Stubbs, 1995). Cook et al. (1993a) failed to observe that autoantibodies to serotonin receptors (5HT1A and 5HT2), alpha2-adrenergic, D1 and D2 receptors and/or associated membrane proteins are of importance in autistic children.

Exposure to influenza epidemics during gestation was not found to be associated with autism (Dassa et al., 1995). In addition, several studies were performed to investigate the existence of excesses of births of autistic children in certain seasons (speculations range from exposure to infections to nutrition or other effects). Gillberg (1990) found an excess for March births, as did Mouridsen et al. (1994) and Barak et al. (1995) for March and August births. Bolton et al. (1992) could not replicate earlier findings of any seasonal birth effects.

There are a few known medical conditions with importance to autism, namely Rett's syndrome, the fragile X syndrome and tuberous scleroses. Rett's syndrome in girls shows autistic like symptomatology, and there are also differences after the preschool years (Olsson & Rett, 1990). Several reports initially indicated a strong association of the fragile X chromosomal anomaly with autism (Watson et al., 1984; Blomquist et al., 1985; Cohen et al., 1991), whereas others did not support this finding (Venter et al., 1984; Einfeld et al., 1989; Bailey et al., 1993a). With knowledge of the FMR-1 gene responsible for the fragile X syndrome (Oberlé et al., 1991; Verkerk et al., 1991; Yu et al., 1991) and the possibility of a more exact molecular genetic analysis, the nature of association of fragile X and autism was clarified (Hallmayer et al., 1994). Discrepancies between the various studies appear to be due to differences in ascertainment strategy and diagnostic criteria for autism and varying thresholds for the cytogenetic diagnosis of fragile X at Xq27.3. Klauck et al. (1997) performed Southern blot analysis with a FMR-1 specific probe. No significant changes were found in 139 patients (99%) from 122 families other than the normal variations in the population. In the case of one multiplex family with three children showing no dysmorphic features of the fragile X syndrome (one male meeting three of four ADI-algorithm criteria, one normal male with slight learning disability but negative ADI-R testing and one full autistic female) FRAXA full mutation specific CCG repeat expansion in the genotype was not subsequently correlated with the autism phenotype. Further analysis revealed a mosaic pattern of methylation at the FMR-1 gene locus I5in the two sons of the family, indicating at least a partly functional gene. Therefore, an association of autism with fragile X at Xq27.3 does not exist and excludes this location as a candidate gene region for autism.

According to the prevalence studies of Hunt & Shepherd (1993) and Gillberg et al. (1994) tuberous sclerosis and autism are suggested to be strongly associated. Smalley et al. (1992) reported significantly more frequent seizures and more severe mental retardation in children with tuberous sclerosis and autism compared with tuberous sclerosis without autism. Those with both conditions were predominantly males.

There are two contrasting views in relation to the aetiology of autism (Bailey, 1993) which have wide implications for neurobiological research and interpretation. Gillberg & Coleman (1992) on the one hand are convinced that autism is not a homogenous disease, but has several different pathogenic pathways analogous to other disorders with a stable course like, for example, cerebral palsy. Different syndromes are associated with autism (in 37% of the cases with autism after intensive neurobiological investigation; Gillberg, 1992) and, the significant psychopathology of autism or severity of mental retardation are not different from idiopathic cases. The search for autism specific causes is therefore misleading in their view but assessment requires neuropsychiatric assessment, including laboratory examination with lumbar punctures, CFS protein electrophoresis to rule out progressive encephalopathy, and others in the clinical routine.

On the other hand, Rutter et al. (1994) in reviewing the literature on the relation between autism and different medical conditions found the rate of such underlying known conditions in autism to be around 10%, depending on the severity of mental retardation and being much more common in cases with profound mental retardation. Furthermore, the strength of association between autism and known medical conditions is seldom brought into consideration in studying them within groups (to compare the frequency of the association stemming from autism in relation to a certain condition versus the condition in relation to autism). Obviously no consistent aetiological pattern has been found to date.

ACKNOWLEDGEMENTS

Parts of the manuscript were prepared by Dorothea Rühl, MD, and

Bettina Bieber-Martig, MD. This work was also partly supported by the Deutsche Forschungsgemeinschaft (grant no. Po 255/4-3).

REFERENCES

Ahlsen, G., Rosengren, L., Belfrage, M., Palm, A., Haglid, K., Hamberger, A. & Gillberg, C. (1993). Glial fibrillary acidic protein in the cerebrospinal fluid of children with autism and other neuropsychiatric disorders. *Biological Psychiatry*, **33**, 734–43.

Aman, M. G., Van Bourgondien, M. E., Wolford, P. L. & Sarphare, G. (1995). Psychotropic and anticonvulsant drugs in subjects with autism: prevalence and patterns of use. *Journal of the American Academy of Child and Adolescent Psychiatry*, **34**, 1672–81.

Anderson, G. M., Freedman, D. X., Cohen, D. J., Volkmar, F. R., Hoder, E. L., McPhedran, P., Minderaa, R. B., Hansen, C. R. & Young, J. G. (1987). Whole blood serotonin in autistic and normal subjects. *Journal of Child Psychology and Psychiatry*, **28**, 885–900.

Anderson, G. M., Ross, D. L., Klykylo, W., Feibel, F. C. & Cohen, D. J. (1988). Cerebrospinal fluid indoleacetic acid in autistic subjects. *Journal of Autism and Developmental Disorders*, **18**, 259–62.

Anneren, G., Dahl, N., Uddenfeldt, U. & Janols, L. O. (1995). Asperger's syndrome in a boy with a balanced de novo translocation: t(17;19)(p13. 3;p11). *American Journal of Medical Genetics*, **56**, 330–1.

Arrieta, M. I., Martinez, B., Criado, B., Simon, A., Salazar, L. & Lostao, C. M. (1990). Dermatoglyphic analysis of autistic Basque children. *American Journal of Medical Genetics*, **35**, 1–9.

Bailey, A., Bolton, P., Butler, L., Le Couteur, A., Murphy, M., Scott, S., Webb, T. & Rutter, M. (1993a). Prevalence of the fragile X anomaly amongst autistic twins and singletons. *Journal of Child Psychology and Psychiatry*, **34**, 673–88.

Bailey, A., Le Couteur, A., Gottesman, I., Bolton, P., Simonoff, E., Yuzda, E. & Rutter, M. (1995). Autism as a strong genetic disorder: evidence from a British twin study. *Psychological Medicine*, **25**, 63–77.

Bailey, A., Luthert, P., Bolton, P., Le Couteur, A., Rutter M. & Harding, B. (1993b). Autism and megalencephaly. *Lancet*, **341**, 854, 1225–6.

Bailey, A. J. (1993). The biology of autism [editorial] *Psychological Medicine*, **23**, 7–11.

Barak, Y., Ring, A., Sulkes, J., Gabbay, U. & Elizur, A. (1995). Season of birth and autistic disorder in Israel. *American Journal of Psychiatry*, **152**, 798–800.

Barber, J. C., Ellis, K. H., Bowles, L. V., Delhanty, J. D., Ede, R. F., Male, B. M. & Eccles, D. M. (1994). Adenomatous polyposis coli and a cytogenetic deletion of chromosome 5 resulting from a maternal intrachromosomal insertion. *Journal of Medical Genetics*, **31**, 312–16.

Baron-Cohen, S. (1994). Recognition of mental state terms. Clinical findings in children with autism and functional neuroimaging of normal adults. *British Journal of Psychiatry*, **165**, 640–9.

Baron-Cohen, S., Ring, H., Moriarty, J., Schmitz, B., Costa, D. & Ell, P. (1994). Recognition of mental state terms. Clinical findings in children with autism and a functional neuroimaging study of normal adults. *British Journal of Psychiatry*, **165**, 640–9.

Barthelemy, C., Bruneau, N., Cottet-Eymard, J. M., Domenech-Jouve, J., Garreau, B., Lelord, G., Muh, J. P. & Peyrin, L. (1988). Urinary free and conjugated catecholamines and metabolites in autistic children. *Journal of Autism and Developmental Disorders*, **18**, 583–91.

Bauman, M. L. (1991). Microscopic neuroanatomic abnormalities in autism. *Pediatrics*,

87, 791–6.

Bauman, M. L. & Kemper, T. L. (1994). Neuroanatomical observations of the brain in autism. In *The Neurobiology of Autism*, ed. M. L. Bauman & T. L. Kemper, pp. 119–45. Baltimore: The Johns Hopkins University Press.

Bauman, M. & Kemper, T. L. (1985). Histoanatomic observations of the brain in early infantile autism. *Neurology*, 35, 866–74.

Bay, C., Mauk, J., Radcliffe, J. & Kaplan, P. (1993). Mild Brachmann-de Lange syndrome. Delineation of the clinical phenotype, and characteristic behaviors in a six-year-old boy. *American Journal of Medical Genetics*, 47, 965–8.

Berthier, M. L., Starkstein, S. E. & Leiguarda, R. (1990). Developmental cortical anomalies in Asperger's syndrome: neuroradiological findings in two patients. *Journal of Neuropsychiatry and Clinical Neurosciences*, 2, 197–201.

Bieber-Martig, B., Werner, K. & Poustka, F. (1996). Die Rolle von prä- und perinatalen Faktoren in der Ätiologie des Autismus und neurologische Dysfunktion. Zeitschrift für Kinder- und Jugendpsychiatrie.

Blackman, J. A., Selzer, S. C., Patil, S. & Van Dyke, D. C. (1991). Autistic disorder associated with an iso-dicentric Y chromosome. *Developmental Medicine and Child Neurology*, 33, 162–6.

Blomquist, H. K., Bohman, M., Edvinsson, S. O., Gillberg, C., Gustavson, K. H., Holmgren, G. & Wahlström, J. (1985). Frequency of the fragile X syndrome in infantile autism. *Clinical Genetics*, 27, 113–17.

Bolton, P., Pickles, A., Harrington, R., Macdonald, H. & Rutter, M. (1992). Season of birth: issues, approaches and findings for autism. *Journal of Child Psychology and Psychiatry*, 33, 509–30.

Bolton, P. & Holland, A. (1994). Chromosomal abnormalities. In *Child and Adolescent Psychiatry: Modern Approaches* 3rd edn, ed. M. Rutter, M. Taylor & I. Hersh, pp. 152–71. Oxford: Blackwell Scientific.

Bolton, P., Macdonald, H., Pickles, A., Rios, P., Goode, S., Crowson, M., Bailey, A. & Rutter, M. (1994) A case-control family history study of autism. *Journal of Child Psychology and Psychiatry*, 35, 877–900.

Bolton, P., Murphy, M., Sim, L. et al. (1993). Obstetrical complications in autism: consequences rather than causes of the disorder? Paper presented at the 3rd World Congress of Psychiatric Genetics, New Orleans, 25 October 1993. *Psychiatric Genetics*, 3, 178.

Bolton, P., Powell, J., Rutter, M., Buckle, V., Yates, J. R., Ishikawa-Brush, Y. & Monaco, A. P. (1995). Autism, mental retardation, multiple exostoses and short stature in a female with 46,X,t(X;8)(p22. 13;q22. 1). *Psychiatric Genetics*, 5, 51–5.

Boucher, J., Lewis, V. & Collis, G. (1990). Hand dominance of parents and other relatives of autistic children. *Developmental Medicine and Child Neurology*, 32, 304–13.

Bryson, S. E., Smith, I. M. & Eastwood, D. (1988). Obstetrical suboptimality in autistic children. *Journal of the American Academy of Child and Adolescent Psychiatry*, 27, 418–22.

Buchwald, J. S., Erwin, R., Van Lancker, D., Guthrie, D., Schwafel, J. & Tanguay, P. (1992). Midlatency auditory evoked responses: P1 abnormalities in adult autistic subjects. *Electroencephalography and Clinical Neurophysiology*, 84, 164–71.

Buckle, V. J., Fujita, N., Bateson, A. N., Darlison, M. G. & Barnard, E. A. (1989). Localization of the human GABA-A3 receptor subunit gene to Xq28: a candidate gene for X-linked mental depression. *Cytogenetics and Cell Genetics*, 51, 972.

Bundey, S., Hardy, C., Vickers, S., Kilpatrick, M. W. & Corbett, J. A. (1994). Duplication of the 15q11-13 region in a patient with autism, epilepsy and ataxia. *Developmental*

Medicine and Child Neurology, **36**, 736–42.

Buznikov, G. A. (1984). The action of neurotransmitters and related substances on early embryogenesis. *Pharmacology and Therapeutics*, **25**, 23–59.

Carod, F. J., Prats, J. M., Garaizar, C. & Zuazo, E. (1995). Clinical-radiological evaluation of infantile autism and epileptic syndromes associated with autism. *Revue Neurologique*, **23**, 1203–7.

Chess, S. (1977). Follow-up report on autism in congenital rubella. *Journal of Autism and Childhood Schizophrenia*, **7**, 68–81.

Chiron, C., Leboyer, M., Leon, F., Jambaque, I., Nuttin, C. & Syrota, A. (1995). SPECT of the brain in childhood autism: evidence for a lack of normal hemispheric asymmetry. *Developmental Medicine and Child Neurology*, **37**, 849–60.

Christianson, A. L., Chesler, N., Kromberg, J. G. (1994). Fetal valproate syndrome: clinical and neuro-developmental features in two sibling pairs. *Developmental Medicine and Child Neurology*, **36**, 361–9.

Ciesielski, K. T., Courchesne, E. & Elmasian, R. (1990). Effects of focused selective attention tasks on event-related potentials in autistic and normal individuals. *Electroencephalography and Clinical Neurophysiology*, **75**, 207–20.

Ciesielski, K. T. & Knight, J. E. (1994). Cerebellar abnormality in autism: a nonspecific effect of early brain damage? *Acta Neurobiologiae Experimentalis Warszawa*, **54**, 151–4.

Cohen, I. L., Sudhalter, V., Pfadt, A., Jenkins, E. C., Brown, W. T. & Vietze, P. M. (1991). Why are autism and the fragile-X-syndrome associated? Conceptual and methodological issues. *American Journal of Human Genetics*, **48**, 195–202.

Comings, D. E., Comings, B. G., Muhlemann, D., Dietz, G, Shahbahrami, B., Tast, D., Knell, E., Kocsis, P., Baumgarten, R., Kovacs, B. W., Levy, D. L., Smith, M., Borison, R. L., Evans, D. & Klein, D. N. (1991). The dopamine D2 receptor locus as a modifying gene in neuropsychiatric disorders. *JAMA*, **266**, 1793–800.

Comings, D. E. & Comings, B. G. (1991). Clinical and genetic relationships between autism-pervasive developmental disorder and Tourette syndrome: a study of 19 cases. *American Journal of Medical Genetics*, **39**, 180–91.

Cook, E. H. (1990). Autism: review of neurochemical investigation. *Synapse*, **6**, 292–308.

Cook, E. H. Jr., Arora, R. C., Anderson, G. M., Berry-Kravis, E. M., Yan, S. Y., Yeoh, H. C., Sklena, P. J., Charak, D. A. & Leventhal, B. L. (1993a). Platelet serotonin studies in hyperserotonemic relatives of children with autistic disorder. *Life Sciences*, **52**, 2005–15.

Cook, E. H. Jr., Charak, D. A., Arida, J., Spohn, J. A., Roizen, N. J. & Leventhal, B. L. (1994). Depressive and obsessive-compulsive symptoms in hyperserotonemic parents of children with autistic disorder. *Psychiatry Research*, **52**, 25–33.

Cook, E. H., Courchesne, R., Lord, C., Cox, N. J., Yan, S., Lincoln, A., Haas, R., Courchesne, E. & Leventhal, B. L. (1997). Evidence of linkage between the serotonin transporter and autistic disorder. *Molecular Psychiatry*, **2**, 247–50.

Cook, E. H. & Leventhal, B. L. (1996). The serotonin system in autism. *Current Opinion in Pediatrics*, **81**, 348–54.

Cook, E. H. Jr., Leventhal, B. L., Heller, W., Metz, J., Wainwright, M. & Freedman, D. X. (1990). Autistic children and their first-degree relatives: relationships between serotonin and norepinephrine levels and intelligence. *Journal of Neuropsychiatry Clinical Neurosciences*, **2**, 268–74.

Cook, E. H. Jr., Perry, B. D., Dawson, G., Wainwright, M. S. & Leventhal, B. L. (1993b). Receptor inhibition by immunoglobulins: specific inhibition by autistic children, their relatives, and control subjects. *Journal of Autism and Developmental Disorders*, **23**, 67–78.

Fritz Poustka

Courchesne, E. (1991). Neuroanatomic imaging in autism. *Pediatrics*, **87**, 781–90.

Courchesne, E., Press, G. A. & Yeung-Courchesne, R. (1993). Parietal lobe abnormalities detected with MR in patients with infantile autism. *American Journal of Roentgenology*, **160**, 387–93.

Courchesne, E., Saitoh, O., Yeung-Courchesne, R., Press, G. A., Lincoln, A. J. Haas, R. H. & Schreibman, L. T. I. (1994b). Abnormality of cerebellar vermian lobules VI and VII in patients with infantile autism: identification of hypoplastic and hyperplastic subgroups with MR imaging. *American Journal of Roentgenology*, **162**, 123–30.

Courchesne, E., Townsend, J., Akshoomoff, N. A., Saitoh, O., Yeung-Courchesne, R., Lincoln, A. J., James, H. E., Haas, R. H., Schreibman, L. & Lau, L. (1994c). Impairment in shifting attention in autistic and cerebellar patients. *Behavioural Neuroscience*, **108**, 848–65.

Courchesne, E., Townsend, J. & Saitoh, O. (1994a). The brain in infantile autism: posterior fossa structures are abnormal. *Neurology*, **44**, 214–23.

Courchesne, E., Yeung-Courchesne, R., Press, G. A., Hesslink, J. R. & Jernigan, T. L. (1988). Hypoplasia of cerebellar vermal lobules VI and VII in autism. *New England Journal of Medicine*, **318**, 1349–54.

Cuccaro, M. L., Wright, H. H., Abramson, R. K., Marsteller, F. A. & Valentine, J. (1993). Whole-blood serotonin and cognitive functioning in autistic individuals and their first-degree relatives. *Journal of Neuropsychiatry Clinical Neuroscience*, **5**, 94–101.

Daniels, W. W., Warren, R. P., Odell, J. D., Maciulis, A., Burger, R. A., Warren, W. L. & Torres, A. R. (1995). Increased frequency of the extended or ancestral haplotype B44-SC30-DR4 in autism. *Neuropsychobiology*, **32**, 120–3.

Dassa, D., Takei, N., Sham, P. C. & Murray, R. M. (1995). No association between prenatal exposure to influenza and autism. *Acta Psychiatrica Scandinavica*, **92**, 145–9.

Dawson, G., Klinger, L. G., Panagiotides, H., Lewy, A. & Castelloe, P. (1995). Subgroups of autistic children based on social behavior display distinct patterns of brain activity. *Journal of Abnormal Child Psychology*, **23**, 569–83.

DeLong, R. & Nohria, C. (1994). Psychiatric family history and neurological disease in autistic spectrum disorders. *Developmental Medicine and Child Neurology*, **36**, 441–8.

Derry, J. M. & Barnard, P. J. (1991). Mapping of the glycine receptor alpha 2-subunit gene and the GABAA alpha 3-subunit gene on the mouse X chromosome. *Genomics*, **10**, 593–7.

D'Eufemia, P., Finocchiaro, R., Celli, M., Viozzi, L., Monteleone, D. & Giardini, O. (1995). Low serum tryptophan to large neutral amino acids ratio in idiopathic infantile autism. *Biomedical Pharmacotherapeutics*, **49**, 288–92.

Deykin, E. Y. & MacMahon, B. (1979). The incidence of seizures among children with autistic symptoms. *American Journal of Psychiatry*, **126**, 1310–12.

Deykin, E. Y. & MacMahon, B. (1980). Pregnancy, delivery, and neonatal complications among autistic children. *American Journal of Diseased Children*, **134**, 860–4.

Eaves, R. C. & Milner, B. (1993). The criterion-related validity of the Childhood Autism Rating Scale and the Autism Behavior Checklist. *Journal of Abnormal Child Psychology*, **21**, 481–91.

Egaas, B., Courchesne, E. & Saitoh, O. (1995). Reduced size of corpus callosum in autism. *Archives of Neurology*, **52**, 794–801.

Einfeld, S., Moloney, H. & Hall, W. (1989). Autism is not associated with the fragile X syndrome. *American Journal of Medical Genetics*, **34**, 187–93.

Ekman, G., de Chateau, P., Marions, O., Sellden, H., Wahlund, L. O. & Wetterberg, L. (1991). Low field magnetic resonance imaging of the central nervous system in 15 children with autistic disorder. *Acta Paediatrica Scandinavica*, **80**, 243–7.

Elia, M., Musumeci, S. A., Ferri, R. & Bergonzi, P. (1995). Clinical and neurophysiological aspects of epilepsy in subjects with autism and mental retardation. *American Journal of Mental Retardation,* **100**, 6–16.

Erdmann, J., Shimron-Abarbanell, D., Cichon, S., Albus, M., Maier, W., Lichtermann, D., Minges, J., Reuner, U., Franzek, E., Ertl, M. A., Hebebrand, J., Remschmidt, H., Lehmkuhl, G., Poustka, F., Schmidt, M., Fimmers, R., Körner, J., Rietschel, M., Propping, P. & Nöthen, M. M. (1995). Systematic screening for mutations in the promoter and the coding region of the 5-HT1A gene. *American Journal of Medical Genetics,* **60**, 393–9.

Erwin, R., Van-Lancker, D., Guthrie, D., Schwafel, J., Tanguay, P. & Buchwald, J. S. (1991). P3 responses to prosodic stimuli in adult autistic subjects. *Electroencephalography and Clinical Neurophysiology,* **80**, 561–71.

Fahsold, R., Rott, H. D., Claussen, U. & Schmalenberger, B. (1991). Tuberous sclerosis in a child with de novo translocation t(3.,12) (p26. 3.,q23. 3). *Clinical Genetics,* **40**, 326–8.

Fernell, E., Gillberg, C. & von Wendt, L. (1991). Autistic symptoms in children with infantile hydrocephalus. *Acta Paediatrica Scandinavica,* **80**, 451–7.

Folstein, S. & Rutter, M. (1977). Infantile autism: a genetic study of 21 twin pairs. *Journal of Child Psychology and Psychiatry,* **18**, 297–321.

Fombonne, E. (1992). Diagnostic assessment in a sample of autistic and developmentally impaired adolescents. *Journal of Autism and Developmental Disorders,* **22**, 563–81.

Garnier, C., Comoy, E., Barthelemy, C., Leddet, I., Garreau, B., Muh, J. P. & Lelord, G. (1986). Dopamine-beta-hydroxylase (DBH) and homovanillic acid (HVA) in autistic children. *Journal of Autism and Developmental Disorders,* **16**, 23–9.

Garreau, B., Barthelemy, C., Jouve, J., Bruneau, N., Muh, J. P. & Lelord, G. (1988). Urinary homovanillic acid levels of autistic children. *Developmental Medicine and Child Neurology,* **30**, 93–8.

George, M. S., Costa, D. C., Kouris, K., Ring, H. A. & Ell, P. J. (1992). Cerebral blood flow abnormalities in adults with infantile autism. *Journal of Nervous and Mental Disease,* **180**, 413–17.

Gepner, B., Mestre, D., Masson, G. & de Schonen, S. (1995). Postural effects of motion vision in young autistic children. *Neuroreports,* **6**, 1211–14.

Ghaziuddin, M., Bolyard, B. & Alessi, N. (1994a). Autistic disorder in Noonan syndrome. *Journal of Intellectual Disability Research,* **38**, 67–72.

Ghaziuddin, M., Butler, E., Tsai, L. & Ghaziuddin, N. (1994b). Is clumsiness a marker for Asperger syndrome? *Journal of Intellectual Disability Research,* **38**, 519–27.

Ghaziuddin, M., Sheldon, S., Tsai, L. Y. & Alessi, N. (1993). Abnormalities of chromosome 18 in a girl with mental retardation and autistic disorder. *Journal of Intellectual Disability Research,* **37**, 313–17.

Ghaziuddin, M., Tsai, L. Y. & Ghaziuddin, N. (1992). Autism in Down's syndrome: presentation and diagnosis. *Journal of Intellectual Disability Research,* **36**, 449–56.

Gillberg, C. (1990). Do children with autism have March birthdays? *Acta Psychiatrica Scandinavica,* **82**, 152–6.

Gillberg, C. (1992). The Emanuel Miller Memorial Lecture 1991. Autism and autistic-like conditions. Subclasses among disorders of empathy. *Journal of Child Psychology and Psychiatry,* **33**, 813–42.

Gillberg, C. (1995). Endogenous opioids and opiate antagonists in autism: brief review of empirical findings and implications for clinicians. *Developmental Medicine and Child Neurology,* **37**, 239–45.

Gillberg, C. & Coleman, M. (1992). The Biology of the Autistic Syndromes. Oxford: Blackwell Scientific.

Gillberg, C. & Gillberg, I. C. (1983). Infantile autism: a total population study of reduced optimality in the pre-, peri-, and neonatal period. *Journal of Autism Developmental*

159

Disorders, **13**, 153–66.

Gillberg, I. C. (1991). Autistic syndrome with onset at age 31 years: herpes encephalitis as a possible model for childhood autism. *Developmental Medicine and Child Neurology*, **33**, 920–4.

Gillberg, I. C., Bjure, J., Uvebrant, P., Vestergren, E. & Gillberg, C. (1993). SPECT (single photon emission computed tomography) in 31 children and adolescents with autism and autism like conditions. *European Child and Adolescent Psychiatry*, **2**, 50–9.

Gillberg, I. C., Gillberg, C. & Ahlsen, G. (1994). Autistic behaviour and attention deficits in tuberous sclerosis: a population-based study. *Developmental Medicine and Child Neurology*, **36**, 50–6.

Gillberg, I. C., Gillberg, C. & Kopp, S. (1992). Hypothyroidism and autism spectrum disorders. *Journal of Child Psychology and Psychiatry*, **33**, 531–42.

Goa, J. H., Parsons, L. M., Bower, J. M., Xiong, J., Li, J. & Fox, P. T. (1996). Cerebellum implicated in sensory aquistion and discrimination rather than motor control. *Science*, **272**, 545–7.

Goodman, R. (1990). Technical note: are perinatal complications causes or consequences of autism? *Journal of Child Psychology and Psychiatry*, **31**, 809–12.

Goodman, R. & Minne, C. (1995). Questionnaire screening for comorbid pervasive developmental disorders in congenitally blind children: a pilot study. *Journal of Autism and Developmental Disorders*, **25**, 195–203.

Hallett, M., Lebiedowska, M. K., Thomas, S. L., Stanhope, S. J., Denckla, M. B. & Rumsey, J. (1993). Locomotion of autistic adults. *Archives Neurology*, **50**, 1304–8.

Hallmayer, J., Pintado, E., Lotspeich, L., Spiker, D., McMahon, W., Petersen, P. B., Nicholas, P., Pingree, C., Kraemer, H. C., Wong, D. L., Ritvo, E., Lin, A., Hebert, J., Cavalli-Sforza, L. L. & Ciaranello, R. D. (1994). Molecular analysis and test of linkage between the FMR-1 gene and infantile autism in multiplex families. *American Journal of Human Genetics*, **55**, 951–9.

Harris, S. R., MacKay, L. L. & Osborn, J. A. (1995). Autistic behaviors in offspring of mothers abusing alcohol and other drugs: a series of case reports. *Alcohol Clinics and Experimental Research*, **19**, 660–5.

Hashimoto, T., Murakawa, K., Miyazaki, M., Tayama, M. & Kuroda, Y. (1992a). Magnetic resonance imaging of the brain structures in the posterior fossa in retarded autistic children. *Acta Paediatrica*, **81**, 1030–4.

Hashimoto, T., Tayama, M., Miyazaki, M., Murakawa, K., Sakurama, N., Yoshimoto, T. & Kuroda, Y. (1991). Reduced midbrain and pons size in children with autism. *Tokushima Journal of Experimental Medicine*, **38**, 15–18.

Hashimoto, T., Tayama, M., Miyazaki, M., Murakawa, K., Shimakawa, S., Yoneda, Y. & Kuroda, Y. (1993). Brainstem involvement in high functioning autistic children. *Acta Neurologic Scandinavica*, **88**, 123–8.

Hashimoto, T., Tayama, M., Miyazaki, M., Sakurama, N., Yoshimoto, T., Murakawa, K. & Kuroda, Y. (1992b). Reduced brainstem size in children with autism. *Brain Development*, **14**, 94–7.

Hashimoto, T., Tayama, M., Murakawa, K., Yoshimoto, T., Miyazaki, M., Harada, M. & Kuroda, Y. (1995). Development of the brainstem and cerebellum in autistic patients. *Journal of Autism and Developmental Disorders*, **25**, 1–18.

Heath, M. J. S. & Hen, R. (1995). Genetic insights into serotonin function. *Current Biology*, **5**, 997–9.

Hebebrand, J., Martin, M., Korner, J., Roitzheim, B., de Braganca, K., Werner, W. & Remschmidt, H. (1994). Partial trisomy 16p in an adolescent with autistic disorder and Tourette's syndrome. *American Journal of Medical Genetics*, **54**, 268–70.

Holroyd, S., Reiss, A. L. & Bryan, R. N. (1993). Autistic features in Joubert syndrome: a genetic disorder with agenesis of the cerebellar vermis. *Biological Psychiatry*, **29**,

287–94.

Holttum, J. R., Minshew, N. J., Sanders, R. S. & Phillips, N. E. (1992). Magnetic resonance imaging of the posterior fossa in autism. *Biological Psychiatry*, **32**, 1091–101.

Hoon, A. H. Jr., & Reiss, A. L. (1992). The mesial-temporal lobe and autism: case report and review. *Developmental Medicine and Child Neurology*, **34**, 252–9.

Hotopf, M. & Bolton, P. (1995). A case of autism associated with partial tetrasomy 15. *Journal of Autism and Developmental Disorders*, **25**, 41–9.

Howlin, P., Wing, L. & Gould, J. (1995). The recognition of autism in children with Down's syndrome: implications for intervention and some speculations about pathology. *Developmental Medicine and Child Neurology*, **37**, 406–14.

Hsu, M., Yeung-Courchesne, R., Courchesne, E. & Press, G. A. (1991). Absence of magnetic resonance imaging evidence of pontine abnormality in infantile autism. *Archives of Neurology*, **48**, 1160–3.

Hunt, A. & Shepherd, C. (1993). A prevalence study of autism in tuberous sclerosis. *Journal of Autism and Developmental Disorders*, **23**, 323–39.

Jorde, L. B., Hasstedt, S. J., Ritvo, E. R., Mason Brothers, A., Freeman, B. J., Pingree, C., McMahon, W. M., Petersen, B., Jenson, W. A. & Mo, A. (1991). Complex segregation analysis of autism. *American Journal of Human Genetics*, **49**, 932–8.

Kemner, C., Verbaten, M. N., Cuperus, J. M., Camfferman, G. & van Engeland, H. (1995). Auditory event-related brain potentials in autistic children and three different control groups. *Biological Psychiatry*, **38**, 150–65.

Kemner, C., Verbaten, M. N., Cuperus, J. M., Camfferman, G. & Van Engeland, H. (1994). Visual and somatosensory event-related brain potentials in autistic children and three different control groups. *Electroencephalography and Clinical Neurophysiology*, **92**, 225–37.

Kemper, T. L. & Bauman, M. L. (1992). Neuropathology of infantile autism. In *Neurobiology of Infantile Autism*, ed. H. Naruse & E. M. Ornitz, pp. 43–57. Amsterdam: Elsevier Science Publisher.

Kerbeshian, J., Burd, L., Randall, T., Martsolf, J. & Jalal, S. (1990). Autism, profound mental retardation and atypical bipolar disorder in a 33-year-old female with a deletion of 15q12. *Journal of Mental Deficiency Research*, **34**, 205–10.

Klauck, S. M., Münstermann, E., Bieber-Martig, B., Rühl, D., Lisch, S., Schmötzer, S., Poustka, A. & Poustka, F. (1997). Molecular genetic analysis of the FMR-1 gene in a large collection of autistic patients. *Human Genetics*, **100**, 224–9.

Klauck, S. M., Poustka, F., Benner, A., Lesch, K. -P. & Poustka, A. (1997). Serotonin transporter (5-HTT) gene variants associated with autism. *Human Molecular Biology*, **13**, 2233–38.

Kleiman, M. D., Neff, S. & Rosman, N. P. (1992). The brain in infantile autism: are posterior fossa structures abnormal? *Neurology*, **42**, 753–60.

Klin, A. (1993). Auditory brainstem responses in autism: brainstem dysfunction or peripheral hearing loss? *Journal of Autism and Developmental Disorders*, **23**, 15–35.

Knobloch, H. & Pasamanick, B. (1975). Some etiologic and prognostic factors in early infantile autism and psychosis. *Pediatrics*, **55**, 182–91.

Kohen-Raz, R. (1991). Application of tetra-ataxiametric posturography in clinical and developmental diagnosis. *Perception and Motor Skills*, **73**, 635–56.

Kohen-Raz, R., Volkmar, F. R. & Cohen, D. J. (1992). Postural control in children with autism. *Journal of Autism and Developmental Disorders*, **22**, 419–32.

Kokubun, M., Haishi, K., Okuzumi, H. & Hosobuchi, T. (1995). Factors affecting age of walking by children with mental retardation. *Perception and Motor Skills*, **80**, 547–52.

Lappalainen, J., Zhang, L., Dean, M., Oz, M., Ozaki, N., Yu, D. H., Virkkunen, M., Weight, F., Linnoila, M. & Goldman, D. (1995). Identification, expression, and pharmacology of a Cys23-Ser23 substitution in the human 5-HT2C receptor gene (HTR2C). *Genomics*, **27**, 274–9.

Launay, J. M., Bursztejn, C., Ferrari, P., Dreux, C., Braconnier, A., Zarifian, E., Lancrenon, S. & Fermanian, J. (1987). Catecholamines metabolism in infantile autism: a controlled study of 22 autistic children. *Journal of Autism and Developmental Disorders*, **17**, 333–47.

Lekman, A., Skjeldal, O., Sponheim, E. & Svennerholm, L. (1995). Gangliosides in children with autism. *Acta Paediatrica*, **84**, 787–90.

Lensing, P., Klingler, D., Panksepp, J., Huber, M., Saria, A., Hackenberg, B. & Adam, H. (1992). Opiathypothese zur Genese des fruhkindlichen Autismus und Folgerungen zur Psychopharmakotherapie. [Opiate hypothesis of the origin of early childhood autism and sequelae for psychopharmacotherapy] *Z-Kinder-Jugenpsychiatr.*, **20**, 185–96.

Leventhal, B. L., Cook, E. H. Jr., Morford, M., Ravitz, A. & Freedman, D. X. (1990). Relationships of whole blood serotonin and plasma norepinephrine within families. *Journal of Autism and Developmental Disorders*, **20**, 499–511.

Levy, S., Zoltak, B. & Saelens, T. (1988). A comparison of obstetrical records of autistic and nonautistic referrals for psychoeducational evaluations. *Journal of Autism and Developmental Disorders*, **18**, 573–81.

Lincoln, A. J., Courchesne, E., Harms, L. & Allen, M. (1993). Contextual probability evaluation in autistic, receptive developmental language disorder, and control children: event-related brain potential evidence. *Journal of Autism and Developmental Disorders*, **23**, 37–58.

Lincoln, A. J., Courchesne, E., Harms, L. & Allen, M. (1995). Sensory modulation of auditory stimuli in children with autism and receptive developmental language disorder: event-related brain potential evidence. *Journal of Autism and Developmental Disorders*, **25**, 521–39.

Lisch, S., Rühl, D., Sacher, A., Schmötzer, G., Poustka, A. & Poustka, F. (1993). Beziehungen zwischen autistischem Syndrom und dem FraX-Syndrom. In *Biologische Psychiatrie der Gegenwart*, ed. P. Baumann, pp. 390–8. Wien: Springer.

Lobascher, M. E., Kingerlee, P. E. & Gubbay, S. S. (1970). Childhood autism: an investigation of aetiological factors in twenty five cases. *British Journal of Psychiatry*, **117**, 525–9.

Martineau, J., Barthelemy, C., Jouve, J., Muh, J. P. & Lelord, G. (1992a). Monoamines (serotonin and catecholamines) and their derivatives in infantile autism: age-related changes and drug effects. *Developmental Medicine and Child Neurology*, **34**, 593–603.

Martineau, J., Roux, S., Adrien, J. L., Garreau, B., Barthelemy, C. & Lelord, G. (1992b). Electrophysiological evidence of different abilities to form cross-modal associations in children with autistic behavior. *Electroencephalography and Clinical Neurophysiology*, **82**, 60–6.

Martineau, J., Roux, S., Garreau, B., Adrien, J. L. & Lelord, G. (1992c). Unimodal and crossmodal reactivity in autism: presence of auditory evoked responses and effect of the repetition of auditory stimuli. *Biological Psychiatry*, **31**, 1190–203.

McBride, P. A., Anderson, G. M., Hertzig, M. E. Sweeney, J. A., Kream, J., Cohen, D. J. & Mann, J. J. (1989). Serotonergic responsivity in male young adults with autistic disorder. Results of a pilot study. *Archives of General Psychiatry*, **46**, 213–321.

McDougle, C. J., Naylor, S. T., Cohen, D. J., Aghajanian, G. K., Heninger, G. R. & Price, L. H. (1996). Effects of tryptophan depletion in drug-free adults with autistic disorder. *Archives of General Psychiatry*, **53**, 993–1000.

McKelvey, J. R., Lambert, R., Mottron, L. & Shevell, M. I. (1995). Right-hemisphere dysfunction in Asperger's syndrome. *Journal of Child Neurology*, **10**, 310–14.

Miladi, N., Larnaout, A., Kaabachi, N., Helayem, M. & Ben-Hamida, M. (1992).

Phenylketonuria: an underlying etiology of autistic syndrome. A case report. *Journal of Child Neurology*, **7**, 22–3.

Miller, G. (1989). Minor congenital anomalies and ataxic cerebral palsy. *Archives of Disease in Childhood*, **64**, 557–62.

Minderaa, R. B., Anderson, G. M., Volkmar, F. R., Akkerhuis, G. W. & Cohen, D. J. (1987). Urinary 5-hydroxyindoleacetic acid and whole blood serotonin and tryptophan in autistic and normal subjects. *Biological Psychiatry*, **22**, 933–40.

Minderaa, R. B., Anderson, G. M., Volkmar, F. R., Akkerhuis, G. W. & Cohen, D. J. (1994). Noradrenergic and adrenergic functioning in autism. *Biological Psychiatry*, **36**, 237–41.

Minshew, N. J. (1991). Indices of neural function in autism: clinical and biological implications. *Pediatrics*, **31**, 774–80.

Minshew, N. J. & Dombrowski, S. M. (1994). In vivo neuroanatomy of autism: neuroimaging studies. In *The Neurobiology of Autism*, ed. M. L. Bauman & T. L. Kemper, pp. 66–85. Baltimore: The Johns Hopkins University Press.

Minshew, N. J., Goldstein, G., Dombrowski, S. M., Panchalingam, K. & Pettegrew, J. W. (1993). A preliminary 31P MRS study of autism: evidence for undersynthesis and increased degradation of brain membranes. *Biological Psychiatry*, **33**, 762–73.

Morrow, J. D., Whitman, B. Y. & Accardo, P. J. (1990). Autistic disorder in Sotos syndrome: a case report. *European Journal of Pediatrics*, **149**, 567–9.

Mountz, J. M., Tolbert, L. C., Lill, D. W., Katholi, C. R. & Liu, H. G. (1955). Functional deficits in autistic disorder: characterization by technetium-99m-HMPAO and SPECT. *Journal of Nuclear Medicine*, **36**, 1156–62.

Mouridsen, S. E., Nielsen, S., Rich, B. & Isager, T. (1994). Season of birth in infantile autism and other types of childhood psychoses. *Child Psychiatry and Human Development*, **25**, 31–43.

Myrianthopoulos, N. C. & Melnick, M. (1977). Malformations in monozycotic twins: a possible example of environmental influence on the developmental genetic clock. In *Gene Environment Interaction in Common Diseases*, ed. E. Inouye & H. Nishimura, pp. 206–20. Tokyo: University of Tokyo Press.

Naffah-Mazzacoratti, M. G., Rosenberg, R., Fernandes, M. J., Draque, C. M., Silvestrini, W., Calderazzo, L., Cavalheiro, E. A. (1993). Serum serotonin levels of normal and autistic children. *Brazilian Journal of Medical and Biological Research*, **26**, 309–17.

Nagamitsu, S. (1993). CSF beta-endorphin levels in pediatric neurologic disorders. *Kurume Medical Journal*, **40**, 233–41.

Narayan, M., Srinath, S., Anderson, G. M. & Meundi, D. B. (1993). Cerebrospinal fluid levels of homovanillic acid and 5-hydroxyindoleacetic acid in autism. *Biological Psychiatry*, **33**, 630–5.

Nelson, K. B. & Ellenberg, J. H. (1986). Antecedents of cerebral palsy: multivariate analysis of risk. *New England Journal of Medicine*, **315**, 81–6.

Nowell, M. A., Hackney, D. B., Muraki, A. S. & Coleman, M. (1990). Varied MR appearance of autism: fifty-three pediatric patients having the full autistic syndrome. *Magnetic Resonance Imaging*, **8**, 811–16.

Oades, R. D. & Eggers, C. (1993). Childhood autism: an appeal for an integrative and psychobiological approach. *European Child and Adolescent Psychiatry*, **3**, 159–75.

Oades, R. D., Stern, L. M., Walker, M. K., Clark, C. R. & Kapoor, V. (1990). Event-related potentials and monoamines in autistic children on a clinical trial of fenfluramine. *International Journal of Psychophysiology*, **8**, 197–212.

Oberlé, I., Rousseau, F., Heitz, D., Kretz, C., Devys, D., Hanauer, A., Boué, J., Bertheas, M. F. & Mandel, J. L. (1991). Instability of a 550-base pair DNA segment and abnormal methylation in fragile X syndrome. *Science*, **252**, 1097–102.

Olsson, B. & Rett, A. (1990). A review of the Rett syndrome with a theory of autism.

Fritz Poustka

Brain and Development, **12**, 11–15.

Ornitz, E. M. (1978). Biological Homogeneity or Heterogeneity. In *Autism: A Reapprais-al of Concepts and Treatments*, ed. M. Rutter & E. Schopler, pp. 243–50. New York: Plenum Press.

Perry, B. D., Cook, E. H. Jr., Leventhal, B. L., Wainwright, M. S. & Freedman, D. X. (1991). Platelet 5-HT2 serotonin receptor binding sites in autistic children and their first-degree relatives. *Biological Psychiatry*, **30**, 121–30.

Peterson, B. S. (1995). Neuroimaging in child and adolescent neuropsychiatric disorders. *Journal of the American Academy of Child and Adolescent Psychiatry*, **34**, 1560–76.

Piven, J., Arndt, S., Bailey, J., Havercamp, S., Andreasen, N. C. & Palmer, P. (1995). An MRI study of brain size in autism. *American Journal of Psychiatry*, **152**, 1145–9.

Piven, J., Berthier, M. L., Starkstein, S. E., Nehme, E., Pearlson, G. & Folstein, S. (1990). Magnetic resonance imaging evidence for a defect of cerebral cortical development in autism. *American Journal of Psychiatry*, **147**, 734–9.

Piven, J., Nehme, E., Simon, J., Barta, P., Pearlson, G. & Folstein, S. E. (1992). Magnetic resonance imaging in autism: measurement of the cerebellum, pons, and fourth ventricle. *Biological Psychiatry*, **31**, 491–504.

Piven, J., Tsai, G. C., Nehme, E., Coyle, J. T., Chase, G. A. & Folstein, S. E. (1991). Platelet serotonin, a possible marker for familial autism. *Journal of Autism and Developmental Disorders*, **21**, 51–9.

Poustka, F. & Lisch, L. (1993). Autistic behavior domains and their relation to self injury behavior. *Acta Paedopsychiatrica*, **56**, 69–73.

Prechtl, H. F. R. (1980). The optimality concept (editorial). *Early Human Development*, **4**, 201–5.

Rantakallio, P. & Von Wendt, L. (1985). Risk factors for mental retardation. *Archives of Disease in Childhood*, **60**, 946–52.

Rao, P. N., Klinepeter, K., Stewart, W., Hayworth, R., Grubs, R. & Pettenati, M. J. (1994). Molecular cytogenetic analysis of a duplication Xp in a male: further delineation of a possible sex influencing region on the X chromosome. *Human Genetics*, **94**, 149–53.

Raymond, G. V., Bauman, M. L. & Kemper, T. L. (1989a). Hippocampus in autism: Golgi analysis. *Annals of Neurology*, **26**, 483–4.

Raymond, G. V., Bauman, M. L. & Kemper, T. L. (1989b). Hippocampus in autism: a Golgi analysis. *Acta Neuropatholoque Berlin*, **91**, 117–19.

Realmuto, G. M., Jensen, J. B., Reeve, E. & Garfinkel, B. D. (1990). Growth hormone response to L-dopa and clonidine in autistic children. *Journal of Autism and Developmental Disorders*, **20**, 455–65.

Reiss, A. L., Aylward, E., Freund, L., Joshi, P. K. & Bryan, R. N. (1991). Neuroanatomy in fragile X syndrome: the posterior fossa. *Annals of Neurology*, **29**, 26–32.

Reiss, A. L., Patel, S., Kumar, A. J. & Freund, L. (1988). Preliminary communication: neuroanatomical variations of the posterior fossa in men with the fragile X (Martin Bell) syndrome. *American Journal of Medical Genetics*, **31**, 407–14.

Richdale, A. L. & Prior, M. R. (1992). Urinary cortisol circadian rhythm in a group of high-functioning children with autism. *Journal of Autism and Developmental Disorders*, **22**, 433–47.

Risch, N. (1990a). Linkage strategies for genetically complex traits. I. Multilocus models. *American Journal of Human Genetics*, **46**, 222–8.

Risch, N. (1990b). Linkage strategies for genetically complex traits. II. The power of affected relative pairs. *American Journal of Human Genetics*, **46**, 229–41.

Ritvo, E. R., Freeman, B. J., Scheibel, A. B., Duong, T., Robinson, H., Guthrie, D. & Ritvo, A. (1986). Lower Purkinje cell counts in the cerebella of four autistic subjects:

initial findings of the UCLA-NSAC autopsy research report. *American Journal of Psychiatry*, **143**, 862–6.

Ritvo, E. R., Ritvo, R., Yuwiler, A., Brothers, A., Freeman, B. J. & Plotkin, S. (1993). Elevated daytime melatonin concentrations in autism: a pilot study. *European Child and Adolescent Psychiatry*, **2**, 75–8.

Rolf, L. H., Haarmann, F. Y., Grotemeyer, K. H. & Kehrer, H. (1993). Serotonin and amino acid content in platelets of autistic children. *Acta Psychiatrica Scandinavica*, **87**, 312–16.

Root-Bernstein, R. S. & Westall, F. C. (1990). Serotonin binding sites. II. Muramyl dipeptide binds to serotonin binding sites on myelin basic protein, LHRH, and MSH-ACTH 4-10. *Brain Research Bulletin*, **25**, 827–41.

Rosengren, L. E., Ahlsen, G., Belfrage, M., Gillberg, C., Haglid, K. G. & Hamberger, A. (1992). A sensitive ELISA for glial fibrillary acidic protein: application in CSF of children. *Journal of Neuroscience Methods*, **44**, 113–19.

Rossi, P. G., Parmeggiani, A., Bach, V., Santucci, M. & Visconti, P. (1995). EEG features and epilepsy in patients with autism. *Brain and Development*, **17**, 169–74.

Rutter, M. (1984). Autistic children growing up. *Developmental Medicine and Child Neurology*, **26**, 122–9.

Rutter, M. (1988). Biological basis to autism: implications for intervention. In *Preventive and Curative Interventions in Mental Retardation*, ed. F. J. Menolascino & J. A. Stark, pp. 265–94. Baltimore: Brookes Publishing.

Rutter, M., Bailey, A., Bolton, P., Le Couteur, A. (1994). Autism and known medical conditions: myth and substance. *Journal of Child Psychology and Psychiatry*, **35**, 311–22.

Rutter, M. & Redshaw, J. (1991). Annotation: growing up as a twin: twin-singleton differences in psychological development. *Journal of Child Psychology and Psychiatry*, **32**, 885–95.

Saitoh, O., Courchesne, E., Egaas, B., Lincoln, A. J. & Schreibman, L. (1995). Cross sectional area of the posterior hippocampus in autistic patients with cerebellar and corpus callosum abnormalities. *Neurology*, **45**, 317–24.

Sameroff, A. J., Seifer, R. & Zax, M. (1982). Early development of children at risk for emotional disorder. *Monographs of the Society for Research in Child Development*, **47**, 1–82.

Schaefer, G. B., Thompson, J. N., Bodensteiner, J. B., McConnell, J. M., Kimberling, W. J., Gay, C. T., Dutton, W. D., Hutchings, D. C. & Gray, S. B. (1996). Hypoplasia of the cerebellar vermis in neurogenetic syndromes. *Annals of Neurology*, **39**, 382–5.

Schain, R. J. & Freedman, D. X. (1961). Studies on 5-hydroxyindole metabolism in autistic and mentally retarded children. *Journal of Pediatrics*, **58**, 315–20.

Schifter, T., Hoffman, J. M., Hatten, H. P. Jr., Hanson, M. W., Coleman, R. E. & DeLong, G. R. (1994). Neuroimaging in infantile autism. *Journal of Child Neurology*, **9**, 155–61.

Schinzel, A. (1990). Autistic disorder and additional inv dup(15)(pter---q13) chromosome. *American Journal of Medical Genetics*, **35**, 447–8.

Schmamann, J. D. (1991). An emerging concept. The cerebellar contribution to higher function. *Archives of Neurology*, **271**, 153–84.

Sersen, E. A., Heaney, G., Clausen, J., Belser, R. & Rainbow, S. (1990). Brainstem auditory-evoked responses with and without sedation in autism and Down's syndrome. *Biological Psychiatry*, **15**, 834–40.

Seshadri, K., Wallerstein, R. & Burack, G. (1992). 18q- chromosomal abnormality in a phenotypically normal 2 1/2-year-old male with autism. *Developmental Medicine and Child Neurology*, **34**, 1005–9.

Shaffer, L. G., McCaskill, C., Hersh, J. H., Greenberg, F. & Lupski, J. R. (1996). A clinical and molecular study of mosaicism for trisomy 17. *Human Genetics*, **97**, 69–72.

Shannon, M. & Graef, J. W. (1996). Lead intoxication in children with pervasive developmental disorders. *Journal of Toxicology and Clinical Toxicology*, **34**, 177–81.

Siegel, B. V. Jr., Asarnow, R., Tanguay, P., Call, J. D., Abel, L., Ho, A., Lott, I. & Buchsbaum, M. S. (1992). Regional cerebral glucose metabolism and attention in adults with a history of childhood autism. *Journal of Neuropsychiatry Clinical Neuroscience*, **4**, 406–14.

Siegel, B. V. Jr., Nuechterlein, K. H., Abel, L., Wu, J. C. & Buchsbaum, M. S. (1995). Glucose metabolic correlates of continuous performance test performance in adults with a history of infantile autism, schizophrenics, and controls. *Schizophrenia Research*, **17**, 85–94.

Singh, V. K., Warren, R. P., Odell, J. D. & Cole, P. (1993). Changes of soluble interleukin-2, interleukin-2 receptor, T8 antigen, and interleukin-1 in the serum of autistic children. *Clinical Immunology and Immunopathology*, **61**, 448–55.

Singh, V. K., Warren, R. P. & Singh, E. A. (1990). Binding of [3H]serotonin to lymphocytes in patients with neuropsychiatric disorders. *Molecular Chemistry and Neuropathology*, **13**, 167–73.

Smalley, S. L., Tanguay, P. E., Smith, M. & Gutierrez, G. (1992). Autism and tuberous sclerosis. *Journal of Autism and Developmental Disorders*, **22**, 339–55.

Steffenburg, S., Gillberg, C., Hellgren, L., Andersson, L., Gillberg, C., Jakobsson, G. & Bohman, M. (1989). A twin study of autism in Denmark, Finland, Iceland, Norway and Sweden. *Journal of Child Psychology and Psychiatry*, **30**, 405–16.

Steffenburg, S., Gillberg, C. & Steffenburg, U. (1996). Psychiatric disorders in children and adolescents with mental retardation and active epilepsy. *Archives of Neurology*, **53**, 904–12.

Stone, R. L., Aimi, J., Barshop, B. A., Jaeken, J., Van den Berghe, G., Zalkin, H. & Dixon, J. E. (1992). A mutation in adenylosuccinate lyase associated with mental retardation and autistic features. *Nature Genetics*, **1**, 59–63.

Strandburg, R. J., Marsh, J. T., Brown, W. S., Asarnow, R. F., Guthrie, D. & Higa, J. (1993). Event related potentials in high functioning adult autistics: linguistic and nonlinguistic visual information processing tasks. *Neuropsychologia*, **31**, 413–34.

Stromland, K., Nordin, V., Miller, M., Akerstrom, B. & Gillberg, C. (1994). Autism in thalidomide embryopathy: a population study. *Developmental Medicine and Child Neurology*, **36**, 351–6.

Stubbs, G. (1995). Interferonemia and autism. *Journal of Autism and Developmental Disorders*, **25**, 71–3.

Sverd, J. (1991). Tourette syndrome and autistic disorder: a significant relationship. *American Journal of Medical Genetics*, **39**, 173–9.

Szatmari, P. (1992). A review of the DSM-III-R criteria for autistic disorder. *Journal of Autism and Developmental Disorders*, **22**, 507–23.

Tantam, D., Evered, C. & Hersov, L. (1990). Asperger's syndrome and ligamentous laxity. *Journal of the American Academy of Child and Adolescent Psychiatry*, **29**, 892–6.

Thivierge, J., Bedard, C., Cote, R. & Maziade, M. (1990). Brainstem auditory evoked response and subcortical abnormalities in autism. *American Journal of Psychiatry*, **147**, 1609–13.

Todd, R. D., Hickok, J. M., Anderson, G. M. & Cohen, D. J. (1988). Antibrain antibodies in infantile autism. *Biological Psychiatry*, **23**, 644–7.

Tordjman, S., Anderson, G. M., McBride, P. A., Hertzig, M. E., Snow, M. E., Hall, L. M., Ferrari, P. & Cohen, D. J. (1995). Plasma androgens in autism. *Journal of Autism and*

Developmental Disorders, **25**, 295–304.

Tsai, L. Y. & Stewart, M. A. (1983). Etiological implication of maternal age and birth order in infantile autism. *Journal of Autism and Developmental Disorders*, **13**, 57–65.

Tsai, L. Y., Tsai, M. C. & August, G. J. (1985). Brief report: implication of EEG diagnoses in the subclassification of infantile autism. *Journal of Autism and Developmental Disorders*, **15**, 339–44.

Tuchman, R. F., Rapin, I. & Shinnar, S. (1991). Autistic and dysphasic children. II. Epilepsy. *Pediatrics*, **88**, 1219–25.

Tuchman, R. F., Rapin, I. & Shinnar, S. (1992). Autistic and dysphasic children. II. Epilepsy. (published erratum appears in *Pediatrics*, **90** (2 Pt 1): 264.

Venter, P. A., Op't Hof, J., Coetzee, D. J., Van der Walt, C. & Retief, A. E. (1984). No marker (X) syndrome in autistic children. *Human Genetics*, **67**, 107.

Verkerk, A. J. M. H., Pieretti, M., Sutcliffe, J. S., Fu, Y. -H., Kuhl, D. P. A., Pizzuti, A., Reiner, O., Richards, S., Victoria, M. F., Zhang, F., Eussen, B. E., van Ommen, G. J. B., Blonden, L. A. J., Riggins, G. J., Chastain, J. L., Kunst, C. B., Galjaard, H., Caskey, C. T., Nelson, D. L., Oostra, B. A. & Warren, S. T. (1991). Identification of a gene (*FMR*-1) containing a CGG repeat coincident with a breakpoint cluster region exhibiting length variation in fragile X syndrome. *Cell*, **65**, 905–14.

Volkmar, F. R., Cicchetti, D. V., Bregman, J. & Cohen, D. J. (1992). Three diagnostic systems for autism: DSM-III, DSM-III-R, and ICD-10. *Journal of Autism and Developmental Disorders*, **22**, 483–92.

Volkmar, F. R. & Cohen, D. J. (1988). Diagnosis of pervasive developmental disorders. In *Advances in Clinical Child Psychology*, ed. B. Lahey & A. Kazdin, pp. 249–84. New York: Plenum Press.

Volkmar, F. R., Klin, A., Siegel, B., Szatmari, P., Lord, C., Campbell, M., Freeman, B. J., Cicchetti, D., Rutter, M. & Members of the DSM-IV Autism/PDD Field Trial Group: DSM-IV Autism/Pervasive Developmental Disorders Field Trial. (1994). *American Journal of Psychiatry*, **151**, 1361–7.

Volkmar, F. R. & Nelson, D. S. (1990). Seizure disorders in autism. *Journal of the American Academy of Child and Adolescent Psychiatry*, **29**, 127–9.

Warren, R. P., Burger, R. A., Odell, D., Torres, A. R. & Warren, W. L. (1994). Decreased plasma concentrations of the C4B complement protein in autism. *Archives of Pediatric and Adolescent Medicine*, **148**, 180–3.

Warren, R. P., Singh, V. K., Cole, P., Odell, J. D., Pingree, C. B., Warren, W. L. & White, E. (1991). Increased frequency of the null allele at the complement C4b locus in autism. *Clinical and Experimental Immunology*, **83**, 438–40.

Warren, R. P., Yonk, J., Burger, R. W., Odell, D. & Warren, W. L. (1995). DR-positive T cells in autism: association with decreased plasma levels of the complement C4B protein. *Neuropsychobiology*, **31**, 53–7.

Watson, M. S., Leckman, J. F., Annex, B., Breg, W. R., Boles, D., Volkmar, F. R. & Cohen, D. J. (1984). Fragile X in a survey of 75 autistic males. *New England Journal of Medicine*, **310**, 1462.

Willemsen-Swinkels, S. H., Buitelaar, J. K., Nijhof, G. J. & van England, H. (1995). Failure of naltrexone hydrochloride to reduce self-injurious and autistic behavior in mentally retarded adults. Double-blind placebo-controlled studies. *Archives of General Psychiatry*, **52**, 766–73.

Williams, R. S., Hauser, S. L., Purpura, D. P., Delong, G. R. & Swisher, C. W. (1980). Autism and mental retardation. *Archives of Neurology*, **37**, 749–53.

Wolman, S. R., Campbell, M., Marchi, M. L., Deutsch, S. I. & Gershon, T. D. (1990). Dermatoglyphic study in autistic children and controls. *Journal of the American Academy of Child and Adolescent Psychiatry*, **29**, 878–84.

Wong, V. (1993). Epilepsy in children with autistic spectrum disorder. *Journal of Child Neurology*, **8**, 316–22.

Wong, V. & Wong, S. N. (1991). Brainstem auditory evoked potential study in children with autistic disorder. *Journal of Autism and Developmental Disorders*, **21**, 329–40.

Yu, S., Pritchard, M., Kremer, E., Lynch, M., Nancarrow, J., Baker, E., Holman, K., Mulley, J. C., Warren, S. T., Schlessinger, D., Sutherland, G. R. & Richards, R. I. (1991). Fragile X genotype characterized by an unstable region of DNA. *Science*, **252**, 1179–81.

Yuwiler, A., Shih, J. C., Chen, C. H., Ritvo, E. R., Hanna, G., Ellison, G. W. & King, B. H. (1992). Hyperserotoninemia and antiserotonin antibodies in autism and other disorders. *Journal of Autism and Developmental Disorders*, **22**, 33–45.

Zilbovicius, M., Garreau, B., Samson, Y., Remy, P., Barthelemy, C., Syrota, A. & Lelord, G. (1995). Delayed maturation of the frontal cortex in childhood autism. *American Journal of Psychiatry*, **152**, 248–52.

Zilbovicius, M., Garreau, B., Tzourio, N., Mazoyer, B., Bruck, B., Martinot, J. L., Raynaud, C., Samson, Y., Syrota, A. & Lelord, G. (1992). Regional cerebral blood flow in childhood autism: a SPECT study. *American Journal of Psychiatry*, **149**, 924–30.

Fritz Poustka

6

Psychopharmacology

Christopher J. McDougle

INTRODUCTION

While research over the past 35 years has shown the aetiology of autism to be multifactorial (Ciaranello & Ciaranello, 1995), direct and indirect lines of evidence suggest that certain neurochemical systems are of particular relevance to the pathophysiology of autism (Cook, 1990). The use of drugs targeted toward these specific neural systems can often reduce aggression, self-injury and interfering repetitive behaviour, as well as improving some aspects of social relatedness in children, adolescents and adults with the autistic syndrome. Combined with a comprehensive individualized treatment programme, appropriate pharmacotherapy can enhance the autistic person's ability to benefit from educational and behaviour modification interventions (McDougle et al., 1994). This chapter reviews psychopharmacology research in pervasive developmental disorder(s) (PDD(s)) from the perspective of specific neurochemical systems. When relevant, differences in drug treatment response between the *Diagnostic and Statistical Manual of Mental Disorders*, Fourth Edition (DSM-IV) (American Psychiatric Association, 1994) subtypes of PDD, including autistic disorder, Rett's syndrome, childhood disintegrative disorder, Asperger's syndrome and PDD not otherwise specified (NOS), will be highlighted.

Christopher J. McDougle

DRUGS AFFECTING SEROTONIN FUNCTION

While little is definitively known regarding the pathophysiology of the syndrome of autism, abnormalities in the serotonin (5-hydroxytryptamine (5-HT)) neurotransmitter system have been identified in a subset of patients. Schain and Freedman first reported elevated levels of whole blood 5-HT in the peripheral vascular system of autistic children in 1961 (Schain & Freedman, 1961). Others have replicated this finding in groups of autistic children compared with normal controls (Anderson et al., 1987). Antibodies against human brain 5-HT receptors were identified in the blood and cerebrospinal fluid (CSF) of a child with autism (Todd & Ciaranello, 1985), although subsequent studies found no difference in the degree of immunoglobulin inhibition of binding of the 5-HT1A agonist [^{3}H]-8-hydroxy-N,N-dipropyl-2-aminotetralin(DPAT) to 5-HT1A receptors between autistic patients and controls (Yuwiler et al., 1992; Cook et al., 1993). Blunted neuroendocrine responses to pharmacological probes of the 5-HT system have been observed in autistic children (Hoshino et al., 1984) and adults (McBride et al., 1989) compared with normal subjects. Finally, acute dietary depletion of the 5-HT precursor tryptophan has been associated with an exacerbation of behavioural symptoms in drug-free autistic adults (McDougle et al., 1996a). Based upon evidence implicating a dysregulation in 5-HT function in some patients with autism, drugs which affect this system have been studied.

Fenfluramine

Fenfluramine is an indirect 5-HT receptor agonist which releases 5-HT presynaptically and blocks its reuptake from 5-HT neurons. Although fenfluramine increases 5-HT neurotransmission acutely, ongoing administration results in a reduction in brain 5-HT.

Enthusiasm for the drug as a potential treatment for autism was generated following a report in 1982 describing its effects in three hyperserotonaemic autistic boys (Geller et al., 1982). To follow up these preliminary findings, a large multicentre single-blind study of fenfluramine was conducted at 18 sites. Following a 2 week open placebo baseline period, patients received 4 additional weeks of placebo, 16 weeks of fenfluramine (1.5 mg/kg in two divided doses) and 8 weeks of placebo. Ritvo et al. (1983) published a report describing their centre's experience with 14 autistic patients in this study. A significant decrease in abnormal motor

170

movements was found and improvement was seen on scales measuring social and sensory function. No adverse reactions or clinically significant side effects were reported.

In a subsequent report, results from nine of the participating centres were described (Ritvo et al., 1986). Data from 64 boys and 17 girls with autism, ranging in age from 33 months to 24 years (mean age 8.8 years) were presented. The mean values of the overall motor, social and sensory scales of the Ritvo–Freeman Real-Life Rating Scale (Freeman et al., 1986) showed significant improvement with fenfluramine. Mean changes on the affect and language scales did not reach significance. IQ testing showed slight but statistically significant increases during drug treatment. On categorical measures of patient response, 27 (33%) were 'strong responders', 42 (52%) were 'moderate responders' and 12 (15%) were 'nonresponders'. Lethargy and irritability were the most frequently reported side effects.

In contrast, more recent controlled studies of fenfluramine in autism have not been as encouraging. Employing a double blind, placebo controlled parallel groups design, Campbell et al. (1988b) studied the effects of fenfluramine on the core symptoms of autism and discrimination learning. The sample included 28 hospitalized children with autism (22 boys, six girls, mean age 4.6 years), whose intelligence ranged from severely mentally retarded to dull normal. Following a 2 week placebo baseline period, patients were randomly assigned to fenfluramine (mean dose 1.7 mg/kg per day; maximum dose 50 mg/day) or placebo for 8 weeks. Fenfluramine was associated with a significant decrease in fidgetiness and withdrawal, although no difference between fenfluramine and placebo was found for ratings of stereotypy or the core symptoms of autism. Furthermore, fenfluramine had a retarding effect on discrimination learning. The most common side effects were weight loss, excessive sedation, loose stools and irritability. Additional double blind, placebo controlled crossover studies of fenfluramine for 4 weeks (15 autistic children) (Sherman et al., 1989), 5–12 weeks (11 children with autism) (Duker et al., 1991), and 16 weeks (20 children with autism) (Ekman et al., 1989) failed to show significant drug–placebo differences.

Fenfluramine has been shown to lead to significant reductions in brain 5-HT content and to produce potentially irreversible changes in 5-HT neurons in certain regions of the brain in rats, guinea pigs and rhesus monkeys (Schuster et al., 1986). In addition, Leventhal et al. (1993) found that plasma norepinephrine (noradrenaline) levels were decreased as long as 8 weeks after fenfluramine treatment in autistic children. Based on the potential risk of long term, possibly irreversible changes in 5-HT and possibly catecholaminergic neurons, together with controlled studies demonstrating that fenfluramine is no better than placebo in reducing the core symptoms of autism, this drug cannot be recommended as a routine treatment for most patients with autistic disorder (Campbell, 1988).

Buspirone

Buspirone is a 5-HT1A receptor partial agonist which has been shown in preclinical studies to increase 5-HT function with chronic administration (Blier et al., 1990). It is marketed in the USA for the treatment of generalized anxiety disorder. A 4 week open label study of buspirone was conducted in four autistic children (three boys, one girl), aged 9–10 years, in doses of 15 mg/day (Realmuto et al., 1989). Two children showed a reduction in hyperactivity, one a reduction in stereotypic behaviour and the fourth showed no significant change. No adverse effects were observed.

In an open label study of buspirone in 14 developmentally disabled, self-injurious adults (three with autism) (age range 23–63 years), nine showed some improvement with the drug (Ratey et al., 1989). The dose of buspirone ranged from 15 to 45 mg/day, and of the nine responders, seven were on concomitant psychoactive medication. The authors stated that the effect of buspirone allowed for the reduction or discontinuation of neuroleptics and facilitated a more adaptive existence for many of the patients. No controlled studies of buspirone in patients with PDD have been published.

Clomipramine

Clomipramine is a nonselective tricyclic agent that has been shown in double blind, placebo controlled trials to be efficacious in the treatment of depression and obsessive–compulsive disorder (OCD) (Greist et al., 1995a). Although clomipramine affects norepinephrine and dopamine neuronal uptake, its most potent action is to inhibit 5-HT uptake.

Reports have described the potential usefulness of clomipramine in the treatment of children and adults with autistic disorder. In the first published controlled study of clomipramine in autism, Gordon et al. (1993) found clomipramine (152 ± 56 mg/day) to be superior to the relatively selective norepinephrine uptake inhibitor desipramine (127 ± 52 mg/day) and placebo in a 10 week (5 weeks on each drug or placebo), randomized, crossover study in children with autism (mean age 9.6 years). In the comparison of clomipramine with placebo, significant improvement was found in the core symptoms of autism: anger/uncooperativeness, hyperactivity and obsessive–compulsive symptoms. When clomipramine was compared with desipramine, significant changes in the core symptoms of autism: anger/uncooperativeness and obsessive–compulsive symptoms, were also observed. There was no significant difference between the two drugs in the treatment of hyperactivity. Adverse effects from clomipramine included prolongation of the corrected QT interval, tachycardia and grand mal seizure, whereas irritability, temper outbursts and uncharacteristic aggression were seen with desipramine.

The Yale group found that four of five young adults with a DSM-III-R (American Psychiatric Association, 1987) diagnosis of autism presenting with disturbances in social relatedness, repetitive thoughts and behaviour, and/or impulsive aggression had a significant improvement in symptomatology with open label clomipramine treatment (McDougle et al., 1992). The fifth patient remained unchanged. Up to 12 weeks of treatment with clomipramine was necessary in some cases before appreciable change occurred. The dose of clomipramine in the four responders ranged from 75 to 250 mg/day, with a mean dose of 185 mg/day. Other than dry mouth in two cases, the patients tolerated the drug well and had no adverse effects.

We recently completed the first systematic study of clomipramine in adults with PDDs, including autism (Brodkin et al., 1997). Thirty-five subjects, 24 men and 11 women, who met DSM-IV criteria for PDD (autistic disorder $n = 15$, Asperger's syndrome $n = 8$, PDD-NOS $n = 12$) entered a 12 week open label trial of clomipramine. The mean age of the group was 30.2 years (range 18–44 years). Of the 33 patients who completed the 12 week trial, 18 (55%) were responders based on the Clinical Global Impression (CGI) Scale (Guy, 1976) scores of 'much' or 'very much improved'. Improvement was seen in repetitive thoughts and behaviour, aggression and social relatedness. The mean dose of clomipramine for the group was 139.4 ± 50.4 mg/day. Some variability in symptom presentation between patients with different diagnostic subtypes of PDD was identified in the study. Those patients with Asperger's syndrome had a higher mean total Yale–Brown Obsessive Compulsive Scale (Y-BOCS) (Goodman et al., 1989a,b) score, a higher mean Y-BOCS obsession subscale score and fewer symptoms of language impairment (as measured by subscale V of the Ritvo–Freeman Scale) compared with patients with autistic disorder and PDD-NOS. These findings may reflect the Asperger's syndrome patients' relatively preserved language development and superior capability of reporting repetitive thoughts. As measured by the Ritvo–Freeman subscale II (Social Relationship to People), patients with Asperger's syndrome were less impaired than those with autistic disorder and PDD-NOS. There were no significant differences among the three diagnostic subtypes in the pattern of symptomatic change or in global treatment response to clomipramine. Two patients had grand mal seizures and one had an exacerbation of absence seizures. No adverse cardiac events occurred. These preliminary data suggest that clomipramine may be effective in reducing interfering behaviours in many adults with PDDs, but that careful monitoring for the induction or exacerbation of seizures is necessary.

Fluvoxamine

Fluvoxamine is a potent and selective 5-HT uptake inhibitor that has little or no affinity for 5-HT, dopamine, adrenergic, histaminic or muscarinic receptors, and no known clinically active metabolites (Benfield & Ward, 1986). Its in vitro potency for blocking 5-HT uptake is equivalent to that of clomipramine, and it causes minimal inhibition of dopamine or norepinephrine uptake. Fluvoxamine has been shown to be effective in the treatment of OCD (Goodman et al., 1989c). Importantly, a recent controlled study found fluvoxamine more effective than placebo in the treatment of social phobia (van Vliet et al., 1994), a disorder that may occur more frequently in first degree relatives of autistic probands than in relatives of control probands (Smalley et al., 1995).

In the first report to describe the use of a 5-HT uptake inhibitor in autistic disorder, McDougle et al. (1990) found fluvoxamine to be effective in the treatment of a 30 year old man with autism and comorbid OCD. Subsequently, they completed the first double blind, placebo controlled investigation of fluvoxamine in patients with autistic disorder (McDougle et al., 1996b). The sample consisted of 27 men and three women, aged 18–53 years (mean age 30.1 years) with a diagnosis of autistic disorder based on DSM-III-R criteria. One male patient had fragile X syndrome, whereas none of the other patients had a diagnosed genetic, metabolic or neurological aetiology for their syndrome.

After baseline behavioural ratings were obtained, patients were randomized to 12 weeks of double blind treatment with fluvoxamine or placebo. The drug was started at 50 mg every night and the dosage was then increased by 50 mg daily every 3 or 4 days to a maximum dosage of 300 mg/day. Thus, the maximum dosage of fluvoxamine was attained within 3 weeks and patients received this dose for a minimum of 9 weeks.

Behavioural ratings were obtained every 4 weeks throughout the 12 week study and included the Y-BOCS, the Brown Aggression Scale (Brown et al., 1979), the Ritvo–Freeman Real-Life Rating Scale and the Vineland Adaptive Behaviour Scale (Sparrow et al., 1984) Maladaptive Behaviour Subscales (Part 1 and Part 2). Finally, the CGI global improvement item (7 = 'very much worse' to 1 = 'very much improved') was recorded at each rating session following the baseline period. Treatment response was determined by scores obtained at the end of the last week of the study on the CGI. Patients with CGI scores of 'much improved' or 'very much improved' were categorized as responders.

There was no significant difference in dosage between patients randomized to fluvoxamine (276.7 $\pm$ 41.7 mg/day) versus placebo (283.3 $\pm$ 36.2 mg/day). The fluvoxamine group (age 30.1 $\pm$ 7.1 years) contained two women and 13 men, whereas the placebo group (age 30.1 $\pm$ 8.4 years) consisted of one woman and 14 men. There were no significant differences in age, gender distribution or full scale IQ scores between the two groups.

Ratings on the CGI showed fluvoxamine superior to placebo beginning at week 4 and continuing at weeks 8 and 12. Eight of 15 (53%) of the fluvoxamine patients were categorized as responders compared with 0 of 15 in the placebo group. Treatment response was not correlated with age or full scale IQ. As measured by reduction in total Y-BOCS scores, fluvoxamine was superior to placebo in the treatment of repetitive thoughts and behaviour beginning at week 8 and continuing at week 12 of treatment. On the Brown Aggression Scale and the Vineland Maladaptive Behaviour Subscales, fluvoxamine was more effective than placebo beginning at week 4 and continuing through weeks 8 and 12. Fluvoxamine was superior to placebo in improving the behavioural symptoms of autistic disorder as measured by the Ritvo–Freeman Scale overall score. In particular, fluvoxamine was superior to placebo in improving language usage (subscale V) beginning at week 4 and continuing at weeks 8 and 12.

Fluvoxamine was well tolerated, with no medically significant adverse events. Four patients reported nausea (three on active drug, one on placebo) during the first 2 weeks, but they developed tolerance and were able to continue. Three different patients developed moderate sedation (two on active drug, one on placebo), which also resolved. No anticholinergic side effects developed and no significant changes in pulse or sitting and standing blood pressure occurred. No laboratory or electrocardiographic changes could be attributed to fluvoxamine. No dyskinesias, adverse cardiovascular events or seizures occurred.

Fluoxetine

Fluoxetine is a potent and selective 5-HT uptake inhibitor that has been shown in double blind, placebo controlled investigations to be effective in the treatment of depression and OCD (Tollefson et al., 1994). Preliminary open label studies and case reports suggest that fluoxetine may be useful in the treatment of some patients with autistic disorder (Mehlinger et al., 1990; Ghaziuddin et al., 1991; Hamdan-Allen, 1991; Todd, 1991; Cook et al., 1992).

Mehlinger et al. (1990) reported that fluoxetine 20 mg every other day was useful in reducing ritualistic behaviour and in improving mood in a 26 year old autistic women. Hamdan-Allen (1991) described marked improvement in trichotillomania in an 18 year old man with autism who had been resistant to a 6 month trial of imipramine at therapeutic blood levels. Todd (1991) reported that three of four patients with autism showed a significant reduction in ritualistic behaviour or increased tolerance of changes in routine with fluoxetine treatment. Ghaziuddin et al. (1991) found fluoxetine 20–40 mg/day effective in reducing depressive symptoms in adolescents with autistic disorder, although many of the core features of autism remained unchanged.

In a larger open label case series, Cook et al. (1992) found that fluoxetine in doses ranging from 20 mg every other day to 80 mg/day led to significant improvement in subjects with autistic disorder (mean age 15.9 years) and in subjects with mental retardation without autism (mean age 21 years). Subjects had been treated with fluoxetine for approximately 6 months at the time of rating. In subjects with autistic disorder, fluoxetine led to an improvement in CGI severity scale scores in 15 of 23 subjects. Ten of 16 mentally retarded subjects had an improvement of one point or more on CGI overall severity ratings including improvement in impulse control, attention span and ability to tolerate frustration. Six of 23 subjects with autism and three of 16 subjects with mental retardation had side effects which consisted primarily of restlessness, hyperactivity, agitation, decreased appetite and insomnia.

Sertraline

Sertraline is a potent and selective 5-HT uptake inhibitor that has been shown in double blind, placebo controlled studies to be effective in the treatment of depression and OCD (Greist et al., 1995a). Preliminary results from our group suggest that sertraline may be useful for improving aggression and repetitive behaviour in some adults with PDDs, including autism (McDougle et al., 1998). In an open label study, 24 of 42 (57%) adults were rated as 'much' or 'very much improved' on the global improvement item of the CGI following 12 weeks of treatment with sertraline (50–200 mg/day). Five patients ended the trial prematurely due to the emergence of interfering anxiety ($n = 3$), syncope ($n = 1$) and noncompliance ($n = 1$), respectively. No other significant side effects or adverse reactions occurred.

In summary, while further controlled research is necessary to determine if potent 5-HT uptake inhibitors and other drugs affecting 5-HT function have efficacy for improving the interfering behavioural symptoms of autism, the data reviewed above suggest that this line of approach warrants further investigation. In support of this, indirect evidence from related areas of preclinical and clinical research supports a role for central 5-HT in the neuromodulation of many of the clinical characteristics of autism, including aggression, social dysfunction, and repetitive thoughts and behaviour. For example, CSF levels of 5-hydroxyindoleacetic acid (5-HIAA) are reduced in children with conduct and other aggressive behavioural disorders (Kruesi et al., 1990, 1992). Fluvoxamine (McDougle et al., 1996b), fluoxetine (Markowitz, 1992), sertraline (Kelley et al., 1993) and paroxetine (Snead et al., 1994), as well as clomipramine (Garber et al., 1992), all of which increase synaptic 5-HT in the brain, have been reported to reduce aggression and self-injurious behaviour in patients with autism and other developmental disabilities.

Many consider the core disturbance in autistic disorder to be impaired reciprocal verbal and nonverbal social interaction (Volkmar, 1987). Central 5-HT has been found to contribute to the regulation of social behaviour and social hierarchies in animals. For example, the tryptophan hydroxylase enzyme inhibitor *p*-chlorophenylalanine (PCPA) resulted in decreased grooming, approaching, resting and eating behaviour, and increased locomotion, being solitary, being vigilant and avoiding when administered to vervet monkeys; fluoxetine, tryptophan and the 5-HT receptor agonist quipazine had the opposite effect (Raleigh et al., 1980). The autistic patients' improvement with 5-HT uptake inhibitors suggests that enhancement of central 5-HT function may be important for facilitating certain aspects of social interaction in some patients.

Brain 5-HT has also been hypothesized to be involved in modulating repetitive thoughts and behaviour. Although the types, frequency and quality of repetitive thoughts and behaviour of age and sex matched adults with OCD and autistic disorder have been shown to be different

177

(McDougle et al., 1995b), these interfering symptoms often improve with 5-HT uptake inhibitor treatment in both diagnostic groups (McDougle et al., 1996b; Goodman et al., 1989c).

DRUGS AFFECTING DOPAMINE FUNCTION

Evidence from clinical neurobiological studies and drug treatment response data suggest that dopamine function may be increased in some patients with autistic disorder. Gillberg et al. (1983) found that mean basal CSF concentrations of homovanillic acid (HVA), the primary metabolite of brain dopamine, were elevated in 13 medication free autistic children compared with matched controls. In addition, the indirect dopamine receptor agonist amphetamine has been shown to exacerbate stereotypic motor symptoms and hyperactivity in some autistic children, whereas controlled studies of dopamine receptor antagonists have found these drugs to be effective in improving some of the behavioural symptoms associated with autistic disorder.

Haloperidol

The dopamine receptor antagonist haloperidol has been extensively studied in controlled clinical trials in children with autistic disorder. Campbell et al. (1978) completed a 12 week, double blind, placebo controlled study of haloperidol in 40 hospitalized autistic children (32 boys and eight girls, mean age 4.5 years). Patients were randomly assigned to one of four treatment groups based upon drug (haloperidol versus placebo) and level of concomitant language training (response-contingent reinforcement versus response-independent (placebo) reinforcement). Following a 2 week drug free period, haloperidol 0.5 mg or placebo was given in identical appearing tablets. Dosage was increased twice weekly during the first 3 weeks to a maximum of 4 mg/day (mean optimal dose 1.65 mg/day) depending upon therapeutic response or the development of untoward side effects. Haloperidol was found to be superior to placebo in reducing stereotypies and withdrawal, particularly for children above 4.5 years of age. In addition, the combination of haloperidol and behavioural language training was more effective than haloperidol or behavioural therapy alone in facilitating the imitation of new words in training sessions. Twelve children experienced dose dependent sedation and two had acute dystonic reactions.

In an attempt to replicate the findings of the first study, Cohen et al. (1980) conducted a double blind, placebo controlled within subjects reversal (A-B-A-B) design study of haloperidol. Ten hospitalized autistic children (six girls and four boys, mean age 4.7 years), who were mildly to profoundly retarded completed the study. Following a 2 week placebo period, patients were randomly assigned to alternating treatment periods of haloperidol or placebo at 2 week intervals. The mean optimal dose of haloperidol was 1.65 mg/day during the initial administration period and 1.90 mg/day upon repeat administration. Eight of ten children experienced excessive sedation during haloperidol treatment and one had two episodes of acute dystonia relieved by diphenhydramine 25 mg intramuscularly. Haloperidol was effective in reducing stereotypies and in helping the children to orient attention to a rater's requests. As in the initial study, the older children responded better to haloperidol than the younger patients.

Anderson et al. (1984) conducted a 12 week follow up study to determine if learning was facilitated because haloperidol reduced stereotypies and withdrawal, or because of a direct effect on attentional mechanisms. Following a 2 week placebo period, 40 autistic children (29 boys, 11 girls, mean age 4.6 years), entered a double blind crossover study of haloperidol versus placebo. The maximum dose of haloperidol was 4.0 mg/day and the optimal dose was 1.1 mg/day. The most frequent side effects were excessive sedation and increased irritability, although these were reported to occur only during dosage adjustment or above optimal doses. Acute dystonic reactions occurred in 11 children. Haloperidol led to a significant decrease in symptoms of withdrawal, stereotypies, hyperactivity, abnormal object relations, fidgetiness, negativism, angry affect and lability of mood. Furthermore, haloperidol produced greater facilitation and retention of discrimination learning in a structured laboratory setting. These findings led the authors to suggest that the effect of haloperidol on learning was not a function of its decreasing maladaptive behaviours but rather a direct effect on attentional mechanisms.

As longer term administration of medication is often needed in moderately to severely affected autistic children, Perry et al. (1989) studied the effects of haloperidol given for 6 months in a large group of children with autism. Sixty children with autistic disorder (48 boys, 12 girls, mean age 5.1 years), who had previously shown clinically significant improvement on haloperidol, completed the study as outpatients. The children were randomly assigned to two groups: group I received haloperidol on a continuous basis and group II on a discontinuous schedule consisting of 5 days of haloperidol alternating with 2 days of placebo. Following the 6 month treatment period, both groups were placed on placebo for 4 weeks. Haloperidol doses ranged from 0.5 to 4.0 mg/day (mean optimal dose 1.23 mg/day). At these doses, sedation and parkinsonian side effects were not observed. Twelve children developed haloperidol related dyskinesias, three during haloperidol administration and nine upon discontinuation. Long term haloperidol administration was found to be effective in reducing maladaptive symptoms in these autistic children. Improvement was seen in 71.5% of children, 20% showed no improvement and 8.5% were rated as worse. The discontinuous drug administration did not reduce the efficacy of haloperidol and there was no difference in side effects between children who received continuous versus discontinuous treatment. Fifty-nine per cent of the children had a significant return of symptoms during the 4 week placebo period.

In an attempt to more carefully define the occurrence of drug related dyskinesias in this patient group, Campbell et al. (1988a) conducted a prospective study of 82 autistic children whose ages ranged from 2.3 to 8.2 years at the time of entry into the study. Patients received haloperidol 0.25–10.5 mg/day (mean 0.054 mg/kg per day) for 0.8–78.5 months (mean 18.1 months). Twenty-four of the 82 children developed dyskinesias, 21% during haloperidol administration and 79% during drug withdrawal. The dyskinesias tended to occur in the orofacial muscles, the tongue and the upper extremities, and females showed a trend toward greater risk. While all of the dyskinesias were reversible, the time course for this to occur varied from 7 days to 7.5 months.

Pimozide

Like haloperidol, pimozide is a dopamine receptor antagonist which has received attention as a potential treatment for autistic disorder. In a multicentre investigation, Naruse et al. (1982) conducted a double blind crossover study of pimozide, haloperidol and placebo in children with behaviour disorders. The patients ranged in age from 3 to 16 years and included 34 autistic children. The doses of pimozide ranged from 1 to 9 mg/day. A significant reduction occurred in some types of aggression, including 'injury and violence to others' and 'breaking furniture', although self-mutilation was not significantly improved.

In an open label pilot study, Ernst et al. (1992) found pimozide in doses of 3–6 mg/day (mean 4.9 mg/day) to be helpful in hospitalized autistic children. Eight moderately to profoundly retarded boys (mean age 5.7

years) completed the 3 week study. Untoward side effects were minimal and transient, and clinical improvement was found on global measures of behavioural change.

Stimulants

Stimulant medications, such as dextroamphetamine and methylphenidate, affect a number of neurotransmitter systems, although their most potent effect is to enhance dopamine neurotransmission. Reports describing the efficacy of stimulants for treating symptoms of hyperactivity in autistic children are equivocal. Campbell et al. (1976) found that levoamphetamine worsened negativism in eight of 11 autistic children although five of seven subjects who had hyperactivity showed a reduction of that symptom. Strayhorn et al. (1988) described a 6 year old autistic boy who showed improvement in attention and motor hyperactivity, and a reduction in destructive behaviour and stereotyped movements on methylphenidate 10 mg twice a day. In addition to these positive effects, however, the child became more depressed and had an increase in temper tantrums. More recently, Quintana et al. (1995) described results from a double blind, crossover trial of methylphenidate 10 or 20 mg twice a day in ten children with autistic disorder. A statistically significant reduction in measures of hyperactivity was observed without an increase in stereotypic behaviour. Controlled studies of stimulants in larger numbers of autistic children are needed to determine if a reduction in inattentiveness and hyperactivity can be consistently attained, and if these effects outweigh potential increases in negativism and dysphoria.

ATYPICAL NEUROLEPTIC AGENTS

Risperidone

Risperidone is a highly potent dopamine D2/5-HT2 receptor antagonist (Leysen et al., 1988) that has been shown in controlled clinical trials to have efficacy in improving both the positive and negative symptoms of schizophrenia (Chouinard et al., 1993). In addition, its side effect profile appears superior to those of typical neuroleptics (Moller et al., 1991). A recent controlled study found risperidone significantly better than placebo in reducing persistent behavioural disturbances when added to existing medication in patients with severe to profound mental retardation (Vanden

Borre et al., 1993). A robust and sustained clinical improvement in several adults with autism-spectrum disorders treated with open label risperidone has been observed (McDougle et al., 1995a). In addition, Purdon et al. (1994) described the favourable clinical response to risperidone in two adult males with PDD and mental retardation. A 30 year old man showed a marked decrease in ritualistic behaviours, facial grimacing, verbal perseveration and obsessive preoccupation on a combination of risperidone 8 mg/day, methotrimeprazine 37.5 mg/day and clonazepam 1 mg/day. The other patient, a 29 year old man, exhibited a marked decline in psychomotor agitation, self-directed speech, rocking and facial stereotypies on a combination of risperidone 6 mg/day and clomipramine 50 mg/day.

Risperidone has been shown to improve the negative symptoms of schizophrenia, including blunted affect, emotional withdrawal, poor rapport, passive/apathetic social withdrawal, difficulty in abstract thinking, lack of spontaneity and flow of conversation, and stereotyped thinking (Chouinard et al., 1993), which is of interest with regard to the impairment in reciprocal social interaction that characterizes autism. It has been hypothesized that the unique ratio of 5-HT2 to dopamine D2 receptor antagonism which characterizes risperidone may account for its efficacy in improving the negative symptoms of schizophrenia and its lack of prominent acute (dystonia, akathisia) and chronic (tardive dyskinesia) extrapyramidal side effects (Moller et al., 1991).

In addition to impaired social relatedness, it is not uncommon for autistic patients to have interfering repetitive thoughts and behaviour. Risperidone addition has recently been reported to improve repetitive thoughts and behaviour in OCD patients unresponsive to fluvoxamine alone (McDougle et al. 1995c). Importantly, risperidone may be effective in reducing these symptoms in adults with PDDs.

Prospective double blind, placebo controlled trials of risperidone are necessary to determine its efficacy in the treatment of patients with autism and other PDDs. These preliminary results suggest that continued investigation into the role of dopamine and 5-HT in the pathophysiology and treatment of autism are warranted.

DRUGS AFFECTING NOREPINEPHRINE FUNCTION

Studies investigating norepinephrine function and the response to drugs that affect this system suggest that norepinephrine may not be significantly involved in the pathophysiology and treatment of autistic disorder (Minderaa et al., 1994). Although Lake et al. (1977) found elevated levels of plasma norepinephrine in autistic patients compared with age matched controls, not all of these patients were drug free at the time of the study. Furthermore, Young et al. (1981) showed that levels of plasma free 3-methoxy-4-hydroxyphenethylene glycol (MHPG), the principal metabolite of brain norepinephrine, were no different between autistic patients and normal controls. Moreover, Gillberg et al. (1983) found no difference in MHPG levels in the CSF of autistic children compared with control subjects. As mentioned previously, Gordon et al. (1993) found the 5-HT uptake inhibitor clomipramine to be superior to the norepinephrine uptake inhibitor desipramine in the treatment of autistic children. Additional studies of drugs that affect norepinephrine function are reviewed below.

Beta blockers

Beta blockers are drugs that block norepinephrine receptors and reduce overall norepinephrine neurotransmission. Ratey et al. (1987a,b) described a reduction in aggressive, impulsive and self-injurious behaviour and an improvement in speech and socialization in eight hospitalized adults with autism treated with open label propranolol or nadolol. Seven of the eight patients were receiving concomitant neuroleptic or mood stabilizing drugs during the trial. Patients were started on propranolol or nadolol 40 mg/day and the dose was increased weekly or biweekly in 40 mg increments until clinical effect or hypotension occurred. Final doses of propranolol ranged from 100 to 420 mg/day (mean 225 mg/day). The mean duration of treatment at the time of assessment was 14.2 months. All eight patients showed a moderate to marked reduction in aggressivity, six of eight improved their social skills and sought more human contact, and four of eight improved their speech. Five patients were able to have their dose of neuroleptic reduced and one patient was able to discontinue the neuroleptic. The authors speculated that the observed clinical improvement was a result of a decrease in chronic hyperarousal.

Clonidine

Clonidine is an alpha-2 noradrenergic receptor agonist that has been shown to decrease norepinephrine neurotransmission. In a double blind, placebo controlled crossover study, clonidine was given to eight autistic boys (mean age 8.1 years) who demonstrated symptoms of inattention, impulsivity and hyperactivity which limited the effectiveness of educational and behavioural interventions (Jaselskis et al., 1992). All the children had been previously treated with methylphenidate, neuroleptic or desipramine without effect. Clonidine (0.15–0.20 mg/day) or placebo was given three times a day for 6 weeks, and following a 1 week washout, the alternate treatment was given for 6 weeks. Teacher and parent ratings showed modest improvement of hyperactivity and irritability during clonidine treatment. Clinician ratings of behaviour during videotaped sessions, however, were not significantly different between clonidine and placebo. Sedation and decreased blood pressure were the most frequent side effects. In addition, many of the patients eventually developed tolerance to the therapeutic effects of clonidine, as well as an associated increase in irritability. The authors concluded that because of these factors, the use of clonidine to treat symptoms of hyperactivity in autistic children may be limited.

DRUGS AFFECTING NEUROPEPTIDE FUNCTION

To date, the opioid system has been the most extensively studied peptidergic system with respect to autistic disorder. Weizman et al. (1984) found significantly decreased blood levels of endorphin H in autistic and schizophrenic patients compared with controls. Gillberg et al. (1985) identified elevated CSF endorphin fraction II levels in autistic children in comparison with controls. The 55% of patients with autism who had CSF endorphin levels above the highest control value also demonstrated decreased pain sensitivity. Ross et al. (1987) found elevated CSF beta endorphin levels in autistic children compared with controls and hypothesized that a defect in the maturation of brain endorphin systems may underlie some of the symptoms of autism. Adrenocorticotrophic hormone (ACTH) analogues have also received attention as potential treatments for some symptoms of autism.

Naltrexone

In an open label study, Campbell et al. (1989) evaluated the safety and efficacy of the opiate receptor antagonist naltrexone in ten hospitalized autistic boys (mean age 5.0 years). Following a 2 week baseline period during which behavioural ratings were obtained, patients received single oral doses of naltrexone 0.5 mg/kg per day, 1.0 mg/kg per day and 2.0 mg/kg per day in ascending order, once a week. Seven children showed mild sedation and one became hypoactive. No changes in liver function tests, electrocardiograms or vital signs occurred. Naltrexone resulted in a reduction in withdrawal across all three doses, increased verbal production at the 0.5 mg/kg per day dose, and reduced stereotypies at the 2.0 mg/kg per day dose. At baseline, eight of ten children displayed mild to severe aggression and five of ten self-injurious behaviour. The authors clinical impression was that there was only a slight reduction in these behaviours with naltrexone. Overall, eight of ten children were judged to show a positive response to naltrexone.

Borghese et al. (1991) studied the acute effects of naltrexone (0.5, 1.0, 1.5 and 2.0 mg/kg) in 13 autistic children. Scores on the Childhood Autism Rating Scale (CARS) were significantly lower in response to the 1.0, 1.5 and 2.0 mg/kg doses of naltrexone in comparison with placebo; however, a detailed assessment of eye contact and social avoidance showed no difference between naltrexone and placebo. The authors concluded that these data failed to confirm the hypothesis of opioid involvement in the social dysfunction characteristic of autism. In a study of similar design, this same research group demonstrated that naltrexone was more effective than placebo in reducing the locomotor hyperactivity characteristic of many autistic children (Asleson et al., 1991).

In a double blind, randomized study, Leboyer et al. (1992) administered naltrexone 0.5 mg/kg per day, 1.0 mg/kg per day and 2.0 mg/kg per day and placebo for 1 week each to four autistic children (three boys, one girl), aged 4, 12, 12 and 19 years. All four children had self-injurious behaviour. Three patients had elevated levels of blood beta endorphin at baseline, and each of these children demonstrated a significant improvement in symptoms at the lowest and highest doses of naltrexone. The one patient who had a normal blood level of beta endorphin showed no clinical improvement. There was no change in behaviour during placebo for any of the children, and there were no adverse effects during naltrexone administration. The three responders showed increased socialization, improved eye contact, increased verbalization, increased attentiveness and decreased restlessness and self-injurious behaviour.

In a double blind, placebo controlled study in 41 autistic children, Campbell et al. (1993) found naltrexone useful only for symptoms of hyperactivity with no effect on discrimination learning. The authors reported that there was a suggestion that naltrexone had a beneficial effect on self-injurious behaviour, but that further study would be necessary. Untoward effects of naltrexone were mild and transient.

Willemsen-Swinkels et al. (1995) described a 4 week, double blind, placebo controlled trial of naltrexone 50 mg/day or 150 mg/day in 32 adult subjects (seven with autism, 16 with autism and self-injurious behaviour and nine with self-injurious behaviour alone). Naltrexone had no therapeutic effects on autistic symptoms or self-injurious behaviour, and increased the incidence of stereotypic behaviour. In summary, most controlled studies suggest that the core symptoms of autism and self-injurious behaviour are not significantly affected by naltrexone. A reduction of motor hyperactivity may occur in some autistic children who receive the drug.

Adrenocorticotrophic hormone (ACTH) analogue (Org 2766)

In a double blind, placebo controlled crossover study, Buitelaar et al. (1990) studied Org 2766, a synthetic analogue of ACTH 4-9, in 14 children with autism. Following a 2 week single blind, placebo period, Org 2766 20 mg/day or placebo was given for 4 weeks in a randomized manner. Patients were then crossed over to the alternate treatment. Org 2766 seemed to have an activating and stimulating effect on behaviour, as evidenced by increases in locomotion, changing toys and talkativeness. A decrease in stereotypic behaviour was also observed. Parents rated 11 of 14 patients as improved and investigators rated eight of 14 patients as showing improvement with Org 2766. No adverse events or side effects were observed. In a subsequent report, the same investigators documented an improvement in the coordination of gaze behaviours resulting in increased eye contact, an increase in mutual smiling and a decrease in the interactional role of stereotyped behaviours with Org 2766 administration (Buitelaar et al., 1992).

SUMMARY

Preliminary evidence suggests that drugs that increase 5-HT neurotransmission, such as the 5-HT uptake inhibitors clomipramine, fluvoxamine, fluoxetine, sertraline and paroxetine, as well as 5-HT receptor agonists such as buspirone, may be useful in reducing interfering repetitive behaviour and aggression and in improving social relatedness in some children and adults with autistic disorder. To date, only two controlled studies have been conducted with these drugs. Clomipramine was found to be more effective than desipramine, a relatively selective norepinephrine uptake inhibitor, and placebo for improving the core symptoms of autism, anger and obsessive–compulsive symptoms in children with autism. Fluvoxamine was superior to placebo for reducing aggressive impulsivity and interfering repetitive thoughts and behaviour and for enhancing social relatedness, particularly language usage, in adults with autism. Clomipramine can lower the seizure threshold and affect cardiac conduction making it imperative that close monitoring for these adverse effects be utilized. Otherwise, these medications are generally well tolerated and are not associated with significant short- or long-term side-effects. Double blind, placebo controlled trials of clomipramine in autistic adults and fluvoxamine in autistic children and adolescents are necessary to evaluate the impact of brain developmental changes in response to these drugs. Controlled studies of fluoxetine, sertraline, paroxetine and buspirone have yet to be published in children, adolescents or adults with autism.

Well designed controlled studies have demonstrated that dopamine receptor antagonists such as haloperidol are effective in reducing many of the maladaptive behaviours of autistic children. As there is a relatively high percentage of drug induced and withdrawal related dyskinesias associated with this class of drugs, safer agents are needed. The recent development of alternative drugs which modulate dopamine transmission with significantly lower risks of extrapyramidal side effects and tardive dyskinesia (e.g. risperidone) may prove useful in some patients with autistic disorder. Controlled studies of risperidone in children and adults with autism are currently underway. The role of stimulants, such as dextroamphetamine and methylphenidate, for treating symptoms of hyperactivity in autistic children needs to be clarified. While clinical lore has suggested that these agents typically exacerbate restlessness and impulsivity, recent reports describe more favourable results. As distractibility and hyperactivity are often prominent interfering symptoms in autistic children, controlled studies of stimulants in larger numbers of patients appear warranted.

Investigations of drugs that affect norepinephrine function have not suggested a primary role for these agents in treating the core symptoms of autism. Controlled studies of beta blockers have not been conducted to determine if these drugs are useful for reducing aggression and self-injury in patients with autistic disorder. Beta blockers currently have a limited role in the pharmacotherapy of autism because of the potential for adverse cardiac effects and the present availability of safer agents. Studies of the alpha-2 receptor agonist clonidine have suggested that symptoms of hyperactivity might show initial improvement, but that tolerance and irritability often develop with ongoing treatment.

The opiate receptor antagonist naltrexone has been shown to be useful in reducing hyperactivity in some children with autism, although recent evidence indicates that its prosocial effects and ability to improve self-injurious and aggressive behaviour may be minimal. Preliminary findings suggest that ACTH analogues may play some role in the treatment of impaired social relatedness. Speculation about the prosocial effects of the nonapeptide oxytocin (Insel, 1992) may warrant further thought with respect to autism (Panksepp, 1993).

ACKNOWLEDGEMENTS

The author thanks Elizabeth Kyle for preparing the manuscript. This work was supported by a National Alliance for Research on Schizophrenia and Depression Independent Investigator Award (Dr McDougle), a Theodore and Vada Stanley Foundation Research Award (Dr McDougle) the State of Connecticut Department of Mental Health and Addiction Services, the Korczak Foundation for Autism and Related Disorders, and National Institutes of Health grants M01 RR06022-33, P50 MH30929-18, HD 03008-27 and a Research Unit on Pediatric Psychopharmacology (RUPP) grant to Indiana University (Dr McDougle).

REFERENCES

American Psychiatric Association. (1987). *Diagnostic and Statistical Manual of Mental Disorders*, 3rd edn-revised (DSM-III-R). Washington, DC: American Psychiatric Association.

American Psychiatric Association. (1994). *Diagnostic and Statistical Manual of Mental Disorders*, 4th edn (DSM-IV). Washington, DC: American Psychiatric Association.

Anderson, L., Campbell, M., Grega, D., Perry, R., Small, A. & Green, W. (1984). Haloperidol in the treatment of infantile autism: effects on learning and behavioral symptoms. *American Journal of Psychiatry*, **141**, 1195–202.

Anderson, G. M., Freedman, D. X., Cohen, D. J., Volkmar, F. R., Hoder, E. L., McPhedran, P., Minderaa, R. B., Hansen, C. R. & Young, J. G. (1987). Whole blood serotonin in autistic and normal subjects. *Journal of Child Psychology and Psychiatry*, **28**, 885–900.

Asleson, G. S., Herman, B. H., Borghese, I. F., Allen, R. P. & Arthur-Smith, A. (1991). Effects of acute naltrexone on locomotor activity in autistic children. *Society for Neuroscience Abstracts*, **17**, 1346.

Benfield, P. & Ward, A. (1986). Fluvoxamine: a review of its pharmacodynamic and pharmacokinetic properties, and therapeutic efficacy in depressive illness. *Drugs*, **32**, 313–34.

Blier, P., de Montigny, C. & Chaput, Y. (1990). A role for the serotonin system in the mechanism of action of antidepressant treatments: preclinical evidence. *Journal of Clinical Psychiatry*, **51**, 14–20.

Borghese, I. F., Herman, B. H., Asleson, G. S., Chatoor, I., Benoit, M. B., Papero, P. & McNulty, G. (1991). Effects of acutely administered naltrexone on social behaviour of autistic children. *Society for Neuroscience Abstracts*, **17**, 1252.

Brodkin, E. S., McDougle, C. J., Naylor, S. T., Cohen, D. J. & Price, L. H. (1997). Clomipramine in adults with pervasive developmental disorders: a prospective open-label investigation. *Journal of Child and Adolescent Psychopharmacology*, **7**, 109–21.

Brown, G. L., Goodwin, F. K., Ballenger, J. C., Goyer, P. F. & Major, L. F. (1979). Aggression in humans correlates with cerebrospinal fluid amine metabolites. *Psychiatry Research*, **1**, 131–9.

Buitelaar, J. K., van Engeland, H., van Ree, J. M. & de Wied, D. (1990). Behavioral effects of Org 2766, a synthetic analog of the adrenocorticotrophic hormone (4-9), in 14 outpatient autistic children. *Journal of Autism and Developmental Disorders*, **20**, 467–78.

Buitelaar, J. K., van Engeland, H., de Kogel, K. H., de Vries, H., van Hooff, J. A. R. A. M. & van Ree, J. M. (1992). The use of adrenocorticotrophic hormone (4-9) analog ORG 2766 in autistic children: effects on the organization of behavior. *Biological Psychiatry*, **31**, 1119–29.

Campbell, M. (1988). Fenfluramine treatment of autism. *Journal of Child Psychology and Psychiatry*, **29**, 1–10.

Campbell, M., Adams, P., Perry, R., Spencer, E. K. & Overall, J. E. (1988a). Tardive and withdrawal dyskinesia in autistic children: a prospective study. *Psychopharmacology Bulletin*, **24**, 251–5.

Campbell, M., Adams, P., Small, A. M., Curren, E. L., Overall, J., Anderson, L. T., Lynch, N. & Perry, R. (1988b). Efficacy and safety of fenfluramine in autistic children. *Journal of the American Academy of Child and Adolescent Psychiatry*, **27**, 434–9.

Campbell, M., Anderson, L., Meier, M., Cohen, I., Small, A., Samit, C. & Sachar, E. (1978). A comparison of haloperidol and behavior therapy and their interaction in autistic children. *Journal of the American Academy of Child and Adolescent Psychiatry*, **17**, 640–55.

Campbell, M., Anderson, L. T., Small, A. M., Adams, P., Gonzalez, N. M. & Ernst, M. (1993). Naltrexone in autistic children: behavioral symptoms and attentional learning. *Journal of the American Academy of Child and Adolescent Psychiatry*, **32**, 1283–91.

Campbell, M., Overall, J. E., Small, A. M., Sokol, M. S., Spencer, E. K., Adams, P., Foltz, R. L., Monti, K. M., Perry, R., Nobler, M. & Roberts, E. (1989). Naltrexone in autistic children: an acute open dose range tolerance trial. *Journal of the American Academy of Child and Adolescent Psychiatry*, **28**, 200–6.

Campbell, M., Small, A. M., Collins, P. J., Friedman, E., David, R. & Genieser, N. (1976). Levodopa and levoamphetamine: a crossover study in young schizophrenic children. *Current Therapeutic Research*, **19**, 70–83.

Chouinard, G., Jones, B., Remington, G., Bloom, D., Addington, D., MacEwan, G. W., Labelle, A., Beauclair, L. & Arnott, W. (1993). A Canadian multicenter placebo-controlled study of fixed doses of risperidone and haloperidol in the treatment of chronic schizophrenic patients. *Journal of Clinical Psychopharmacology*, **13**, 25–40.

Ciaranello, A. L. & Ciaranello, R. D. (1995). The neurobiology of infantile autism. *Annual Review of Neuroscience*, **18**, 101–28.

Cohen, I. L., Campbell, M., Posner, D., Small, A. M., Triebel, D. & Anderson, L. T. (1980). Behavioral effects of haloperidol in young autistic children. *Journal of the*

American Academy of Child and Adolescent Psychiatry, **19**, 665–77.

Cook, E. H. (1990). Autism: review of neurochemical investigation. *Synapse*, **6**, 292–308.

Cook, E. H., Rowlett, R., Jaselskis, C. & Leventhal, B. L. (1992). Fluoxetine treatment of children and adults with autistic disorder and mental retardation. *Journal of the American Academy of Child and Adolescent Psychiatry*, **31**, 739–45.

Cook, E. H. Jr., Perry, B. D., Dawson, G., Wainwright, M. S. & Leventhal, B. L. (1993). Receptor inhibition by immunoglobulins: specific inhibition by autistic children, their relatives, and control subjects. *Journal of Autism and Developmental Disorders*, **23**, 67–78.

Duker, P., Welles, K., Seys, D., Rensen, H. & Vis, A. (1991). Brief report: effects of fenfluramine on communicative, stereotypic, and inappropriate behaviors of autistic-type mentally handicapped individuals. *Journal of Autism and Developmental Disorders*, **21**, 355–63.

Ekman, G., Miranda-Linné, F., Gillberg, C., Garle, M. & Wetterberg, L. (1989). Fenfluramine treatment of twenty children with autism. *Journal of Autism and Developmental Disorders*, **19**, 511–32.

Ernst, M., Magee, H. J., Gonzalez, N. M., Locascio, J. J., Rosenberg, C. R. & Campbell, M. (1992). Pimozide in autistic children. *Psychopharmacology Bulletin*, **28**, 187–91.

Freeman, B. J., Ritvo, E. R., Yokota, A. & Ritvo, A. (1986). A scale for rating symptoms of patients with the syndrome of autism in real life settings. *Journal of the American Academy of Child and Adolescent Psychiatry*, **25**, 130–6.

Garber, H. J., McGonigle, J. J., Slomka, G. T. & Monteverde, E. (1992). Clomipramine treatment of stereotypic behaviors and self-injury in patients with developmental disabilities. *Journal of the American Academy of Child and Adolescent Psychiatry*, **31**, 1157–60.

Geller, E., Ritvo, E., Freeman, B. & Yuwiler, A. (1982). Preliminary observations on the effect of fenfluramine on blood serotonin and symptoms in three autistic boys. *New England Journal of Medicine*, **307**, 165–9.

Ghaziuddin, M., Tsai, L. & Ghaziuddin, N. (1991). Fluoxetine in autism with depression. *Journal of the American Academy of Child and Adolescent Psychiatry*, **30**, 3 (letter).

Gillberg, C., Svennerholm, L. & Hamilton-Hellberg, C. (1983). Childhood psychosis and monoamine metabolites in spinal fluid. *Journal of Autism and Developmental Disorders*, **13**, 383–96.

Gillberg, C., Terenius, L. & Lonnerholm, G. (1985). Endorphin activity in childhood psychosis. *Archives of General Psychiatry*, **42**, 780–3.

Goodman, W. K., Price, L. H., Rasmussen, S. A., Delgado, P. L., Heninger, G. R. & Charney, D. S. (1989a). Efficacy of fluvoxamine in obsessive–compulsive disorder: a double-blind comparison with placebo. *Archives of General Psychiatry*, **46**, 36–43.

Goodman, W. K., Price, L. H., Rasmussen, S. A., Mazure, C., Fleischmann, R., Hill, C., Heninger, G. R. & Charney, D. S. (1989b). The Yale–Brown Obsessive Compulsive Scale (Y-BOCS): Part I. Development, use, and reliability. *Archives of General Psychiatry*, **46**, 1006–11.

Goodman, W. K., Price, L. H., Rasmussen, S. A., Mazure, C., Delgado, P., Heninger, G. R. & Charney, D. S. (1989c). The Yale–Brown Obsessive Compulsive Scale (Y-BOCS): Part II. Validity. *Archives of General Psychiatry*, **46**, 1012–16.

Gordon, C. T., State, R. C., Nelson, J. E., Hamburger, S. D. & Rapoport, J. L. (1993). A double-blind comparison of clomipramine, desipramine, and placebo in the treatment of autistic disorder. *Archives of General Psychiatry*, **50**, 441–7.

Greist, J. H., Chouinard, G., DuBoff, E., Halaris, A., Kim, S. W., Koran, L., Liebowitz, M., Lydiard, R. B., Rasmussen, S., White, K. & Sikes, C. (1995a). Double-blind parallel comparison of three dosages of sertraline and placebo in outpatients with obsessive–compulsive disorder. *Archives of General Psychiatry*, **52**, 289–95.

Greist, J. H., Jefferson, J. W., Kobak, K. A., Katzelnick, D. J. & Serlin, R. C. (1995b). Efficacy and tolerability of serotonin transport inhibitors in obsessive–compulsive disorder. *Archives of General Psychiatry*, **52**, 53–60.

Guy, W. (1976). *ECDEU assessment manual for psychopharmacology*. Publication 76-338, Washington, DC: National Institute of Mental Health, US Department of Health, Education and Welfare.

Hamdan-Allen, G. (1991). Brief report: trichotillomania in an autistic male. *Journal of Autism and Developmental Disorders*, **21**, 79–82.

Hoshino, Y., Tachibana, J. R., Watanabe, M., Murata, S., Yokoyama, F., Kaneko, M., Yashima, Y. & Kumoshiro, H. (1984). Serotonin metabolism and hypothalamic-pituitary function in children with infantile autism and minimal brain dysfunction. *Japanese Journal of Psychiatry and Neurology*, **26**, 937–45.

Insel, T. R. (1992). Oxytocin: a neuropeptide for affiliation. Evidence from behavioral, receptor autoradiographic, and comparative studies. *Psychoneuroendocrinology*, **17**, 3–35.

Jaselskis, C. A., Cook, E. H. Jr., Fletcher, K. E. & Leventhal, B. L. (1992). Clonidine treatment of hyperactive and impulsive children with autistic disorder. *Journal of Clinical Psychopharmacology*, **12**, 322–7.

Kelley, L. A., Hellings, J. A., Gabrielli, W. F. & Kilgore, E. (1993). Sertraline response in mentally retarded adults. *American Psychiatric Association New Research Abstracts*, **NR173**, 103.

Kruesi, M. J., Hibbs, E. D., Zahn, T. P., Keysor, C. S., Hamburger, S. D., Bartko, J. J. & Rapoport, J. L. (1992). A 2-year prospective follow-up study of children and adolescents with disruptive behavior disorders: prediction by cerebrospinal fluid 5-hydroxyindoleacetic acid, homovanillic acid, and autonomic measures? *Archives of General Psychiatry*, **49**, 429–35.

Kruesi, M. J., Rapoport, J. L., Hamburger, S., Hibbs, E., Potter, W. Z., Lenane, M. & Brown, G. L. (1990). Cerebrospinal fluid monoamine metabolites, aggression, and impulsivity in disruptive behavior disorders of children and adolescents. *Archives of General Psychiatry*, **47**, 419–26.

Lake, C. R., Ziegler, M. G. & Murphy, D. L. (1977). Increased norepinephrine levels and decreased dopamine-β-hydroxylase activity in primary autism. *Archives of General Psychiatry*, **34**, 553–6.

Leboyer, M., Bouvard, M. P., Launay, J. -M., Tabuteau, F., Waller, D., Dugas, M., Kerdelhue, B., Lensing, P. & Panksepp, J. (1992). Brief report: a double-blind study of naltrexone in infantile autism. *Journal of Autism and Developmental Disorders*, **22**, 309–19.

Leventhal, B. L., Cook, E. H. Jr., Morford, M., Ravitz, A. J., Heller, W. & Freedman, D. X. (1993). Fenfluramine: clinical and neurochemical effects in children with autism. *Journal of Neuropsychiatry and Clinical Neurosciences*, **5**, 307–15.

Leysen, J. E., Gommeren, W., Eens, A., De Chaffoy De Courcelles, D., Stoof, J. C. & Janssen, P. A. J. (1988). Biochemical profile of risperidone, a new antipsychotic. *Journal of Pharmacology and Experimental Therapeutics*, **247**, 661–70.

Markowitz, P. I. (1992). Effect of fluoxetine on self-injurious behavior in the developmentally disabled: a preliminary study. *Journal of Clinical Psychopharmacology*, **12**, 27–31.

McBride, P. A., Anderson, G. M., Hertzig, M. E., Sweeney, J. A., Kream, J., Cohen, D. J. & Mann, J. J. (1989). Serotonergic responsivity in male young adults with autistic disorder: results of a pilot study. *Archives of General Psychiatry*, **46**, 213–21.

McDougle, C. J., Brodkin, E. S., Naylor, S. T., Carlson, D., Cohen, D. J. & Price, L. H. (1998). Sertraline in adults with pervasive developmental disorders: a prospective open-label investigation. *Journal of Clinical Pharmacology*. (In press.)

Christopher J. McDougle

McDougle, C. J., Brodkin, E. S., Yeung, P. P., Naylor, S. T., Cohen, D. J. & Price, L. H. (1995a). Risperidone in adults with autism or pervasive developmental disorder. *Journal of Child and Adolescent Psychopharmacology*, **5**, 273–82.

McDougle, C. J., Kresch, L., Goodman, W. K., Naylor, S. T., Volkmar, F. R., Cohen, D. J. & Price, L. H. (1995b). A case-controlled study of repetitive thoughts and behavior in adults with autistic disorder and obsessive–compulsive disorder. *American Journal of Psychiatry*, **152**, 772–7.

McDougle, C. J. Fleischmann, R. L., Epperson, C. N., Wasylink, S., Leckman, J. F. & Price, L. H. (1995c). Risperidone addition in fluvoxamine-refractory obsessive compulsive disorder: three cases. *Journal of Clinical Psychiatry*, **56**, 526–8.

McDougle, C. J., Naylor, S. T., Cohen, D. J., Aghajanian, G. K., Heninger, G. R. & Price, L. H. (1996a). Effects of tryptophan depletion in drug-free adults with autism. *Archives of General Psychiatry*, **53**, 993–1000.

McDougle, C. J., Naylor, S. T., Cohen, D. J., Volkmar, F. R., Heninger, G. R. & Price, L. H. (1996b). A double-blind, placebo-controlled study of fluvoxamine in adults with autistic disorders. *Archives of General Psychiatry*, **53**, 1001–8.

McDougle, C. J., Price, L. H. & Goodman, W. K. (1990). Fluvoxamine treatment of coincident autistic disorder and obsessive compulsive disorder: a case report. *Journal of Autism and Developmental Disorders*, **20**, 537–43.

McDougle, C. J., Price, L. H., Volkmar, F. R., Goodman, W. K., Ward-O'Brien, D., Nielsen, J., Bregman, J. & Cohen, D. J. (1992). Clomipramine in autism: preliminary evidence of efficacy. *Journal of the American Academy of Child and Adolescent Psychiatry*, **31**, 746–50.

McDougle, C. J., Price, L. H. & Volkmar, F. R. (1994). Recent advances in the pharmacotherapy of autism and related conditions. In *Child and Adolescent Psychiatric Clinics of North America*, **3**, *Psychoses and Pervasive Developmental Disorders*, ed. F. R. Volkmar, pp. 71–89. Philadelphia: W. B. Saunders.

Mehlinger, R., Scheftner, W. A. & Poznanski, E. (1990). Fluoxetine and autism. *Journal of the American Academy of Child and Adolescent Psychiatry*, **29**, 985 (letter).

Minderaa, R. B., Anderson, G. M., Volkmar, F. R., Akkerhuis, G. W. & Cohen, D. J. (1994). Noradrenergic and adrenergic functioning in autism. *Biological Psychiatry*, **36**, 237–41.

Moller, H. J., Pelzer, E., Kissling, W., Riehl, T. & Wernicke, T. (1991). Efficacy and tolerability of a new antipsychotic compound (risperidone): results of a pilot study. *Pharmacopsychiatry*, **24**, 185–9.

Naruse, H., Nagahata, M., Nakane, Y., Shirahashi, K., Takesada, M. & Yamazaki, K. (1982). A multi-center double-blind trial of pimozide (Orap), haloperidol and placebo in children with behavior disorders, using cross-over design. *Acta Paedopsychiatrica*, **48**, 173–84.

Panksepp, J. (1993). Commentary on the possible role of oxytocin in autism. *Journal of Autism and Developmental Disorders*, **23**, 567–9 (letter).

Perry, R., Campbell, M., Adams, P., Lynch, N., Spencer, E. K., Curren, E. L. & Overall, J. E. (1989). Long-term efficacy of haloperidol in autistic children: continuous versus discontinuous drug administration. *Journal of the American Academy of Child and Adolescent Psychiatry*, **28**, 87–92.

Purdon, S. E., Lit, W., Labelle, A. & Jones, D. W. (1994). Risperidone in the treatment of pervasive developmental disorder. *Canadian Journal of Psychiatry*, **39**, 400–5.

Quintana, H., Birmaher, B., Stedge, D., Lennon, S., Freed, J., Bridge, J. & Greenhill, L. (1995). Use of methylphenidate in the treatment of children with autistic disorder. *Journal of Autism and Developmental Disorders*, **25**, 283–94.

Raleigh, M. J., Brammer, G. L., Yuwiler, A., Flannery, J. W., McGuire, M. T. & Geller, E. (1980). Serotonergic influences on the social behavior of vervet monkeys (*Cer-*

copithecus aethiops sabaeus). *Experimental Neurology*, **68**, 322–4.

Ratey, J. J., Bemporad, J., Sorgi, P., Bick, P., Polakoff, S., O'Driscoll, G. & Mikkelsen, E. (1987a). Brief report: open trial effects of beta-blockers on speech and social behaviors in 8 autistic adults. *Journal of Autism and Developmental Disorders*, **17**, 439–46.

Ratey, J. J., Mikkelsen, E., Sorgi, P., Zuckerman, H. S., Polakoff, S., Bemporad, J., Bick, P. & Kadish, W. (1987b). Autism: the treatment of aggressive behaviors. *Journal of Clinical Psychopharmacology*, **7**, 35–41.

Ratey, J. J., Sovner, R., Mikkelsen, E. & Chmielinski, H. E. (1989). Buspirone therapy for maladaptive behavior and anxiety in developmentally disabled persons. *Journal of Clinical Psychiatry*, **50**, 382–4.

Realmuto, G. M., August, G. J. & Garfinkel, B. D. (1989). Clinical effect of buspirone in autistic children. *Journal of Clinical Psychopharmacology*, **9**, 122–5.

Ritvo, E. R., Freeman, B. J., Geller, E. & Yuwiler, A. (1983). Effects of fenfluramine on 14 outpatients with the syndrome of autism. *Journal of the American Academy of Child and Adolescent Psychiatry*, **22**, 549–58.

Ritvo, E. R., Freeman, B. J., Yuwiler, A., Geller, E., Schroth, P., Yokota, A., Mason-Brothers, A., August, G. J., Klykylo, W., Leventhal, B., Lewis, K., Piggott, L., Realmuto, G., Stubbs, E. G. & Umansky, R. (1986). Fenfluramine treatment of autism: UCLA collaborative study of 81 patients at nine medical centers. *Psychopharmacology Bulletin*, **22**, 133–40.

Ross, D. L., Klykylo, W. M. & Hitzemann, R. (1987). Reduction of elevated CSF beta-endorphin by fenfluramine in infantile autism. *Pediatric Neurology*, **3**, 83–6.

Schain, R. J. & Freedman, D. X. (1961). Studies on 5-hydroxyindole metabolism in autistic and other mentally retarded children. *Journal of Pediatrics*, **58**, 315–20.

Schuster, C., Lewis, M. & Seiden, L. (1986). Fenfluramine: neurotoxicity. *Psychopharmacology Bulletin*, **22**, 148–51.

Sherman, J., Factor, D., Swinson, R. & Darjes, R. (1989). The effects of fenfluramine (hydrochloride) on the behaviors of fifteen autistic children. *Journal of Autism and Developmental Disorders*, **19**, 533–43.

Smalley, S. L., McCracken, J. & Tanguay, P. (1995). Autism, affective disorders, and social phobia. *American Journal of Medical Genetics* (*Neuropsychiatric Genetics*), **60**, 19–26.

Snead, R. W., Boon, R. & Presberg, J. (1994). Paroxetine for self-injurious behavior. *Journal of the American Academy of Child and Adolescent Psychiatry*, **33**, 909–10 (letter).

Sparrow, S. S., Balla, D. A. & Cicchetti, D. V. (1984). *Vineland Adaptive Behavior Scales* (A revision of the Vineland Social Maturity Scale by Edgar A. Doll). Circle Pines, Minnesota: American Guidance Service.

Strayhorn, J. M., Rapp, N., Donina, W. & Strain, P. S. (1988). Randomized trial of methylphenidate for an autistic child. *Journal of the American Academy of Child and Adolescent Psychiatry*, **27**, 244–7.

Todd, R. D. (1991). Fluoxetine in autism. *American Journal of Psychiatry*, **148**, 1089 (letter).

Todd, R. D. & Ciaranello, R. D. (1985). Demonstration of inter- and intraspecies differences in serotonin binding sites by antibodies from an autistic child. *Proceedings of the National Academy of Sciences USA*, **82**, 612–16.

Tollefson, G. D., Rampey, A. H. Jr., Potvin, J. H., Jenike, M. A., Rush, A. J., Dominguez, R. A., Koran, L. M., Shear, M. K., Goodman, W. & Genduso, L. A. (1994). A multicenter investigation of fixed-dose fluoxetine in the treatment of obsessive–compulsive disorder. *Archives of General Psychiatry*, **51**, 559–67.

van Vliet, I. M., den Boer, J. A. & Westenberg, H. G. M. (1994). Psychopharmacological treatment of social phobia: a double-blind placebo-controlled study with flu-

Christopher J. McDougle

voxamine. *Psychopharmacology*, **115**, 128–34.

Vanden Borre, R., Vermote, R., Buttiëns, M., Thiry, P., Dierick, G., Geutjens, J., Sieben, G. & Heylen, S. (1993). Risperidone as add-on therapy in behavioural disturbances in mental retardation: a double-blind placebo-controlled cross-over study. *Acta Psychiatrica Scandinavia*, **87**, 167–71.

Volkmar, F. R. (1987). Social development. In *Handbook of Autism and Pervasive Developmental Disorders*, ed. D. Cohen & A. Donnellan, pp. 41–60. New York: John Wiley.

Weizman, R., Weizman, A., Thano, S., Szekely, G., Weissman, B. A. & Sarne, Y. (1984). Humoral-endorphin blood levels in autistic, schizophrenic and healthy subjects. *Psychopharmacology*, **82**, 368–70.

Willemsen,-Swinkels, S. H. N., Buitelaar, J. K., Nijhof, G. J. & van Engeland, H. (1995). Failure of naltrexone hydrochloride to reduce self-injurious and autistic behavior in mentally retarded adults: double-blind placebo-controlled studies. *Archives of General Psychiatry*, **52**, 766–73.

Young, J. G., Cohen, D. J., Kavanagh, M. E., Landis, H. D., Shaywitz, B. A. & Maas, J. W. (1981). Cerebrospinal fluid, plasma, and urinary MHPG in children. *Life Sciences*, **28**, 2837–45.

Yuwiler, A., Shih, J. C., Chen, C. -H., Ritvo, E. R., Hanna, G., Ellison, G. W. & King, B. H. (1992). Hyperserotoninemia and antiserotonin antibodies in autism and other disorders. *Journal of Autism and Developmental Disorders*, **22**, 33–45.

7

Behavioural and educational approaches to the pervasive developmental disorders

Sandra L. Harris

INTRODUCTION

The past quarter century has witnessed major advances in treatment for children and adults with pervasive developmental disorders (PDDs). The recognition that these are biologically based conditions (Rimland, 1964) and the rejection of the psychoanalytic concept of parental blame (Bettelheim, 1967) as an explanatory mechanism created an intellectual context in which behavioural and educational interventions could take root. Beginning with demonstrations by Ferster (1961), Lovaas et al., (1966) and Bartak & Rutter (1971) that behavioural principles influenced the behaviour of these clients, there developed an appreciation of highly structured, carefully planned interventions to meet the needs of people with autistic disorder and related conditions. Since the mid-1960s the teaching technology for this population has grown increasingly sophisticated and effective.

This chapter reviews the 'state of the art' in behavioural and educational treatments for people with PDDs. The focus is on assessment and treatment of skill deficits, especially language and social skills, and intervention with dangerous or disruptive behaviours such as self-injury or aggression. The behavioural technology for early intervention is addressed, as are the controversial treatment approaches of facilitated communication and auditory integration therapy. Finally, the need to consider the family context in which treatment takes place is discussed.

This chapter is based on research with people diagnosed as exhibiting autistic disorder, Asperger's syndrome and pervasive developmental disorder – not otherwise specified (PDD-NOS). In some cases they are described as 'autistic' or demonstrating 'autistic behaviours'. These variations in language reflect the changing state of the diagnostic art as well as variation among client populations.

BEHAVIOURAL ASSESSMENT

Behavioural assessment is integral to behaviour therapy. Von Houten et al. (1988) call for an initial behavioural assessment and ongoing evaluation as every client's basic right. This assessment approaches each client as a unique person, and examines the learning history, biological factors and current setting in which that person functions. The evaluator explores such questions as 'What are the conditions under which the maladaptive behaviour occurs?', 'Is it possible to change environmental cues to reduce the likelihood of triggering a problem behaviour?', or 'What existing skills may be engaged to assist this client in learning a new skill?' It is important for this assessment to continue over time. Typically, one carries out an initial assessment, tries an intervention and, based on the outcome, either continues the treatment or changes it. Changes in treatment strategy should be data based.

Behavioural assessment also examines the generalization and maintenance of a target behaviour. When we teach a new skill we intend that it be used in every appropriate setting (generalization) and that its use continues over time (maintenance). If a child only speaks to her teacher, or uses the term 'ball' only for a single blue ball, the skill has limited generalization. If the skill drops away over time, it has shown poor maintenance. Both generalization of skills to new persons, places and objects, and maintenance of skills over time are vital if a behaviour is to have adaptive value for the client.

Many clients come for treatment presenting a variety of concerns. For example, if a child with autistic disorder has severe tantrums, is not toilet trained and does not speak, one needs to decide where to begin treatment. The educator or clinician chooses from among several presenting problems those which merit immediate intervention, and those to be addressed later. In their discussion of this decision making process Mash & Terdal (1988) note that some behaviours such as those that are physically dangerous, or keep the client from access to naturally reinforcing environmental events, would be more urgent than behaviours that do not pose an immediate crisis or isolate the client from the community. For example, treating self-injury is usually more urgent than toilet training, although both are important to a client's long term functioning. Developing an intervention hierarchy is typically carried out by the clinician in consultation with the client's family and teachers. Clients of normal intellectual functioning, such as the person with Asperger's syndrome, may have their own treatment priorities.

A good behavioural assessment considers the developmental appropriateness of the targeted skill (Harris & Ferrari, 1983). Both chronological age and mental age should be considered in a treatment plan. Although a person may not be capable of fully mastering the skills being acquired by normally developing peers, it is important to bring him or her as close as possible to that goal. An adolescent with autistic disorder and mental retardation may not 'surf the net', but can probably learn to play some video games.

TEACHING NEW SKILLS

Teaching new, adaptive skills to persons with PDDs is at the heart of the educational enterprise. These disorders, defined in part by deficits in language and social skills, have challenged professionals to generate creative interventions. There are repeated demonstrations that when properly taught, persons with autistic disorder, Asperger's syndrome and PDD-NOS can markedly improve their expressive and receptive language, social awareness and performance on academic, life skills and vocational tasks.

Language

Teaching language to people with PDDs was one of the earliest accomplishments of behaviour therapists. Beginning with the demonstration by Lovaas et al. (1966) that previously mute children could acquire rudimentary speech, there has been continuing research on speech and language. Initially this work used operant techniques in relatively artificial settings to teach specific grammatical forms including nouns (Guess et al., 1968), prepositions (Frisch & Schumaker, 1974) and interrogative sentences (Twardosz & Baer, 1973). Gradually there was a shift toward teaching language in the natural world. This shift was motivated by the discovery that skills learned in a restrictive setting were not automatically generalized to the student's natural environment and the observation that if skills were to be functional they had to be taught in ways that facilitate generalized use (Harris, 1975).

Currently most research on speech and language concerns helping the student acquire spontaneous, socially adaptive speech. This shift from the teaching cubicle to the larger world is reflected in a child's earliest programmes and continues over the years. For example, Koegel et al. (1987) use a natural language teaching paradigm with young children. They offer a variety of interesting toys, and rely primarily on the reinforcement inherent in use of the toys and the natural interaction between child and adult. The child is reinforced for attempts to communicate and the learning opportunities are embedded in the playful context. Their research has yielded important findings including the observation that reinforcing a child's attempts to speak, regardless of the quality of the attempt, results in more speech than using an approach in which only closer and closer approximation of a goal are accepted for reinforcement (Koegel et al., 1988).

The value of teaching in a naturalistic setting was also demonstrated with adolescents who learned receptive labels for food preparation items more readily when these were embedded in the motivating context of lunch preparation, rather than taught in isolation (McGee et al., 1983). An increase in spontaneous speech may be achieved by a time delay procedure in which adult prompts for responding are delayed for increasingly longer periods of time, thus encouraging the child to initiate rather than simply to imitate (Charlop et al., 1985). Taylor & Harris (1995) taught young children with autism to engage in the spontaneous 'curious' behaviour of asking question about unfamiliar objects.

Although current technology enables many people to speak who would previously have been mute, there are still some persons for whom limited speech remains a major barrier to community life. Increasingly for these persons there is a reliance on augmentative communication devices (Harris, 1995). In its simplest version this may be a board with pictures or words to which a person can point, and its most sophisticated form is a small, hand held electronic device which provides a printed message, or functions as a voice synthesizer. With this equipment a person without speech can order a meal in a restaurant, or ask for an item in a store.

SOCIAL SKILLS

Deficits in social skills characterize the PDDs. These problems range from the profound lack of social engagement shown by some persons with autistic disorder and co-occurring mental retardation, to a relatively subtle but nonetheless serious problem in empathic understanding exhibited by a highly intelligent person with Asperger's syndrome. Social skills programmes should be part of the treatment agenda for nearly every person in this diagnostic grouping. Interest in social skills deficits has stirred both theoretical research on 'theory of mind' (Leslie, 1987; Hobson, 1993; Happe, 1995), and applied work on specific interventions to help persons with PDDs become more socially adept.

Countless social skills are necessary to be a competent adult in an industrialized society. For example, one needs to greet other people, keep an appropriate physical distance, make purchases in a store and recognize emotions. To be an active member of the community many other skills are required such as participating in leisure activities, sharing resources, exchanging compliments and so forth. Most of us learned these skills through informal lessons, but for the person with a PDD they must be painstakingly taught. Among the interventions for teaching social behaviours are programmes for playing a game with another person (Coe et al., 1990), expressing affection to another child (McEvoy et al., 1988) offering assistance (Harris et al., 1990), showing appropriate affective behaviour (Gena et al., 1996) and engaging in symbolic (Stahmer, 1995) and sociodramatic play (Thorp et al., 1995).

Social skills may best be taught in groups. Both Mesibov (1984) and Williams (1989) describe programmes to help young people learn some of these complex behaviours. Their training groups use such techniques as role play of interactions, modelling by more skillful peers or group leader, and rehearsal of behaviours to be used in the community. The skills include voice modulation, initiating and terminating interactions, flexibility in unexpected situations, a sense of humour and recognizing and responding to other people's emotions.

Peer modelling is a potent tool for teaching social skills. Research on the benefits of exposure to competent peers has been carried out primarily with preschool aged children (Odom et al., 1985; Odom & Strain, 1986), with a few studies looking at older children (Lord & Hopkins, 1986; Sasso & Rude, 1987) including junior high school youngsters (Haring & Breen, 1992). The early research in this area relied heavily on adult intervention (Strain & Timm, 1974; Strain et al., 1976). More recent work has taught normally developing peers how to engage the child with a PDD (McGee et al., 1992; Pierce & Schreibman, 1995). A promising line of work teaches the child with autism to initiate social interactions (Belchic & Harris, 1994; Zanolli et al., 1996). In clinical practice one is not confined to a single intervention; the teacher may prompt behaviour as needed, peers may be taught skills for initiating play and the child with autism may learn to initiate and respond to social bids. Several studies have demonstrated that classwide interventions involving peer tutoring and cooperative learning groups can improve the academic progress of an entire class, including children with autistic disorder (Kamps et al., 1994; Dugan et al., 1995).

DECREASING MALADAPTIVE BEHAVIOUR

Another area of recent major gains has addressed teaching persons with PDDs greater self-control over disruptive and maladaptive behaviours. As the field has grown more sophisticated in teaching adaptive skills, it has been possible to teach appropriate alternatives to disruptive behaviour and to minimize the use of aversive interventions. One key to the shift from aversive to nonaversive techniques has been the increased effectiveness of methods of assessing the underlying causes of maladaptive responding. This research shows that if one does a careful assessment, teaches the client alternative ways to communicate needs and alters controlling environmental variables, it is possible to reduce the frequency of many intrusive behaviours such as aggression, self-injury and stereotyped behaviour (Wacker et al., 1990; Durand & Carr, 1991). It is essential that this assessment be tailored to each client's needs. For example, Goh et al. (1995) found that although ten of 12 persons who engaged in hand mouthing did so for the sensory properties of the behaviour, for two participants the behaviour was maintained by social variables. Similarly, although many people engage in stereotyped behaviour such as hand flapping for the stimulation inherent in the behaviour (Aiken & Salzberg, 1984), for some people an interpersonal component may maintain the behaviour (Durand & Carr, 1987). One cannot make assumptions about the motivating factors in disruptive behaviour without an assessment.

Many of the studies examining the relation between environmental or contextual events and maladaptive behaviour have focused on two patterns: escape motivated behaviour and attention seeking behaviour (Carr & Durand, 1985). These two variables account for many of the disruptive behaviours emitted by persons with PDDs. Among the other environmental factors that may influence maladaptive behaviours are providing opportunities to make choices (Dyer et al. 1990), certain kinds of verbal reprimands (Fisher et al., 1996), brief breaks from work (Zarcone et al., 1996), giving warnings before changing activities (Tustin, 1995) and meal schedules (Wacker et al., 1996). Physical factors such as middle ear infections, allergies and sleep disruption must also be considered in a comprehensive assessment (O'Neill et al., 1990). It may be important to perform a functional assessment in more than a single setting. Haring & Kennedy (1990) reported that disruptive behaviour in an instructional setting was controlled by different factors than that same behaviour in leisure time.

Once a functional analysis is carried out, and the controlling variables have been identified, it is often possible to provide functional communication training to teach the client an alternative response. For example, a person who engages in a high frequency of self-injury to avoid work may be taught to ask for a break (Bird et al., 1989; Lalli et al., 1995), and a client whose disruptive behaviour is reinforced by attention may learn to ask for his supervisor's approval (Durand, 1990).

EARLY INTERVENTION

Early intervention with children who have PDDs can in some cases markedly alter their developmental trajectory. Some of these children can enter a regular kindergarten or first grade following an intensive preschool experience. The most dramatic demonstration of the benefits of early intervention was offered by Lovaas (1987) in his report that nearly half of his young participants with autistic disorder achieved normal intellectual and educational functioning by first grade. Birnbrauer & Leach (1993) found that four of the nine children they studied were approaching normal levels of functioning after 24 months, while only one of five control children made similar progress. Harris et al. (1991) reported a 19 point increase in Stanford Binet IQ after 1 year in an intensive preschool programme for children with autistic disorder.

A number of factors characterize some of the most effective early intervention programmes (Harris & Handleman, 1994). One feature is individualized, comprehensive programming. As noted above, one of the things behavioural technology does well is to study each child and identify the specific strengths and deficits of that child, as well as the contextual variables that influence the child's behaviour. This assessment, when linked to a comprehensive curriculum that meets a range of needs, serves children with PDDs well. The highly effective programmes also emphasize identifying children as early as possible, and working with them in a very favourable teacher to child ratio, often one to one in the early stages. Most effective programmes also have a highly systematic approach to helping children with autistic disorder and related conditions learn to interact with peers, and function in the natural environment of childhood. As discussed above, peers can play an integral role in this treatment.

CONTROVERSIAL TREATMENTS

Perhaps because we do not fully understand the aetiologies of the PDDs and are not effective at treating every person with these disorders, there continue to be reports of controversial treatments. Were the PDDs as minor as the common cold or as responsive to treatment as many bacterial infections, few parents or professionals would adopt alternative treatments without rigorous supporting data. One must be cautious of uncontrolled case reports of dramatic changes in persons with PDDs. Skepticism is especially in order when these reports make no sense on theoretical grounds or in terms of our knowledge of PDDs, or when disinterested scientists can not replicate the finding. Those principles are part of the 'common sense' of science, but still get brushed aside by some.

Facilitated communication

One current controversial treatment is facilitated communication (Biklen, 1990). Following a great deal of attention in the media, extensive empirical effort was directed toward facilitated communication, a method that provides the nonverbal person with autism an opportunity to communicate through graduated physical guidance at a keyboard or other communication devise (Jacobson et al., 1995). Initial public response to this method was enthusiastic. For example, based on the sophisticated communications which arose using facilitated communication, children with autistic disorder who had been assumed to have co-occurring mental retardation, were moved from specialized to regular classes and a normative curriculum through the support of their facilitator.

In a major review, Jacobson et al. (1995), note that scores of well controlled studies in independent laboratories failed to find that the communications which arise during facilitated communication can be attributed to the person with a PDD. Equally of concern is the repeated finding that it is the facilitator, and not the client, who controls the communication (Montee et al., 1995). Thus, there is reason to question whether children are benefiting from their new educational placements, and whether in fact they are being denied the opportunity to learn essential skills for later life.

Based on their research, Montee et al. (1995: 198) recommend that facilitated communication not be used. They suggest that if individuals are committed to the continuing use of this approach, in spite of the lack of validation, it is essential that ' . . . every communication produced through facilitated communication should be verified through another means . . . ', and that informed consent be required when facilitated communication is attempted. Smith (1996) urges that service providers who rely on facilitated communication be avoided. Given the lack of supporting data and the potential danger of failing to provide an appropriate education, a rigorous assessment of the benefits of facilitated communication for any individual client should be routine if a parent or educator insists upon applying the techniques. The experimental literature has countless models for such an assessment.

Auditory integration training

Auditory integration training (AIT) was initially based on the idea that hypersensitive hearing causes some of the maladaptive behaviours of people with PDDs. It was argued that decreasing this sensitivity by systematic exposure to problematic sound frequencies led to improved behaviour (Stehli, 1991). It is no longer clear whether hypersensitivity plays a major role in predicting response to this treatment (Rimland & Edelson, 1994). During AIT people listen to music electronically modulated, and sometimes filtered, to create what are believed to be therapeutic sounds. Interestingly, questions have been raised about whether filtered sounds are required for the beneficial effects (Rimland & Edelson, 1994; Bettison, 1996). At present this method is still experimental and there are too few data to be certain whether the approach benefits people with PDDs. Some of those who advocate AIT, however, are studying whether and when it might be helpful (Rimland & Edelson, 1995). In the absence of consistently demonstrated benefits it is essential that if AIT is used, data be collected to determine whether a client is benefiting. Unlike facilitated communication, there is no reason to believe that AIT interferes with effective education.

ROLE OF THE FAMILY

Once it was recognized that poor parenting did not cause a child to have a PDD, it became possible to think about parents as partners in a treatment process, rather than as part of the child's problem (Schopler & Reichler, 1971; Lovaas et al., 1973). It was evident that family support was essential if a child's newly learned skills were to be maintained and generalized (Lovaas et al., 1973). Recognition of the crucial role of parents led to research on the most effective ways to teach them behavioural technology (Harris, 1983, 1989; Koegel et al., 1984). That work shows that parents can master essentially any behavioural skill and that their application of these skills can be highly effective, especially when the family is provided with ongoing programming support (Harris, 1986).

Every family which includes a child with a PDD should learn the behavioural teaching strategies to support their child's education; however, it is also important to recognize that being the parent of a child with a PDD is inherently stressful. As a result, parents may require considerable formal and informal support in dealing with the demands imposed on them by their child's unusual needs (Bristol, 1984; Gill & Harris, 1991).

CONCLUSIONS

In the past 25 years there have been major advances in our ability to meet the needs of people with PDDs. Early intervention is especially potent for many young children, but older children, adolescents and adults can also experience a markedly improved quality of life through behavioural technology. One of the challenges facing the field is disseminating this technology as widely as possible to ensure that every young child who requires early intervention, and every older child and adult who needs longer term education and training, has those resources available. Education dollars spent early in the life of a person with a PDD can yield major benefits in both human and economic terms over a lifetime.

REFERENCES

Aiken, J. M. & Salzberg, C. L. (1984). The effects of a sensory extinction procedure on stereotypic sounds of two autistic children. *Journal of Autism and Developmental Disorders*, **14**, 291–9.

Bartak, L. & Rutter, M. (1971). Educational treatment of autistic children. In *Infantile Autism: Concepts, Characteristics and Treatment*, ed. M. L. Rutter, pp. 258–9. Baltimore: Williams & Wilkins.

Belchic, J. K. & Harris, S. L. (1994). The use of multiple peer exemplars to enhance the generalization of play skills to the siblings of children with autism. *Child and Family Behavior Therapy*, **16**, 1–25.

Bettelheim, B. (1967). *The Empty Fortress*. New York: The Free Press.

Bettison, S. (1996). The long-term effects of auditory training on children with autism. *Journal of Autism and Developmental Disorders*, **26**, 361–74.

Biklen, D. (1990). Communication unbound: autism and praxis. *Harvard Educational Review*, **62**, 291–314.

Bird, F., Dores, P. A., Moniz, D. & Robinson, J. (1989). Reducing severe aggressive and self-injurious behaviors with functional communication training. *American Journal on Mental Retardation*, **94**, 37–48.

Birnbrauer, J. S. & Leach, D. J. (1993). The Murdoch early intervention program after 2 years. *Behaviour Change*, **10**, 63–74.

Bristol, M. M. (1984). Family resources and successful adaptation to autistic children. In *The Effects of Autism on the Family*, ed. E. Schopler & G. B. Mesibov, pp. 289–310. New York: Plenum Press.

Carr, E. G. & Durand, V. M. (1985). Reducing behaviour problems through functional communication training. *Journal of Applied Behavior Analysis*, **18**, 111–26.

Charlop, M. H., Schreibman, L. & Thibodeau, M. G. (1985). Increasing spontaneous verbal responding in autistic children using a time delay procedure. *Journal of Applied Behavior Analysis*, **18**, 155–66.

Coe, D., Matson, J., Fee, V., Manikam, R. & Linarello, C. (1990). Training nonverbal and verbal play skills to mentally retarded and autistic children. *Journal of Autism and Developmental Disorders*, **20**, 177–87.

Dugan, E., Kamps, D., Leonard, B., Watkins, N., Rheinberger, A. S. & Stackhaus, J. (1995). Effects of cooperative learning groups during social studies for students with autism and fourth-grade peers. *Journal of Applied Behavior Analysis*, **28**, 175–88.

Durand, V. M. (1990). *Severe Behavior Problems. A Functional Communication Training Approach*. New York: Guilford Press.

Durand, V. M. & Carr, E. G. (1987). Social influences on 'self-stimulatory' behavior: analysis and treatment application. *Journal of Applied Behavior Analysis*, **20**, 119–32.

Durand, V. M. & Carr, E. G. (1991). Functional communication training to reduce challenging behavior: maintenance and application in new settings. *Journal of Applied Behavior Analysis*, **24**, 251–64.

Dyer, K., Dunlap, G. & Winterling, V. (1990). Effects of choice making on the serious problem behaviors of students with severe handicaps. *Journal of Applied Behavior Analysis*, **23**, 515–24.

Ferster, C. B. (1961). Positive reinforcement and behavioral deficits of autistic children. *Child Development*, **32**, 437–56.

Fisher, W. W., Ninness, H. A. C., Piazza, C. C. & Owen-DeSchryver, J. S. (1996). On the reinforcing effects of the content of verbal attention. *Journal of Applied Behavior Analysis*, **29**, 235–8.

Frisch, S. A. & Schumaker, J. B. (1974). Training generalized receptive prepositions in retarded children. *Journal of Applied Behavior Analysis*, **7**, 611–21.

Gena, A., Krantz, P. J., McClannahan, L. E. & Poulson, C. L. (1996). Training and generalization of affective behavior displayed by youths with autism. *Journal of Applied Behavior Analysis*, **29**, 291–304.

Gill, M. J. & Harris, S. L. (1991). Hardiness and social support as predictors of psychological discomfort in mothers of children with autism. *Journal of Autism and Developmental Disorders*, **21**, 407–16.

Goh, H. L., Iwata, B. A., Shore, B. A., DeLeon, I. G., Lerman, D., Ulrich, S. M. & Smith, R. G. (1995). An analysis of the reinforcing properties of hand mouthing. *Journal of Applied Behavior Analysis*, **28**, 269–83.

Guess, D., Sailor, W., Rutherford, G. & Baer, D. M. (1968). An experimental analysis of linguistic development: the productive use of the plural morpheme. *Journal of Applied Behavior Analysis*, **1**, 297–306.

Happe, F. (1995). *Autism. An Introduction to Psychological Theory.* Cambridge MA: Harvard University Press.

Haring, T. G. & Breen, C. G. (1992). A peer-mediated social network intervention to enhance the social integration of persons with moderate and severe disabilities. *Journal of Applied Behavior Analysis,* **25,** 319–33.

Haring, T. G. & Kennedy, C. H. (1990). Contextual control of problem behaviors in students with severe disabilities. *Journal of Applied Behavior Analysis,* **23,** 235–43.

Harris, S. L. (1975). Teaching language to nonverbal children: with emphasis on problems of generalization. *Psychological Bulletin,* **82,** 564–80.

Harris, S. L. (1983). *Families of the Developmentally Disabled: a Guide to Behavioral Intervention.* Elmsford, New York: Pergamon Press.

Harris, S. L. (1986). Parents as teachers: a four to seven year follow up of parents of children with autism. *Child and Family Behavior Therapy,* **8,** 39–47.

Harris, S. L. (1989). Training parents of children with autism: an update on models. *Behavior Therapist,* **12,** 219–21.

Harris, S. L. (1995). Educational strategies in autism. In *Learning and Cognition in Autism,* ed. E. Schopler & G. B. Mesibov, pp. 293–309. New York: Plenum.

Harris, S. L. & Ferrari, M. (1983). Developmental factors in child behavior therapy. *Behavior Therapy,* **14,** 54–72.

Harris, S. L. & Handleman, J. S. (eds) (1994). *Preschool Education Programs for Children with Autism.* Austin TX: Pro-Ed.

Harris, S. L., Handleman, J. S. & Alessandri, M. (1990). Teaching youths with autism to offer assistance. *Journal of Applied Behavior Analysis,* **23,** 297–305.

Harris, S. L., Handleman, J. S., Gordon, R., Kristoff, B. & Fuentes, F. (1991). Changes in cognitive and language functioning of preschool children with autism. *Journal of Autism and Developmental Disorders,* **21,** 281–90.

Hobson, P. (1993). *Autism and the Development of Mind.* Hillsdale, New Jersey: Lawrence Earlbaum Associates.

Jacobson, J. W., Mulick, J. A. & Schwartz, A. A. (1995). A history of facilitated communication. Science, pseudoscience, and antiscience. Science working group on facilitated communication. *American Psychologist,* **50,** 750–65.

Kamps, D. M., Barbetta, P. M., Leonard, B. R. & Delquadri, J. (1994). Classwide peer tutoring: an integration strategy to improve reading skills and promote peer interactions among students with autism and general education peers. *Journal of Applied Behavior Analysis,* **27,** 49–61.

Koegel, R. L., O'Dell, M. & Dunlap, G. (1988). Producing speech use in nonverbal autistic children by reinforcing attempts. *Journal of Autism and Developmental Disorders,* **18,** 525–38.

Koegel, R. L., O'Dell, M. C. & Koegel, L. K. (1987). A natural language teaching paradigm for nonverbal autistic children. *Journal of Autism and Developmental Disorders,* **17,** 187–200.

Koegel, R. L., Schreibman, L., Johnson, J., O'Neill, R. E. & Dunlap, G. (1984). Collateral effects of parent training on families of autistic children. In *Parent Training: Foundations of Research and Practice,* ed. R. F. Dangel & R. A. Polster, pp. 358–78. New York: Guilford Press.

Lalli, J. S., Casey, S. & Kates, K. (1995). Reducing escape behavior and increasing task completion with functional communication training, extinction, and response chaining. *Journal of Applied Behavior Analysis,* **28,** 261–8.

Leslie, A. M. (1987). Pretence and representation: the origins of 'theory of mind'. *Psychological Review,* **94,** 412–26.

Lord, C. & Hopkins, J. M. (1986). The social behavior of autistic children with younger and same-age nonhandicapped peers. *Journal of Autism and Developmental Disorders,*

16, 249–62.

Lovaas, O. I. (1987). Behavioral treatment and normal educational and intellectual functioning in young autistic children. *Journal of Consulting and Clinical Psychology*, **55**, 3–9.

Lovaas, O. I., Berberich, J. P., Perloff, B. F. & Schaeffer, B. (1966). Acquisition of imitative speech by schizophrenic children. *Science*, **151**, 705–7.

Lovaas, O. I., Koegel, R. L., Simmons, J. Q. & Long, J. S. (1973). Some generalization and follow-up measures on autistic children in behavior therapy. *Journal of Applied Behavior Analysis*, **6**, 131–66.

McEvoy, M. A., Nordquist, V. M., Twardosz, S., Heckaman, K. A., Wehby, J. H. & Denny, R. K. (1988). Promoting autistic children's peer interactions in an integrated early childhood setting using affection activities. *Journal of Applied Behavior Analysis*, **21**, 193–200.

McGee, G. G., Almeida, M. C., Sulzer-Azaroff, B. & Feldman, R. S. (1992). Prompting reciprocal interactions via peer incidental teaching. *Journal of Applied Behavior Analysis*, **25**, 117–26.

McGee, G. G., Krantz, P. J., Mason, D. & McClannahan, L. E. (1983). A modified incidental-teaching procedure for autistic youth: acquisition and generalization of receptive object labels. *Journal of Applied Behavior Analysis*, **16**, 329–38.

Mash, E. J. & Terdal, L. G. (1988). Behavioral assessment of child and family disturbance. In *Behavioral Assessment of Childhood Disorders*, 2nd edn, ed. E. J. Mash & L. G. Terdal, pp. 3–65. New York: Guilford.

Mesibov, G. B. (1984). Social skills training with verbal autistic adolescents and adults: a program model. *Journal of Autism and Developmental Disorders*, **14**, 395–404.

Montee, B. B., Miltenberger, R. G. & Wittrock, D. (1995). An experimental analysis of facilitated communication. *Journal of Applied Behavior Analysis*, **28**, 189–200.

Odom, S. L., Hoyson, M., Jamieson, B. & Strain, P. S. (1985). Increasing handicapped preschoolers' peer social interactions: cross-setting and component analysis. *Journal of Applied Behavior Analysis*, **18**, 3–16.

Odom, S. L. & Strain, P. S. (1986). A comparison of peer-initiation and teacher-antecedent intervention for promoting reciprocal social interaction of autistic preschoolers. *Journal of Applied Behavior Analysis*, **19**, 59–71.

O'Neill, R. E., Horner, R. H., Albin, R. W., Storey, K. & Sprague, J. R., (1990). *Functional Analysis of Problem Behavior*. Sycamore IL: Sycamore.

Pierce, K. & Schreibman, L. (1995). Increasing complex social behaviors in children with autism: effects of peer-implemented pivotal response training. *Journal of Applied Behavior Analysis*, **28**, 285–95.

Rimland, B. (1964). *Infantile Autism*. New York: Appleton-Century-Crofts.

Rimland, B. & Edelson, S. M. (1994). The effects of auditory integration training on autism. *American Journal of Speech-Language Pathology*, **3**, 16–24.

Rimland, B. & Edelson, S. M. (1995). Auditory integration training in autism: a pilot study. *Journal of Autism and Developmental Disorders*, **25**, 61–70.

Sasso, G. M. & Rude, H. A. (1987). Unprogrammed effects of training high-status peers to interact with severely handicapped children. *Journal of Applied Behavior Analysis*, **20**, 35–44.

Schopler, E. & Reichler, R. J. (1971). Parents as cotherapists in the treatment of psychotic children. *Journal of Autism and Childhood Schizophrenia*, **1**, 87–102.

Smith, T. (1996). Are other treatments effective? In *Behavioral Intervention for Young Children with Autism*, ed. C. Maurice, G. Green & S. C. Luce, pp. 45–59. Austin TX: Pro-Ed.

Stahmer, A. C. (1995). Teaching symbolic play skills to children with autism using pivotal response training. *Journal of Autism and Developmental Disorders*, **25**, 123–41.

Stehli, A. (1991). *The Sound of a Miracle: a Child's Triumph Over Autism.* New York: Doubleday.

Strain, P. S., Shores, R. E. & Kerr, M. M. (1976). An experimental analysis of 'spill over' effects on the social interaction of behaviorally handicapped preschool children. *Journal of Applied Behavior Analysis*, **9**, 31–40.

Strain, P. S. & Timm, M. A. (1974). An experimental analysis of social interaction between a behaviorally disordered preschool child and her classroom peers. *Journal of Applied Behavior Analysis*, **7**, 583–90.

Taylor, B. A. & Harris, S. L. (1995). Teaching children with autism to seek information: acquisition of novel information and generalization of responding. *Journal of Applied Behavior Analysis*, **28**, 3–14.

Thorp, D. M., Stahmer, A. C. & Schreibman, L. (1995). Effects of sociodramatic play training on children with autism. *Journal of Autism and Developmental Disorders*, **25**, 265–82.

Tustin, R. D. (1995). The effects of advance notice of activity transition on stereotypic behavior. *Journal of Applied Behavior Analysis*, **28**, 91–2.

Twardosz, S. & Baer, D. M. (1973). Training two severely retarded adolescents to ask questions. *Journal of Applied Behavior Analysis*, **6**, 655–61.

Van Houten, R. V., Axelrod, S., Bailey, J. S., Favell, J. E., Foxx, R. M., Iwata, B. A. & Lovaas, O. I. (1988). The right to effective behavioral treatment. *Journal of Applied Behavior Analysis*, **21**, 381–4.

Wacker, D. P., Harding, J., Cooper, L. J., Derby, K. M., Peck, S., Asmus, J., Berg, W. K. & Brown, K. A. (1996). The effects of meal schedule and quantity on problematic behavior. *Journal of Applied Behavior Analysis*, **29**, 79–87.

Wacker, D. P., Steege, M. W., Northup, J., Sasso, G., Berg, W., Reimers, T., Cooper, L., Cigrand, K. & Donn, L. (1990). A component analysis of functional communication training across three topographies of severe behavior problems. *Journal of Applied Behavior Analysis*, **23**, 417–29.

Williams, T. I. (1989). A social skills group for autistic children. *Journal of Autism and Developmental Disorders*, **19**, 143–55.

Zanolli, K., Daggett, J. & Adams, T. (1996). Teaching preschool age autistic children to make spontaneous initiations to peers using priming. *Journal of Autism and Developmental Disorders*, **26**, 407–22.

Zarcone, J. R., Fisher, W. W. & Piazza, C. C. (1996). Analysis of free-time contingencies as positive versus negative reinforcement. *Journal of Applied Behavior Analysis*, **29**, 247–50.

8

Outcome in adult life for people with autism and Asperger's syndrome

Patricia Howlin and Susan Goode

ACCOUNTS OF ADULTS WITH AUTISM

Despite the ever increasing numbers of publications on the topic of autism, relatively little has been written about the outcome in adulthood. More-over, the accounts that are available can present a very confusing picture to families seeking to know what may become of their son or daughter as they grow older. On the one hand, the problems shown by adults with autism often feature prominently in books or papers dealing with 'Challenging Behaviours'. Similarly, lurid accounts of crimes committed by individuals with Asperger's syndrome appear from time to time in daily newspapers. In contrast, there are also impressive personal narratives, such as those by Donna Williams (Williams, 1992, 1994) or Temple Grandin (Grandin, 1995; Grandin & Scariano, 1986), documenting how individuals have set out successfully to overcome their early handicaps. Occasionally reports also appear of individuals with autism who, although remaining generally disabled, show remarkable skill in certain specific areas, such as art, music or calculations (Wiltshire, 1987; O'Connor & Hermelin, 1988).

In fact, few individuals with autism fall into any of these categories but families are provided with very little guidance or information on what the future is likely to hold. Many come to dread the onset of adolescence, in particular, fearing that this is certain to bring increased difficulties and almost all parents have serious concerns about the ability of their son or daughter to cope when they are no longer there to care for them.

Over the past few decades there has been a number of studies that have followed up individuals with autism as they reach adolescence or adulthood. Drawing firm conclusions from these studies is not easy because of the limited numbers of studies involved (long term research is costly and fraught with a host of problems), the small sample size and heterogeneity of subjects, and the variability of outcome measures. Despite these caveats, the findings do provide important information for individuals with autism and their families.

The first descriptive studies

In the mid to late 1950s there began to appear a number of studies on prognosis in 'childhood psychosis', 'early childhood schizophrenia' or 'infantile autism'. On reading these reports, it is apparent that many of the subjects involved showed the characteristic symptoms of autism. The heterogeneity of the groups, in terms of age, intellectual level, diagnosis and aetiology, however, made the interpretation of outcome data extremely difficult. Thus, Lotter (1978) reviewing a total of 25 follow up studies of 'psychotic children' concluded that the majority suffered from such serious flaws in research design (including inadequate diagnostic criteria, subjective reporting or very mixed subject groups) that 'very little could be concluded about prognosis'.

One of the earliest reports focusing on children who clearly met diagnostic criteria for autism was that of Eisenberg (1956). Although the account is largely anecdotal, with many cases still in their early teens when assessed, Eisenberg, like many subsequent authors, documented the wide variety of possible outcomes. Many of the individuals described remained very dependent but about one-third were found to have made 'at least a moderate social adjustment', despite the lack of any specialist provision or treatment available at that time. A minority had managed to achieve good independence, although even among this group social impairments remained apparent. As an illustration of this Eisenberg cites the case of one young man who, called upon to speak as a student leader at a football rally, announced (with undeniable accuracy) that his team was going to lose.

In a slightly later report from Britain, Creak (1963) describes 100 cases of 'childhood psychosis'. Again the information is very anecdotal and because the figures do not distinguish clearly between adult and child cases the longer term outcome remains unclear. Out of the total sample, 43 were living in institutional care, 40 remained at home attending school or day centres and 17 were coping with mainstream schooling or employment.

By far the most fascinating and detailed accounts of this period are those of Kanner himself (1943, 1949, 1973). Kanner kept meticulous records of what happened to the children under his care and he followed up many into their twenties and beyond. He, too, noted the great variability in outcome and, like Eisenberg before him, stressed the importance of well developed communication skills and intellectual ability for a good prognosis. Individuals who remained mute had the least favourable outcome. The majority of this group remained highly dependent as they grew older, living either with their parents, in sheltered communities, in state institutions for people with learning disabilities or in psychiatric hospitals. Among cases with better communication skills outcome was rather more positive. Just over half of this group was functioning relatively well at home or in the community, although with varying degrees of support (Kanner & Eisenberg, 1956).

Of special interest is Kanner's account of 96 individuals, first seen before 1953, and in their twenties and thirties when followed up (Kanner, 1973; Kanner & Eisenberg, 1956). Twelve cases were reported to have done remarkably well as they grew older, and as 'mingling, working and maintaining themselves in society'.* Kanner also notes that in the majority of these cases 'a remarkable change took place' around their mid-teens. 'Unlike most other autistic children they became uneasily aware of their peculiarities and began to make a conscious effort to do something about them'. In particular, they tried to improve their interactions with their peers, often using their obsessional preoccupations or special skills 'to open a door for contact'.

Among these more successful individuals, 11 had jobs (ranging from an accountant, a laboratory technician and a meteorologist in the navy, to dishwashing and shelf stacking) and one was still at college. Jobs were often at a lower level than the individuals' qualifications might have predicted. One young woman who was training to be a nurse failed because she would stick rigidly to rules. Thus, having been told that 20 minutes was the usual time it took for breast feeding, she would remove babies from their mothers' breast if they exceeded this. She later succeeded as a hospital laboratory technician. Another individual, with a postgraduate degree in economics, was working as an accounts clerk because he could not cope with the managerial demands of a higher level job. Yet another, with a BA degree in history, had a 'blue collar job' in a horticultural research station and was much disappointed at his failure to work with 'educated people'.

Seven of the group had their own homes and one individual (who was also a successful music composer) was married with a child. The remainder

* Two other cases are also noted. One, formerly attending college, could no longer be traced, and a 'gifted student of mathematics' had been killed in an accident.

lived with their parents. Although many belonged to social groups or clubs (involving singing, hiking, sport, transport, bridge or the church) few had any close or intimate relationships. Several explained this on the grounds that women 'cost too much money' or that it would not be worthwhile to 'waste money on a girl who isn't serious'.

Asperger' accounts

Writing at much the same time as Kanner, Asperger also noted the very variable outcome among the individuals he studied. The least favourable outcome was for those with learning disabilities in addition to their autism and Asperger commented that 'the fate of the latter cases is often very sad'. For those more able individuals who did make progress it was, again, often their special skills or interests that eventually led to social integration. Asperger quotes examples of many individuals who had done remarkably well in later life, including a professor of astronomy, mathematicians, technologist, chemists, high ranking civil servants and an expert in heraldry. Indeed he suggests that:

able autistic individuals can rise to eminent positions and perform with such outstanding success that one may even conclude that *only* such people are capable of certain achievements. It is as if they had compensatory abilities to counterbalance their deficiencies. Their unswerving determination and penetrating intellectual powers . . . their narrowness and single mindedness . . . can be immensely valuable and lead to outstanding achievements in their chosen areas. (For an annotated translation of Asperger's initial paper, see Frith, 1991).

Autobiographical writings

Personal accounts also illustrate the mixture of success and difficulties encountered by individuals with autism. Donna Williams, who now makes an independent living as an author, writes movingly of her journey from *Nobody Nowhere* (1992) to *Somebody Somewhere* (1994). Misunderstood, often mistreated, as a child by her teachers, her family and her peers, in adulthood her great strength and determination, the eventual support of an understanding psychologist and her contacts with individuals similarly affected have resulted in considerable personal and professional success. Nevertheless, it is evident that life remains a continuing battle:

Autism tries to stop me from being free to be myself. Autism tries to rob me of a life, of friendship, of caring, of sharing, of showing interest, of using my intelligence, of being affected . . . it tries to bury me alive.

Temple Grandin, a woman in her mid-forties, has carved out for herself a successful career as an animal psychologist, designing livestock handling facilities for farms and meatpacking plants (Sacks, 1993; Grandin, 1995). Many of her designs have been developed from the 'squeeze machines' that she first began to construct while she was at school. Although she continues to have difficulties in understanding ordinary social relationships and feelings, describing herself in many ways like 'an anthropologist on Mars' (Sacks, 1993) she has clearly come a long way from her confused, withdrawn, noncommunicating early childhood.

For some, however, the struggle against autism seems almost unbearable. Despite successfully obtaining postgraduate qualifications in psychology and living independently, Therese Jolliffe writes:

no one really understands what the emotional suffering of a person with autism is like, and there is no pain killer, injection or operation that can get rid of it or even . . . relieve it a little. Autism affects everything all the time (even) your dreams . . . sometimes it gets too much, then people say they are surprised when I get angry. Life is such a struggle; indecision over things that other people refer to as trivial results in an awful lot of distress . . . I constantly labour, in a cognitive sense, over what may or may not occur . . . It is the confusion that results from not being able to understand the world around me which I think causes all the fear. This fear then brings a need to withdraw. (Jolliffe et al., 1992).

Various other accounts of the personal experience of autism have been published (Bemporad, 1979; Volkmar & Cohen, 1985; Cesaroni & Garber, 1991; Schopler & Mesibov, 1992). Although autobiographical writings by people with autism remain fascinating, partly because they are so unusual and partly because of what they reveal about the ways in which these individuals think, feel and understand, the accounts give little indication of what happens to most people with autism as they grow older. In order to investigate this, larger scale and long term follow up studies are required.

Early follow up reports

Initial studies of the outcome for children with autism were, as noted above, largely anecdotal and unsystematic. Towards the end of the 1960s, Rutter and his colleagues carried out a detailed assessment of 63 individuals, initially diagnosed as autistic at the Maudsley hospital in London in the 1950s and early 1960s. At follow up, 38 individuals were aged 16 years or over. Of these two were still at school, but of the remainder only three had paid jobs. Over half were placed in long stay hospitals, seven were still living with their parents with no outside occupation, three were living in special communities and four attended day centres. Rutter notes that several individuals living at home or in a Special Community could have been capable of employment 'at least in a sheltered setting, had adequate training facilities been available'. General outcome for the adult cases in this study is not differentiated from that for the under 16s, but overall only 14% of the group was said to have made a good social adjustment. Nevertheless, most individuals tended to improve with age, and although there was a number of cases who showed a worsening in certain aspects of behaviour over time 'it was rare to see marked remissions and relapses as in adult psychotic illnesses.' No significant sex differences were found, although girls were somewhat less likely to fall within the good or very poor groups (Rutter & Lockyer, 1967; Rutter et al., 1967; Lockyer & Rutter, 1969, 1970).

Although a number of other follow up studies appeared around this time (Mittler et al., 1966; DeMeyer et al. 1973) most of the individuals involved were still in their early teens, so that they contain little information on later outcome and progress. The first study to look specifically at outcome in an older age group was that of Lotter (1974a,b). Twenty-nine young people between the ages of 16 and 18 years who had been diagnosed as autistic when younger were assessed. In general, the findings were similar to those of Rutter and his colleagues although many more children (24%) were still at school, reflecting improvements in educational provision over the previous decade (less than half of the children seen by Rutter had received as much as 2 year's schooling and many had never attended school at all). Nevertheless, among the 22 individuals who had left school only one had a job. Almost half the sample was in long stay hospital provision; two individuals were living at home and five were attending day training centres. In terms of overall social adjustment, 14% were described as having done well, although the majority were described as having a 'poor' or 'very poor' outcome. Overall, girls did less well, with none being rated as attaining either a good or fair outcome.

Factors related to outcome

In all these early follow up studies three particular factors were consistently associated with later prognosis. The first, noted initially by Eisenberg, was the importance of early language development. For individuals who had developed some useful speech by the age of around 5 years outcome tended to be much more favourable. Only a tiny minority of children who remained without speech after this age made significant improvements. The degree of intellectual impairment was another crucial factor. Children who were either untestable or who had nonverbal IQ scores below the range of 55–60, almost invariably remained highly dependent. The third major factor was that of education. Kanner (1973) noted that admission into hospital care rather than a school placement was 'tantamount to a death sentence' and subsequent studies, particularly those of Rutter and Lotter, also noted the association between years of schooling and later outcome. As educational placement is directly affected by factors such as language and IQ, however, the influence of schooling per se on long term functioning remains somewhat unclear.

The impact of other factors, such as the severity of autistic symptomatology, early behavioural difficulties, family factors or the sex of the child also remains uncertain. Rutter and colleagues found no significant correlation between individual symptoms (other than lack of speech) and later outcome, although there was a significant relation with the total number of major symptoms rated. Thus, hardly surprisingly, the more severe the social and behavioural problems, the worse the ultimate outcome.

The relation with gender is also unclear. Rutter found that girls fell neither in the very good nor very poor categories, although Lotter reported that the outcome for girls was generally worse than for boys. Again the impact of intellectual level needs to be taken into account here as there is some indication from the studies of Catherine Lord and colleagues that females with autism may tend to have a lower IQ than males (Lord & Schopler, 1985).

As far as family factors were concerned, while socio-economic factors and ratings of family adequacy may be correlated with outcome (DeMeyer et al., 1973; Lotter, 1974a), there is little evidence of a direct causal relation between an impoverished or disruptive family background and later outcome, although, as with any other condition, disruption at home is unlikely to be beneficial.

Later follow up studies

Throughout the 1980s and 1990s there has been a number of follow up studies or reports of adults with autism. As many of these have involved subjects who were still relatively young, or have focused more specifically on high functioning individuals, the implications for older people within the wider autistic spectrum are somewhat limited.

Chung et al. (1990), for example, followed up 66 children attending a psychiatric clinic in Hong Kong in the decade from 1976. As in other studies, the best outcome was found for cases who had developed speech before the age of 5 years, and who scored more highly on tests of intellectual and social functioning. As only nine cases were above 12 years old, there is no information about longer term outcome.

Gillberg & Steffenberg (1987) report on a group of 23 individuals aged 16 years or over living in Sweden. Only one person was found to be fully self-supporting at the time of follow up, although the authors suggest that the numbers may increase with time (only one-third of the group was then aged over 20 years). Of the remainder, almost half were described as functioning fairly well, but 11 individuals had a 'poor' or 'very poor' outcome. As in other studies, an IQ above 50 at initial diagnosis and the presence of communicative speech before the age of 6 years were the most important prognostic indicators. In some, but not all cases, the development of epilepsy around puberty seemed to result in a worse outcome. Again, women tended to have a 'very poor' outcome more frequently than men.

A much larger study of young adults with autism (170 males, 31 females), aged between 18 and 33 years, was conducted by Kobayashi and colleagues (1992) in Japan. Outcome was assessed by means of postal questionnaires to parents. The average follow up period was 15 years, during which time four cases, all male, had died (one of encephalopathy age 6; head injury from severe self-injury age 16; nephrotic syndrome age 20; and asthma age 22). Almost half the group was reported as having good or very good communication skills, and over a quarter were described as having a good or very good outcome (i.e. able to live independently or semi-independently and succeeding at work or college). Women tended to have better language outcomes than men but there were no significant differences in social functioning between the sexes.

Forty-three individuals were employed, with a further 11 still attending school or college. Jobs were mostly in food and service industries but several individuals were described as having realized 'their childhood dreams' of being a bus conductor, car mechanic or cook. The highest level of jobs obtained were a physiotherapist, a civil servant, a printer and two office workers. All but three of those with jobs still lived with their parents; one was in a group home and two had their own apartments; none was married.

Approximately one-fifth of the sample had developed epilepsy (usually in their early teens) but this was well controlled in all but three cases. Seventy-three families reported a marked improvement occurring in their children between the ages of around 10–15 years, the period when Kanner too, had remarked on significant change. In 47 cases, however, deterioration in behaviour (such as destructiveness, aggression, self-injury, obsessionality, overactivity, etc.) was noted and these changes also tended to occur around early adolescence. As in other studies, outcome in adulthood was significantly correlated with early language abilities and intellectual functioning in males; however, there was no significant correlation with early language in females, and the correlation with IQ was also small. Generally the outcome for females was less good than for males.

Although, by virtue of its size, this remains a very informative study, reliance on questionnaire data, with little or no direct contact with the autistic individuals themselves, clearly raises problems. Parents' ratings of how well their children are functioning may not always accurately reflect their true status. Moreover, there is no current confirmation of diagnosis, and this is an important omission as diagnostic criteria have changed somewhat since the cases were initially identified.

In a more recent London based study (Goode et al., 1994), parents and individuals were all interviewed independently, diagnostic criteria were reconfirmed and detailed assessments were carried out of language, cognitive, social and academic functioning. Seventy-five individuals aged 21 years or older were involved in total (62 males and 13 females), the average age being 29 years. Eight individuals were living independently or semi-independently, but a third were still with their parents and 40% lived in sheltered communities, mostly specifically for people with autism. Ten individuals were in long stay hospital care.

Despite the fact that one-fifth had obtained some formal qualifications before leaving school (seven had attended college or university) employment levels were generally disappointing. Only seven individuals were in regular, paid employment and one was self-employed; four others worked in a voluntary capacity and a few (15%) were in some form of sheltered occupation. Two-thirds attended day or residential centres where there was little scope for the development of competitive work skills.

In terms of social functioning, a quarter of the group was described as having some friends, with 14 individuals showing evidence of shared enjoyment or closer intimacy. One individual was married, although he later divorced, and another has married more recently. Almost two-thirds had no friends at all.

A composite rating of outcome, based on social interactions, level of independence and occupational status, indicated that 15 individuals could be described as having a 'good' or 'very good' outcome. Most of these had some friends and either had a job or were undergoing training. Even if they still lived at home they had a relatively high level of independence, being largely responsible for their own finances, buying their own clothes or taking independent holidays. Eighteen individuals continued to be moderately dependent on their families or other carers for support, and few in this group had any close friendships. The remainder of the sample was highly dependent, living either in special residential units or long term hospital care. None of those who had 'good' or 'fair' outcomes were women. Preliminary data analyses also indicate that early language and cognitive levels were highly predictive of later success.

Outcome for more able individuals

In recent years, there has been a number of accounts focusing specifically on more able individuals with autism or Asperger's syndrome. Rumsey and his colleagues (Rumsey et al., 1985) followed up 14 young men aged between 18 and 39 years of age, all of whom fulfilled the *Diagnostic and Statistical Manual of Mental Disorders* (DSM-III) criteria for autism, and several of whom had initially been diagnosed by Kanner himself. Nine were described as high functioning, with verbal IQs well within the normal range. In the 'lower functioning' group, three were of normal nonverbal IQ but had continuing language impairments; two were also mildly intellectually impaired.

Socially, all the individuals continued to have marked difficulties. Most were described as 'loners'; none was married and only one had friends (mostly through his church). Even among the intellectually more able, several continued to show socially inappropriate behaviours and half the group exhibited peculiar use of language, such as stereotyped and repetitive speech or talking to themselves.

Academically, those in the 'lower functioning' group had needed specialist education into late adolescence, but all had achieved basic reading, writing and mathematical skills. In the higher ability group, only one had remained in specialist educational provision, five had completed high school and two had attended junior college; several showed good ability in mathematics and two in foreign languages. Nevertheless, assessment of social outcomes, as measured by the Vineland Social Maturity Scale, indicated that their scores here were often 'strikingly' low in relation to IQ. Problems among the more able group were generally related to deficits in the areas of self-direction, socialization and occupational achievements. Similar difficulties were found in those who were less able but they also had additional impairments in communication and independence of travel.

In terms of independent living, six individuals in the more able group still lived with their parents and two were in supervised apartments; only one lived entirely alone. In the less able group none was living independently; three lived with their families, one was in group home and one in a state hospital. With the exception of one person who was unemployed, all the 'lower ability' group were attending a sheltered workshop or special job programme. Among the others, four were in employment (a janitor, a cab driver, a library assistant and a key punch operator); of the remainder, three were in special training or college courses, one was in a sheltered workshop and one was unemployed. Even among those who had jobs, only two had found these independently and generally 'parents played a major role in finding employers willing to give their sons a chance'.

Szatmari et al. (1989b) working in Toronto, studied a group of 12 males and five females aged 17 years or over, with an average IQ over 90. Educationally, half the group had received special schooling but the other half had attended college or university, with six obtaining a degree or equivalent qualification. Two were unemployed and four were in sheltered workshop schemes; three were still studying; one worked in the family business and six were in regular, fulltime employment. One was a librarian, another a physics tutor, two were salesmen with semi-managerial positions, one worked in a factory and one was a library technician. In contrast with some other studies (presumably because the ability range was relatively restricted) little or no relation was found between early measures of language or social behaviour and later functioning although there was a high and significant correlation between current IQ and social functioning as measured by the Vineland.

In terms of independent functioning, ten of the 16 cases still lived at home and one was in a group home but five lived independently and a further three individuals living at home were said by their parents to be completely independent. Only one individual was felt to need constant supervision at home, one required moderate care and six required some minimal supervision. Socially, nine individuals had never had a sexual relationship with anyone of the opposite sex but a quarter of the group had dated regularly or had long term relationships; one was married.

The authors are open about the problems related to the study, including the small sample size (compounded by a high refusal rate) and, because of the group's high IQ, a lack of representativeness for autistic individuals as a whole. Nevertheless, they note that outcome is not necessarily as gloomy as many earlier studies had indicated. They conclude: 'A small percentage of nonretarded autistic children . . . can be expected to recover to a substantial degree. It may take years to occur, and the recovery may not always be complete, but substantial improvement does occur'.

Another Canadian based study (Venter et al., 1992) has also focused on intellectually able children, although the findings concentrate more on intellectual and academic attainments rather than overall functioning. Fifty-eight children (35 males and 23 females) with an average full scale IQ of 79, and a mean age of just under 15 years were involved. The authors found a marked improvement in children's academic attainments compared with the earlier follow up studies of Rutter and Bartak in the mid-1970s (Rutter & Bartak, 1973; Bartak & Rutter, 1978). Thus, even among the lower functioning group, over half could read and do simple arithmetic compared to about one-fifth in the studies conducted 20 years ago.

Twenty-two individuals in the study were aged 18 years or over; of these six were competitively employed and 13 were in sheltered employment or special training programmes. Only three had no occupation. Nevertheless, all those who were employed were in relatively low level jobs and all but one had required special assistance in finding employment. Two of the three individuals not involved in any adult programme were female, and all of the competitively employed people were male. No individual was married, and only two lived alone, one of these with considerable support from his mother. Four people lived in apartments with minimal supervision.

In a further study based at the Maudsley Hospital, London (Mawhood, 1995) the outcome for 19 autistic young men was studied in great detail, as part of a comparative follow up study of individuals with autism and developmental language disorders. Individuals had initially been seen between the ages of 4 and 9 years and all had a nonverbal IQ within the normal range. At follow up, the average performance IQ of the group remained well within the normal range and five individuals had attended college or university. Despite this they showed continuing problems in social relationships, and most remained very dependent. Only three individuals were living independently, one of these in sheltered accommodation; three had jobs (two of these under special arrangements); non had married and only three were described as having close friendships. Almost half the group was said never to have had any friends and about one-third had 'acquaintances' only. Fifteen subjects had never had either a close friendship or a sexual relationship. Thirteen were still described as having moderate to severe behavioural difficulties, associated with obsessional or ritualistic tendencies. A composite rating of outcome, based on communication skills, friendships, levels of independence and behavioural difficulties indicated that overall only three subjects were considered to have a good outcome; two remained moderately impaired and 14 continued to show substantial impairments.

Tantam (1986) describes outcome in 46 individuals with Asperger's syndrome, with an average age of 24 years. Despite being of normal intellectual ability, only two had any education after school and only four were in jobs. One individual was married but most continued to live with their parents or in residential care. A somewhat similar group of 93 young adults was described by Newson and her colleagues in 1982. Unfortunately, formal diagnostic and IQ data are lacking, but rather more had received further education, 22% were in jobs and 7% lived independently. Only one individual was married and although 15% were reported to have had heterosexual relationships, at an average age of 23 years almost three-quarters still lived with their parents.

A summary of the principal follow up studies to date, and the main findings in terms of outcome, are presented in Tables 8.1 and 8.2.

WHAT CAN FOLLOW UP STUDIES TELL US?

Factors related to outcome

Recent studies have tended to confirm the suggestion from early follow up reports that a number of factors related to early development appear to be significantly associated with later outcome. The presence of at least simple communicative language by the age of 5 or 6 years is one of the most important prognostic indicators, as is the ability to score within the mildly retarded range or above on nonverbal tests of ability. There is also some indication from the work of Mawhood (1995) that social development in childhood is related to measures of later social competence.

The presence of relatively good cognitive and communication skills alone does not necessarily guarantee a successful outcome. The presence of additional skills or interests (such as specialized knowledge in particular areas or competence in mathematics, music or computing) which allow individuals to find their own 'niche' in life, and which may enable them to

Table 8.1. *Studies of autism in adult life: 1956–95*

Study	Date	No. of cases	Mean IQ (range)	Mean age (range)
1950–70s				
1. Eisenberg	1956	63	No details	15.0 (9–25)
2. Creak	1963	100	No details	(9–28)
3. Mittler et al.	1966	27	49.7 (24–111)	15.2 (7–27)
4. Rutter et al.	1967	63	72.0	15.7
5. Kanner	1973	96	No details	(?22–39)
6. DeMeyer et al.	1973	126	53.5 (6% 95+; 55% <50)	12.0
7. Lotter	1974a,b	30	71 (55–90)	(16–18)
1980 on				
8. Newson et al.	1982	93	No details	23.0
9. Rumsey et al.	1985	14	97.4 (55–129)	28.0 (18–39)
10. Tantam	1986	46	92.2 VIQ; 86.7 PIQ	24.4
11. Gillberg and Steffenberg	1987	23	26% 70+; 35% 51–70; 39% <51	19.8 (16–23)
12. Szatmari et al.	1989a,b	16	92.4 (68–110)	26.1 (17–34)
13. Chung et al.	1990	66	24% 70+; 56% 35–69; 11% <34	Only 13% >12 years
14. Venter et al.	1992	58	83.31; all >60	14.69
15. Kobayashi et al.	1992	201	24% 70+; 61% 35–69; 16% <34	21.8 (18–33)
16. Goode et al.	1994	75	75	29.8 All 18+
17. Mawhood et al.	1995	19	82.8 (67–117)	23.9 (21–26)

From Howlin (1997).
IQ data generally based on Performance IQ scores.
See notes under Table 8.2.

be more easily integrated into society, also seems to be of prognostic importance (Kanner, 1973).

General outcome and patterns of change over time

Noting that 11–12% of his original sample had done well in the absence of any specialist intervention or support, Kanner speculated that the outcome for people with autism might well improve in future years as recognition of the disorder, and knowledge about causation, and appropriate educational and therapeutic facilities progressed.

Figure 8.1 attempts to summarize the major findings from studies of outcome in adult life. The analysis is split into those studies taking place over the past two decades (i.e. 1980 onwards) and those conducted between 1950 and the end of the 1970s. From this summary it would appear, as Kanner had hoped, that over the years there has been a gradual improvement in the prospects for people with autism.

Comparisons between studies must, of course, be treated with caution. First, the data from the later studies are much more systematic and objective than from earlier ones, and hence it is possible that certain important findings may have been omitted from these. Second, several of the later studies have concentrated on individuals of higher ability and therefore a more favourable outcome would be expected. Nevertheless, there were many individuals in the earlier reports who were of relatively high intellectual ability, and indeed the average nonverbal IQ of subjects in the Rutter and Lotter studies fell just within the normal range (i.e. above 70). Similarly, there were many subjects in the later investigations who were well below average intelligence. Third, overall judgements of whether outcome is 'good', 'moderate' or 'poor' tend to be somewhat subjective, even if attempts are made to quantify what is meant by these terms. (The footnote to Table 8.2 illustrates the very varied ways in which judgements about outcome were reached.) Finally, no doubt because of factors related to the variability in subject selection and assessment, there continue to be considerable differences between studies. Thus, ratings of 'good' to 'fair' outcome range from over 80% to below 30%.

Progress in language

Again, presumably because of the much greater emphasis on the development of communication skills over recent years, there does appear to have been some improvement in this area. Few of the early studies systematically examined language functioning, but in those that did, around 45–50% of cases were reported as having poor or very poor language skills. More recent studies indicate somewhat higher levels of achievement, although again the figures are very variable. Thus, whereas 'good' or 'near normal' language was recorded in over 70% of subjects in the Rumsey study, only 21% of the subjects studied by Mawhood (who were of similar intellectual ability) were rated as achieving this level. Differences are, no doubt, at least partly explained by the different measures used. Ratings in the Rumsey study are based on verbal IQ scores and it is quite possible for able people with autism, even if their conversational skills are limited, to perform well on such tests, as these often involve skills related to general knowledge or memory. Mawhood's data on the other hand, were based on a variety of different measures, including grammatical and pragmatic functions, and were also checked for reliability.

Table 8.2. *Summary of outcomes in follow up studies of autism*

Study	General % good	Outcome fair	Poor[b]	Language % good	Outcome fair	Poor[c]	In job[d] (%)	In own home (%)	In hospital (%)
1950–70s									
1. Eisenberg	5	22	73	—	51	49	—	0	54
2. Creak	17	40	43	—	—	—	—	—	43
3. Mittler	—	26	74	—	—	45	0	0	74
4. Rutter	14	25	61	16	38	46	8	0	53
5. Kanner	11	—	—	—	49	43	11	7	—
6. DeMeyer	10	16	74	6	—	—	0	0	42
7. Lotter	13	23	63	—	—	—	4	0	48
1980–90s									
8. Newson	7	77	16	—	—	—	22	7	—
9. Rumsey	35	35	28	71	14	14	29	21	7
10. Tantam	3	41	53	—	—	—	9	3	—
11. Gillberg	4	48	48	22	48	30	5	5	26
12. Szatmari	38	31	31	50	12	38	47	33	0
13. Chung	32	48	21	—	—	87.5	—	—	0
14. Venter	—	—	—	—	—	—	27	9	0
15. Kobayashi	27	27	46	47	32	21	22	?1	2
16. Goode	20	24	55	—	—	—	23	11	14
17. Mawhood	16	10	74	21	16	63	16	16	5

General Notes to Tables 8.1 and 8.2

— indicates no data available.

[a] IQ data are generally based on Performance IQ scores.

[b] Ratings of Good (or Very good), Fair and Poor (or Very poor) outcomes are generally based on the social outcome criteria suggested by Rutter & Lockyer (1967) and Lotter (1974a) but should be treated with some caution as they are of necessity somewhat subjective and may vary between different studies. Good indicates that the individual is leading a normal or near normal life, with some friendships, and functioning satisfactorily in work. Fair,

indicates that the individual has some degree of independence, although he or she may have no friends and may still be reliant on family for support.

Poor indicates that the individual is heavily dependent on family or is living in residential or hospital care.

cLanguage ratings are based on a variety of different measures (see notes on individual studies). In general, Good indicates useful conversational speech. Fair is some limited use of language to communicate. Poor indicates little or no speech.

dPercentage 'in job' figures are based on subjects over 18 years only.

Notes on individual studies

1, 2 and 5	Accounts are largely anecdotal.
1, 2 and 3	Diagnosis of subjects in these studies subject to some difficulties because strict diagnostic criteria not then established.
2	Two subjects died of neurolipidosis.
4	Percentage figures for those in work or living in an institution are based on the 38 individuals over the age of 16 years. Performance IQ data are based on 29 subjects (Lockyer & Rutter, 1970).
5a and b	One subject died in an accident. Data on follow up of all 96 cases rather sparse. Full details on selected 20 cases only: the original 11 cases seen in 1943, and nine cases later found to be doing particularly well.
6	IQ data based on 87 cases.
7	One subject died of neurological abnormalities.
8	Diagnostic information poor; outcome ratings based on living arrangements only; no data on language/IQ.
9	Outcome ratings based on accounts of occupation and independent living; language ratings based on verbal IQ scores.
10	All diagnosed as having Asperger's syndrome; outcome ratings based on living arrangements only; no data on language.
11	23 other subjects included, but these not clearly autistic; 20 cases over 18 years.
12	Social ratings based on accounts of independence, jobs and social activity; communication based on Vineland scores. 15 cases over 18 years.
13	Percentage in different outcome groups differs from data in original paper because of inconsistencies in the figures. Good/Fair outcome ratings of 80% difficult to reconcile with finding that only 12.5% had a language level over 3 years. Data from this study are omitted from summary figure.
14	22 subjects were aged over 18 years and percentage ratings are based on these cases only.
15	Four subjects had died. Outcome ratings are based on PAL (Present Adaptive Level) scores; Language ratings are based on PLDL (Present Language Developmental Level) scores.
16 and 17	General Outcome and Language ratings based on Composite scores, made up of observational and informant based data, on different aspects of functioning, and with established reliability scores.

The studies of Wolff et al. (1995, 1991) are not included in this summary, because although a number of individuals do seem to have the characteristics of autism or Asperger's syndrome, diagnosis in others is less clear cut.

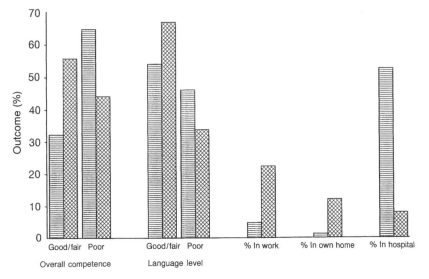

Figure 8.1 Changes in outcome between samples studied pre- and post-1980. Outcome data based only on those studies with adequate information. Study 13 was excluded because of too few adult cases. Percentage totals for good food + fair + poor outcomes do not always equal 100% as some studies were rated on only one of these categories. ☰:pre-1980; ☒: post-1980. From Howlin (1997).

Independent living

Excluding data from the Hong Kong study, because so few subjects had reached adulthood, figures for the proportions in work or living independently also remain very variable. The best outcome was reported in the Canadian study of Szatmari and his coworkers, and although this may be partly understood because of the high ability of the subjects involved, it does not explain why the findings should be considerably better than for the British subjects in the Mawhood study, who were of very similar intellectual levels. It may well be that cultural factors play an important role here as schemes involving supported employment or semi-sheltered living are generally much better established in Canada and the USA than in Britain. The very small number of subjects living independently in the Japanese study is also likely to be related to cultural factors.

One area in which real improvements appear to have taken place is in the proportion of cases placed in long stay hospitals or institutions for people with mental retardation. Over half of all cases studied before 1980 were in long stay hospital provision as adults, whereas in the period after 1980 the figure is around 8%.

There has also been a substantial increase in the numbers of individuals living in their own homes or apartments, either independently or with some minimal supervision. Only Kanner, among the pre-1980 studies, reports on any individuals living in their own homes. In the post-1980 studies an average of around 12% had their own homes. This may not be a particularly high figure but is certainly a great improvement over earlier years.

Work prospects too, seem to have improved, with the average proportion in work rising from around 5% before 1980 to over 20% in the later studies. This figure would be even higher if those in sheltered workshops were also included and very few individuals had no work or training provision of any kind.

Social relationships

Although the quality of relationships has generally not been studied in great detail, in the few investigations to have looked at this crucial aspect of adult life it appears that some individuals are capable of making close relationships. It is true that very few people with autism marry but both Goode and Mawhood found that around 15–20% of subjects were described as having friendships that involved both selectivity and shared enjoyment. A quarter of the subjects studied by Szatmari also had close relationships, and over 40% had had some relationships with members of the opposite sex. Heterosexual relationships were also reported by 15% of subjects studied by Newson and her colleagues.

Are there differences between individuals with autism and Asperger's syndrome?

In reviewing studies of outcome in adult life it did not prove possible systematically to explore differences between these two groups. Diagnostic criteria for Asperger's syndrome tend to differ between studies (for a discussion of diagnostic issues, see Ghaziuddin et al., 1992a; Szatmari et al., 1990; Klin et al., 1995). As Asperger's syndrome was not included as a separate entity in formal classification systems until relatively recently (ICD-10, 1989; DSM-IV, 1994) many earlier studies did not attempt to distinguish between the two conditions. Whether Asperger's syndrome should in the future be distinguished from higher functioning autism remains uncertain. Szatmari et al. (1989b) in an outcome study of 28 children with Asperger's syndrome and 25 high functioning children with autism (mean age 14 and 23 years, respectively) concluded that 'there were no substantive, qualitative differences between the . . . groups'. Klin et al. (1995) remain more cautious and present evidence for a number of possible neuropsychological differences between the two. On the basis of present knowledge, however, there are no data to indicate that outcome does differ between the two groups when IQ is taken into account.

Impact of early intervention on outcome in adult life

Parents of children with autism are faced by bewildering and often conflicting claims about the merits of different interventions. Among the treatments said to have a dramatic impact on outcome are Holding Therapy (Welch, 1988), scotopic sensitivity training (Irlen, 1995), sensory integration (Ayres, 1979), auditory integration (Stehli, 1992), drug and vitamin treatments (Rimland, 1994a,b), music therapy (Alvin & Warwick, 1991), facilitated communication (Biklen, 1990) and intensive behavioural programmes (Lovaas, 1987; McEachin et al., 1993).

Unfortunately, on the whole the more extravagant the promises the more limited are the data on which they are based. Moreover, even when there is evidence of short term gains, reliable information on the impact on adult outcome is generally nonexistent. So far there is no evidence of any cures for autism, any more than there is for other chromosomal or genetically determined conditions such as fragile X or Down's syndrome. The fact that some individuals may be able to attend normal school, or later find jobs or get married, does not mean that they are cured or that the treatment advocated has been responsible for their progress. Many able children do well despite totally inadequate provision and to a great extent eventual outcome is dependent on innate cognitive, linguistic and social abilities. There is little good evidence to suggest that long term outcome can be dramatically improved following the implementation of any particular intervention programme (Howlin & Rutter, 1987). That is not to suggest that appropriate treatment and education have no positive effects. They can make all the difference in helping to minimize or avoid secondary behavioural problems, and can have a significant impact on ensuring that children develop their existing skills to the full. The individuals will continue to be autistic, but the extent to which their social, communication and obsessional difficulties impinge on other areas of functioning, or on family life in general, can be greatly modified.

PSYCHIATRIC DISTURBANCES IN LATER LIFE

Autism and schizophrenia

Despite Kanner's early views on the relation between autism and psycho-sis: 'I do not believe that there is any likelihood that early infantile autism will at any future time have to be separated from the schizophrenias' (1949), later work by Rutter (1972) and Wing (1986) has documented the many crucial differences between the two conditions. Although recent studies by Sula Wolff and her colleagues have again focused on possible links between Asperger's syndrome and schizoid disorders (Wolff & Bar-low, 1979; Wolff, 1991; Wolff & McGuire, 1995) such accounts have been criticized on the grounds that they are 'distressing without being construc-tive' (Wing, 1986).

Of course, there are occasional reports of schizophrenic illness in indi-viduals with autism or Asperger's syndrome. Wolff & McGuire (1995) found that two of 17 girls and two of 32 males with a possible diagnosis of Asperger's syndrome (they were initially diagnosed as 'schizoid') later developed schizophrenia. Clarke and colleagues describe one case of schizophrenia in a group of five young men with autism (Clarke et al., 1989). Wing (1981), in a study of 18 individuals with Asperger's syndrome, describes one with an unconfirmed diagnosis of schizophrenia. Petty et al. (1984) describe three cases in whom early onset schizophrenia seems to have been preceded by autism. There is also a number of single case reports on the comorbidity of the two conditions (Szatmari et al. 1986; Sverd et al., 1993).

As a result of the small size of many of these studies, and the retrospec-tive focus on individuals with psychiatric problems in adulthood, there is little to support claims of 'an excess of schizophrenia in later life' (Wolff & McGuire, 1995). Larger scale follow up studies of children and adolescents with autism have generally failed to find any clear cases of schizophrenia (Chung et al., 1990; Ghaziuddin et al., 1992a). Adult studies have produced similar findings. None of the cases followed up by Kanner over a period of 40 years was reported as showing positive psychiatric symptoms (delusions or hallucinations). Rumsey et al. (1985), in a detailed psychiatric study of 14 young adults, found no evidence of schizophrenia and concluded that 'autistic children do not generally, with any great frequency, develop schizophrenia or other adult psychiatric disorders'. Volkmar & Cohen (1991) found only one individual with an unequivocal diagnosis of schizo-phrenia in a sample of 163 cases. In Goode's study of 74 adults with autism,

229

all over the age of 21 years, none had developed a schizophrenic illness (Goode et al., 1994).

Rates of schizophrenia also appear to be relatively low in studies of more able individuals or those with Asperger's syndrome. Asperger noted that only one of his 200 cases developed schizophrenia (Frith, 1991). Tantam (1991) diagnosed three cases of schizophrenia in 83 individuals with Asperger's syndrome, but notes that this figure is likely to be higher than in an unselected sample because these were all psychiatric referrals. One individual in the Szatmari study of 16 high functioning adults was receiving treatment for chronic schizophrenia (Szatmari et al., 1989b). None of the 19 relatively able subjects in the study by Mawhood (1995) had a schizophrenic disorder. Volkmar & Cohen (1991) concluded that the frequency of schizophrenia in individuals with autism is around 0.6%, which is roughly comparable to that in the general population: 'it does not appear that the two conditions are more commonly observed together than would be expected on a chance basis'.

Autism and other psychotic conditions

Although the presence of first rank schizophrenic symptoms is relatively unusual, cases have been reported of individuals showing a mixture of psychotic symptoms, including paranoid and occasionally delusional thoughts. One young man described by Lorna Wing could not be deterred from his conviction that some day Batman was going to come and take him away as his assistant (Wing, 1981). Clarke et al. (1989) report on another case of delusional disorder and one with an unspecified psychosis. The Szatmari study notes several cases of paranoid thinking or possible hallucinations while Tantam reports on four additional cases with hallucinations, one case with epileptic psychosis and two with obsessive–compulsive disorders. Szatmari et al. (1989a) and Rumsey et al. (1985) also describe a number of cases of obsessional or compulsive disorder in their studies of more able individuals although Szatmari cautions: 'We found it very difficult . . . to distinguish between obsessive ideation and the bizarre preoccupations so commonly seen in autistic individuals'.

Autism and affective disorders

By far the most prevalent psychiatric disturbances reported, either in single case or follow up studies, are those related to anxiety and depression. As early as 1970, Rutter noted the risk of depressive episodes occurring in adolescents or older individuals with autism (Rutter 1970). Other authors have also reported a high frequency of affective disorders (for a review, see Lainhart & Folstein, 1994 and Table 8.3).

Among the larger scale of these studies, Tantam reported a rate of 12% for affective psychosis in a group of adults with Asperger's syndrome. He also noted that in several cases the illness incorporated a delusional content, often linked with the individual's autistic preoccupations. One man, for example, had thrown himself into the Thames because the Government refused to abolish British Summer Time and he believed that watches were damaged by the necessity of being altered twice a year.

In addition to cases with a psychotic disorder, a further 8% suffered from other problems related to depression or anxiety. Similar figures are reported by Wing (1981) who found that 23% of her group of 18 individuals with Asperger's syndrome showed signs of an affective disorder. Two had attempted suicide and one other had talked about doing so although their attempts had not been successful. One young man, who had become very distressed by minor changes in his work routine, tried to drown himself but failed because he was a good swimmer. When he tried to strangle himself the attempt also failed because, as he said, 'I am not a very practical person'. Wolff & McGuire (1995) note that death from suicide was greater in their sample of 'schizoid' men and women (several of whom were probably suffering from Asperger's syndrome) than in the general population (ten of 17 women and 17 of 32 men had attempted suicide). In Rumsey's follow up of 14 relatively high functioning individuals, generalized anxiety problems were found in half the sample. Six individuals also showed occasional outbursts of temper, aggression or destructiveness.

None of these investigations claims to be based on representative samples, so the resulting figures for the prevalence of psychiatric disturbance must be treated with caution. Moreover, the difficulties inherent in making a valid diagnosis of psychosis in people with autism should also be recognized. Impoverished language (Howlin, 1997), literal interpretation of questions (Wing, 1986), concrete thinking (Dykens et al., 1991) and obsessionality (Volkmar & Cohen, 1991) can all give rise to misunderstandings, leading to possible misdiagnosis, even in the case of relatively able individuals. For those with little or no speech, the risks of an incorrect diagnosis (or failure to diagnose when problems do exist) are even higher.

In a preliminary study, Abramson et al. (1992) suggest that the rates of affective disorder may be as high as 33% and Tantam's findings indicate overall rates for mania of 9%, 15% for depression and 7% for clinically

Table 8.3. *Reports of affective disorder in adolescents and adults with autism or Asperger's syndrome*

Author	Age (years)	Sex	Total *n*	Initial diagnosis	Psychiatric disorder
Darr & Worden, 1951	33	F	1	Autism	Low mood; delusions
Reid, 1976	32	F	1	Autism	Depression
Wolff & Chick, 1980	17+	M	22	'Schizoid'/Asperger	2 Depression
					1 Mood swings
					5 Attempted suicide
Wing, 1981	16+	M	18	Asperger	4 Affective disorder
Komoto et al., 1984	13	F	2	Autism	Depression
	13	M			Bipolar illness
Rumsey et al., 1985	18+	M	14	Autism	7 Generalized anxiety disorder
Gillberg, 1985	14	M	1	Asperger	Manic depression
Akuffo et al., 1986	40	F	1	Autism	Manic depression
Steingard & Biederman, 1987	24	M	1	Autism	Manic episodes
Linter, 1987	15	M	1	Autistic like	Manic depression
Kerbeshian & Burd, 1987	13	M	1	Atypical autism	Major depression
Sovner, 1988a, b	25	F	2	Autism	Depression
	26			PDD	Depression
Sovner, 1989	31	M	1	Autistic	Depression
	24	F	1		Manic depression
Clarke et al., 1989	23	M	5	Autistic	1 Major depression
Szatmari et al., 1989a	?	M + F	16	Autistic	4 'Anxiety disorder'
Kerbeshian et al., 1990	33	M	1	Autistic + SLD	Bipolar
Ghaziuddin et al., 1991a, b	17	M	2	Autistic + Down	Depression
	16	F		Autistic	Depression
Tantam, 1991	18+	M	85	Asperger	4 Mania
					4 Bipolar
					2 Depression
					11 Non-psychotic anxiety/depression
Kurita & Nakayasu, 1994	1	M	21	Autism + MR	SADS

From Howlin (1997).

significant anxiety disorders, while the frequency of schizophrenia is probably slightly under 1% (Volkmar & Cohen, 1991). In the absence of larger scale studies, such statistics must remain tentative, but it has become increasingly clear that individuals with autism or Asperger's syndrome may be at particular risk of developi'ng depressive and anxiety related disorders as they grow older (see Table 8.3).

Epilepsy

It is estimated that around one-third of individuals with autism develop epilepsy, with onset often occurring in adolescence or early adulthood. Gillberg (1992) suggests that the most common form of seizure disorder is complex-partial (psychomotor) epilepsy. The incidence tends to be greater in individuals of lower IQ, with the rates being highest in those with severe to profound learning difficulties. If these groups are excluded, the overall rate seems to be around 18–20% (Tantam, 1991; Goode et al. 1994), with there being little difference between those of normal IQ and those with moderate learning disabilities.

Some adolescents or young adults may have one or two isolated fits but no more and because of the disadvantages of giving unnecessary medication, drugs are often not prescribed unless there is evidence of more frequent attacks. There is no evidence to suggest that successful control is particularly difficult to achieve for people with autism although, because individuals are unlikely to report unwanted side effects themselves, careful monitoring of their response to treatment is particularly important.

LEGAL ISSUES

Is there a link between autism and criminality?

Although there is little evidence of an association between autism and criminal offending, occasional and sometimes lurid publicity has led to suggestions that there may be an excess of violent crimes among more able people with autism, particularly those diagnosed as having Asperger's syndrome. In the UK in 1994, for example, the apparently motiveless murder of an 85 year old women on her way to church by a 13 year old boy with Asperger's syndrome led to exaggerated accounts of the potential for violence among this group.

In her original account of people with Asperger's syndrome, Lorna Wing describes the case of one individual, out of a total of 34, who had injured another boy apparently because of his obsession with chemical experiments. Mawson et al. (1985) report on a 44 year old man with Asperger's syndrome who was committed to Broadmoor Special Hospital after attacking a baby. This followed a series of other attacks, including stabbing, on young women or children which had begun in his teens. The attacks seemed to be related to his obsession with getting a girl friend, his dislike of certain styles of dress and the noise of crying. He also had a fascination with poisons.

Baron-Cohen (1988) describes the strange case of a 21 year old man who had, over a period of several years violently assaulted his 71 year old 'girl-friend'. In another report, Chesterman & Rutter (1994) describe a young man with Asperger's syndrome who had been charged with a number of sexual offences; however, these seemed to relate mainly to his obsession with washing machines and women's nightdresses. The case was complicated by the fact that he struck the interviewing police officer when the charge of burglary was raised; as far as he was concerned 'he was merely intending to make use of the occupant's washing machine'.

Everall & Le Couteur (1990) describe a case of firesetting in an adolescent boy with Asperger's syndrome and Tantam (1991) mentions five cases of fire setting, four of which occurred when other people were in the building. He also cites another case in which someone had killed his school mate 'probably as an experiment'. Nevertheless, Tantam notes that violence, in a fight, in an explosion of rage, or in sexual excitement is rare. Among the men with Asperger's syndrome he studied, sexual offending was also unusual, although some got into trouble for indecent exposure. Property offences were also rare except as the 'side effects of the pursuit of a special interest'.

Various other, largely anecdotal, accounts of offending by people with autism or Asperger's syndrome have occurred from time to time (Howlin, 1997). Lack of social understanding or rigid adherence to rules may give rise to problems. Occasionally crimes are unwittingly, or unwillingly, committed at the instigation of others. Obsessional interest may also be involved, and because of this offending may well be of an unusual or bizarre nature, such as attempting to drive away an unattended railway engine because of an obsession with trains, or causing explosions and fires because of an obsessional interest in chemical reaction (Wing, 1986). Rarely, however, does there appear to be a deliberate intention to hurt or harm others.

Estimates of offending by people with autism or Asperger's syndrome

On the basis of their single case report, Mawson et al. (1985) suggest that many people who come to the attention of secure units because of violent offences may have Asperger's syndrome. In fact, evidence in support of such a statement is extremely limited.

Scragg & Shah (1994) assessed the entire male population of Broadmoor Special Hospital, using case notes to identify possible autistic cases. Subsequently, on the basis of personal interviews and the Handicap, Behaviour and Skills schedule of Wing & Gould (1978), they identified three cases with autism and six with Asperger's syndrome, using Gillberg & Gillberg's criteria (1989). Out of a total of 392 patients this represented a prevalence rate of just over 2%. The offences committed included violence or threats of violence (five cases), unlawful killing (three cases, including one of matricide) and firesetting (one case). Solitariness or lack of empathy was noted in each case. Six of the cases had a fascination for topics such as poisons, weapons, murder books or combat. The prevalence of Asperger's syndrome in this special hospital setting was higher than predicted and Scragg and Shah also conclude that there is an association between Asperger's syndrome and violence.

Ghaziuddin, in contrast, points out that the number of reports of violence or other offences by people with autism or Asperger's syndrome is actually very small. In 1991, Ghaziuddin et al. (1991b) reviewed accounts of offending by people with Asperger's syndrome. Out of a total of 132 cases, only three had a clear history of violent behaviour (these are the cases described by Wing, 1981; Baron-Cohen, 1988; Mawson et al., 1985, noted above). The low incidence of violence found by Ghaziuddin is compared with a rate of 7% of violent crimes (rape, robbery and assault) in the 20–24 year age group in the United States (US Bureau of Justice Statistics, 1987). As Scragg & Shah (1994) suggest, there may well be more people with autism in prisons or secure accommodation than is realized, and it is clearly important that such individuals are correctly identified and treated; however, estimates of the prevalence of violence in this group can only be made on the basis of community studies. Until then, speculation on the alleged links between violence and autism or Asperger's syndrome is only likely to increase the stigma and distress of those affected and their families. Currently, there is no reason to suppose that people with autism are more prone to committing offences than anyone else; indeed, because of the very rigid way in which many tend to keep to rules and regulations, they may well be more law abiding than the population generally.

CONCLUSIONS

How far Kanner would have considered these findings fulfil the 'better expectations' he was hoping for as therapeutic and educational provision for individuals with autism improved will never be known. Yet it is clear that at least a minority, although continuing to be affected by their autism, can find work, may live independently and may develop close relationships with others. These achievements do not come easily, however. Jobs are often found only with the support of families, opportunities to live independently depend heavily on local provision, and friendships are often forged through special interests and skills, rather than via spontaneous contacts. Nevertheless, as admissions to hospital care have fallen, and expectations about the future for people with disabilities generally have risen over the years, the outlook seems far less bleak than was once assumed. At least for those individuals who are of relatively high intelligence, and who develop effective communication skills, appropriate education is able to offer them a chance of being accepted, if never quite completely integrated, into society. Encouragement to develop and make use of obsessional interests and special skills is also a significant factor in many cases. Those who achieve most highly tend to view their autism as a challenge to be overcome rather than as a handicap which must be accepted, although the extent to which even they can succeed is likely to depend heavily on the assistance offered by families, teachers and other support systems.

REFERENCES

Abramson, R. K., Wright, H. H., Cuccara, M. L., Lawrence, L. G., Babb, S., Pencarinha, D., Marstellar, F. & Harris, E. C. (1992). Biological liability in families with autism. *Journal of the American Academy of Child and Adolescent Psychiatry*, **31**, 370–1.

Akuffo, E., MacSweeney, D. A. & Gajwani, A. K. (1986). Multiple pathology in a mentally handicapped individual. *British Journal of Psychiatry*, **149**, 377–8.

Alvin, J. & Warwick, A. (1991). *Music Therapy for the Autistic Child*, 2nd edn. New York: Oxford University Press.

American Psychiatric Association. (1994). *Diagnostic and Statistical Manual of Mental Disorders, (DSM-IV)*, 4th edn. Washington, DC.

Asperger, H. (1944). Autistic psychopathy in childhood. Translated and annotated by U. Frith (ed.). In *Autism and Asperger Syndrome*, 1991. Cambridge: Cambridge University Press.

Ayres, J. A. (1979). *Sensory Integration and the Child*. Western Psychology Service. Los Angeles, California.

Baron-Cohen, S. (1988). Assessment of violence in a young man with Asperger's syndrome. *Journal of Child Psychology and Psychiatry*, **29**, 351–60.

Bartak, L. & Rutter, M. (1978). Differences between mentally retarded and normally intelligent autistic children. *Journal of Autism and Childhood Schizophrenia*, **6**, 109–20.

Bemporad, J. R. (1979). Adult recollections of a formerly autistic child. *Journal of Autism and Developmental Disorders*, **9**, 179–97.

Biklen, D. (1990). Communication unbound: autism and praxis. *Harvard Educational Review*, **60**, 291–315.

Cesaroni, L. & Garber, M. (1991). Exploring the experience of autism through first-hand accounts. *Journal of Autism and Developmental Disorders*, **21**, 303–14.

Chesterman, P. & Rutter, S. C. (1994). A case report: Asperger's syndrome and sexual offending. *Journal of Forensic Psychiatry*, **4**, 555–62.

Chung, S. Y., Luk, F. L. & Lee, E. W. H. (1990). A follow-up study of infantile autism in Hong Kong. *Journal of Autism and Developmental Disorders*, **20**, 221–32.

Clarke, D. J., Littlejohns, C. S., Corbett, J. A. & Joseph, S. (1989). Pervasive developmental disorders and psychoses in adult life. *British Journal of Psychiatry,*, **155**, 692–9.

Creak, M. (1963). Childhood psychosis: a review of a 100 cases. *British Journal of Psychiatry*, **10**, 984–9.

Darr, G. C. & Worden, F. G. (1951). Case report twenty eight years after an infantile autistic disorder. *American Journal of Orthopsychiatry*, **21**, 559–69.

DeMyer, M. K., Barton, S., DeMyer, W. E., Norton, J. A., Allan, J. & Steele, R. (1973). Prognosis in autism: a follow-up study. *Journal of Autism and Childhood Schizophrenia*, **3**, 199–246.

Dykens, E., Volkmar, F. & Glick, M. (1991). Thought disorder in high functioning autistic adults. *Journal of Autism and Developmental Disorders*, **21**, 303–14.

Eisenberg, L. (1956). The autistic child in adolescence. *American Journal of Psychiatry*, **1112**, 607–12.

Everall, I. P. & Le Couteur, A. (1990). Fire-setting in an adolescent boy with Asperger's syndrome. *British Journal of Psychiatry,*, **157**, 284–7.

Frith, U. (1991). *Autism and Asperger Syndrome*. Cambridge: Cambridge University Press.

Ghaziuddin, M., & Tsai, L. (1991). Depression in autistic disorder. *British Journal of Psychiatry*, **159**, 721–3.

Ghaziuddin, M., Tsai, L. & Ghaziuddin, N. (1991a). Fluoxetine in autism with depression. *Journal of the American Academy of Child and Adolescent Psychiatry*, **30**, 508–9.

Ghaziuddin, M., Tsai, L. Y. & Ghaziuddin, N. (1991b). Brief report. Violence in Asperger syndrome: a critique. *Journal of Autism and Developmental Disorders*, **21**, 349–54.

Ghaziuddin, M., Tsai, L. Y. & Ghaziuddin, N. (1992a). Brief report: a comparison of the diagnostic criteria for Asperger's syndrome. *Journal of Autism and Developmental Disorders*, **22**, 643–51.

Ghaziuddin, M., Tsai, L. Y. & Ghaziuddin, N. (1992b). Comorbidity of autistic disorder in children and adolescents. *European Journal of Child and Adolescent Psychiatry*, **1**, 209–13.

Gillberg, C. (1985). Asperger's syndrome and recurrent psychosis: a case study. *Journal of Autism and Developmental Disorders*, **15**, 389–97.

Gillberg, C. (1992). Epilepsy. In *The Biology of the Autistic Syndromes*, 2nd edn, ed. C. Gillberg & M. Coleman, pp. 60–73. Oxford: MacKeith Press.

Gillberg, C. & Gillberg, C. (1989). Asperger syndrome: some epidemiological considerations. *Journal of Child Psychology and Psychiatry*, **30**, 631–8.

Gillberg, C. & Steffenberg, S. (1987). Outcome and prognostic factors in infantile autism and similar conditions: a population-based study of 46 cases followed through puberty. *Journal of Autism and Developmental Disorders*, **17**, 272–88.

Goode, S., Rutter, M. & Howlin, P. (1994). A twenty-year follow-up of children with autism. Paper presented at the 13th Biennial Meeting of the *International Society for the Study of Behavioural Development*. Amsterdam, The Netherlands.

Grandin, T. (1995). The learning style of people with autism: an autobiography. In *Teaching Children with Autism: Strategies to Enhance Communication and Socialization*, ed. K. A. Quill, pp. 33–52. New York: Delmar.

Grandin, T. & Scariano, M. (1986). *Emergence Labelled Autistic*. Tunbridge Wells, Kent. Costello. Novato: Arena Press.

Howlin, P. (1997). *Autism: Preparing for Adulthood*. London: Routledge.

Howlin, P. & Rutter, M. (1987). *Treatment of Autistic Children*. Chichester: John Wiley.

Irlen, H. (1995). Viewing the world through rose tinted glasses. *Communication*, **29**, 8–9.

Jolliffe, T., Landsdown, R. & Robinson, T. (1992). *Autism: a Personal Account*. London: The National Autistic Society.

Kanner, L. (1943). Autistic disturbances of affective contact. *Nervous Child*, **2**, 217–50.

Kanner, L. (1949). Problems of nosology and psychodynamics of early infantile autism. *American Journal of Orthopsychiatry*, **19**, 416–26.

Kanner, L. (1973). *Childhood Psychosis: Initial Studies and New Insights*. New York: Winston/Wiley.

Kanner, L. & Eisenberg, L. (1956). Early infantile autism 1943–1955. *American Journal of Orthopsychiatry Psychiatry*, **26**, 55–65.

Kaufmann, B. (1981). *A Miracle to Believe In*. New York: Doubleday.

Kerbeshian, J. & Burd, L. (1987). Are schizophreniform symptoms present in attenuated form in children with Tourette's disorder and other developmental disorders? *Canadian Journal of Psychiatry*, **32**, 123–35.

Kerbeshian, J., Burd, L., Randall, T., Martsolf, J. & Jalal, S. (1990). Autism, profound mental retardation and atypical bipolar disorder in a 33 year old female with a deletion of 15q12. *Journal of Mental Deficiency Research*, **34**, 205–10.

Klin, A., Volkmar, F. R., Sparrow, S. S., Cicchetti, D. V. & Rourke, B. P. (1995). Validity and neuropsychological characterization of Asperger syndrome: convergence with nonverbal learning disabilities syndrome. *Journal of Child Psychology and Psychiatry*, **36**, 1127–40.

Kobayashi, R., Murata, T. & Yashinaga, K. (1992). A follow-up study of 201 children with autism in Kyushu and Yamguchia, Japan. *Journal of Autism and Developmental Disorders*, **22**, 395–411.

Komoto, J., Usui, S. & Hirata, J. (1984). Infantile autism and affective disorder. *Journal of Autism and Developmental Disorders*, **14**, 81–4.

Kurita, H. & Nakayasu, N. (1994). Brief report: an autistic male presenting seasonal affective disorder (SAD) and trichotillomania. *Journal of Autism and Developmental Disorders*, **24**, 687–92.

Lainhart, J. E. & Folstein, S. E. (1994). Affective disorders in people with autism: a review of published cases. *Journal of Autism and Developmental Disorders*, **24**, 587–601.

Linter, C. M. (1987). Short-cycle manic–depressive psychosis in a mentally handicapped child without family history: a case report. *British Journal of Psychiatry*, **151**, 554–5.

Lockyer, L. & Rutter, M. (1969). A five to fifteen year follow-up study of infantile psychosis. III. Psychological aspects. *British Journal of Psychiatry*, **115**, 865–82.

Lockyer, L. & Rutter, M. (1970). A five to fifteen year follow-up study of infantile psychosis. IV. Patterns of cognitive abilities. *British Journal of Social and Clinical Psychology*, **9**, 152–63.

Lord, C. & Schopler, E. (1985). Differences in sex ratios in autism as a function of measured intelligence. *Journal of Autism and Developmental Disorders*, **15**, 185–93.

Lotter, B. (1974a). Factors related to outcome in autistic children. *Journal of Autism and Childhood Schizophrenia*, **4**, 263–77.

Lotter, B. (1974b). Social adjustment and placement of autistic children in Middlesex: a follow-up study. *Journal of Autism and Childhood Schizophrenia*, **4**, 11–32.

Lotter, B. (1978). Follow-up studies. In *Autism: a Reappraisal of Concepts and Treatment*, ed. M. Rutter & E. Schopler, pp. 475–96. New York: Plenum Press.

Lovaas, O. I. (1987). Behavioral treatment and normal educational and intellectual functioning in young autistic children. *Journal of Consulting and Clinical Psychology*, **55**, 3–9.

Mawhood, L. (1995). *Autism and developmental language disorder: implications from a follow-up in early adult life*. Unpublished PhD Thesis, University of London.

Mawson, D., Grounds, A. & Tantam, D. (1985). Violence in Asperger's syndrome: a case study. *British Journal of Psychiatry*, **147**, 566–9.

Mittler, P., Gillies, S. & Jukes, E. (1966). Prognosis in psychotic children: report of a follow-up study. *Journal of Mental Deficiency Research*, **10**, 73–83.

McEachin, J. J., Smith, T. & Lovaas, O. I. (1993). Long-term outcome for children with autism who received early intensive behavioral treatment. *American Journal of Mental Retardation*, **97**, 359–72.

Newson, E., Dawson, M. & Everard, T. (1982). The natural history of able autistic people: their management and functioning in a social context. Unpublished report to the Department of Health and Social Security, London. Summary published in four parts in *Communication*, **19–21** (1984–1985).

O'Connor, M. & Hermelin, B. (1988). Low intelligence and special abilities. *Annotation: Journal of Child Psychology and Psychiatry*, **29**, 391–6.

Petty, L. K., Ornitz, E. M., Michelman, J. D. & Zimmerman, E. G. (1984). Autistic children who become schizophrenic. *Archives of General Psychiatry*, **41**, 129–35.

Reid, A. H. (1976). Psychiatric disturbances in the mentally handicapped. *Proceedings of the Royal Society of Medicine*, **69**, 509–12.

Rimland, B. (1994a). Information pack on drug treatments for autism. *Autism Research Review International*. Information Pack P6.

Rimland, B. (1994b). Information pack on vitamins allergies and nutritional treatments for autism. *Autism Research Review International*. Information Pack P24.

Rumsey, J. M., Rapoport, J. L. & Sceery, W. R. (1985). Autistic children as adults: psychiatric social and behavioural outcomes. *Journal of the American Academy of Child Psychiatry*, **24**, 465–73.

Rutter, M. (1970). Autistic children: infancy to adulthood. *Seminars in Psychiatry*, **2**, 435–50.

Rutter, M. (1972). Childhood schizophrenia reconsidered. *Journal of Autism and Childhood Schizophrenia*, **2**, 315–37.

Rutter, M. & Bartak, L. (1973). Special educational treatment of autistic children: a comparative study. II. Follow-up findings and implications for services. *Journal of Child Psychology and Psychiatry*, **14**, 241–70.

Rutter, M., Greenfield, D. & Lockyer, L. (1967). A five to fifteen year follow-up study of infantile psychosis. II. Social and behavioural outcome. *British Journal of Psychiatry*, **113**, 1183–99.

Rutter, M. & Lockyer, L. (1967). A five to fifteen year follow-up study of infantile psychosis. I. Description of sample. *British Journal of Psychiatry*, **113**, 1169–82.

Sacks, O. (1993). A neurologist's notebook: an anthropologist on Mars. *New Yorker*, 27th December, pp. 106–25.

Schopler, E. & Mesibov, G. B. (1992). *High Functioning Individuals with Autism*. New York: Plenum Press.

Scragg, P. & Shah, A. (1994). Prevalence of Asperger's syndrome in a secure hospital.

British Journal of Psychiatry, **161**, 679–82.

Stehli, A. (1992). *The Sound of a Miracle: a Child's Triumph over Autism*. Fourth Estate Publications, USA.

Steingard, R. & Biederman, J. (1987). Lithium responsive manic-like symptoms in two individuals with autism and mental retardation. *Journal of the American Academy of Child and Adolescent Psychiatry*, **26**, 932–5.

Sovner, R. (1988a). Anticonvulsant drug therapy of neuropsychiatric disorders in mentally retarded persons. In *Use of Anticonvulsants in Psychiatry*, ed. S. McElroy & H. G. Pope, Jr, pp. 169–81. Clinton, NJ. Oxford Health Care.

Sovner, R. (1988b). Behavioral psychopharmacology: a new psychiatric subspeciality. In *Mental Retardation and Mental Health: Classification, Diagnosis, Treatment, Services*, ed. J. Stark, F. J. Menolascino, M. Albarielli et al., pp. 229–42. New York: Springer.

Sovner, R. (1989). The use of valproate in the treatment of mentally retarded persons with typical and atypical bipolar disorders. *Journal of Clinical Psychiatry*, **50** (Suppl. 3), 40–3.

Sverd, J., Montero, G. & Gurevich, N. (1993). Brief report: cases for an association between Tourette's syndrome, autistic disorder and schizophrenia-like disorder. *Journal of Autism and Developmental Disorders*, **23**, 407–14.

Szatmari, P., Bartolucci, G. & Bremner, R. S. (1989a). Asperger's syndrome and autism: a comparison of early history and outcome. *Developmental Medicine and Child Neurology*, **31**, 709–20.

Szatmari, P., Bartolucci, G., Bremner, R. S., Bond, S. & Rich, S. (1989b). A follow-up study of high functioning autistic children. *Journal of Autism and Developmental Disorders*, **19**, 213–26.

Szatmari, P., Bartolucci, G., Finlayson, A. & Krames, L. (1986). A vote for Asperger's syndrome. *Journal of Autism and Developmental Disorders*, **16**, 515–17.

Szatmari, P., Tult, L. & Finlayson, J. A. J. (1990). Asperger's syndrome and autism: neurocognitive aspects. *Journal of the American Academy of Child Psychiatry*, **29**, 130–6.

Tantam, D. (1986). *Eccentricity and Autism*. Unpublished PhD Thesis, University of London.

Tantam, D. (1991). Asperger's syndrome in adulthood. In *Autism and Asperger Syndrome*, ed. U. Frith, pp. 147–83. Cambridge: Cambridge University Press.

US Bureau of Justice Statistics. (1987). *Adolescents* (Fall 1989). Princeton. New Jersey: The Robert Wood Johnson Foundation.

Venter, A., Lord, C. & Schopler, E. (1992). A follow-up study of high functioning autistic children. *Journal of Child Psychology and Psychiatry*, **33**, 489–507.

Volkmar, F. R. & Cohen, D. J. (1985). The experience of infantile autism: a first-person account by Tony W. *Journal of Autism and Developmental Disorders*, **15**, 47–54.

Volkmar, F. R. & Cohen, D. J. (1991). Comorbid association of autism and schizophrenia. *American Journal of Psychiatry*, **148**, 1705–7.

Welch, M. (1988). *Holding Time*. London: Century Hutchinson.

Williams, D. (1992). *Nobody Nowhere*. London: Corgi Books.

Williams, D. (1994). *Somebody Somewhere*. London: Corgi Books.

Wing, L. (1981). Asperger's syndrome: a clinical account. *Psychological Medicine*, **11**, 115–29.

Wing, L. (1986). Clarification on Asperger's syndrome. Letter to the Editor. *Journal of Autism and Developmental Disorders*, **16**, 513–15.

Wing, L. & Gould, J. (1978). Systematic recording of behaviors and skills of retarded and psychotic children. *Journal of Autism and Childhood Schizophrenia*, **8**, 79–97.

Wiltshire, S. (1987). *Drawings: Selected and with an Introduction by Sir Hugh Cassan*. London: Dent.

Wolff, S. (1991). Schizoid personality in childhood and adult life. I. The vagaries of diagnostic labelling. *British Journal of Psychiatry*, **159**, 615–20.

Wolff, S. & Barlow, A. (1979). Schizoid personality in childhood: a comparative study of schizoid, autistic and normal children. *Journal of Child Psychology and Psychiatry*, **20**, 29–46.

Wolff, S. & Chick, J. (1980). Schizoid personality in childhood: a controlled follow-up study. *Psychological Medicine*, **10**, 85–100.

Wolff, S. & McGuire, R. J. (1995). Schizoid personality in girls: a follow-up study. What are the links with Asperger's syndrome? *Journal of Child Psychology and Psychiatry*, **36**, 793–818.

World Health Organization. (1993). *The ICD-10 Classification of Mental and Behavioural Disorders: Diagnostic Criteria for Research*. Geneva: WHO.

9

Autism and the evolution of human social skills

Lynn Waterhouse and Deborah Fein

INTRODUCTION

At present one of the stumbling blocks impeding our understanding of the neural basis of autism is the absence of any integrated model of the biological basis of human social behaviour. There are a number of component theories, but there is no overarching framework describing the brain basis of normal social skills that can be employed as an analytic tool to explore the nature of autistic social impairment. In an effort to draft an initial pro tem proposal for such a framework, this chapter briefly describes five models of evolution and identifies 11 component frameworks for understanding the neurofunctional basis of human social behaviour, linking each of the 11 with one of three viable models of evolution. An integrated framework for coalescing the 11 models is proposed, and the neural dysfunctions proposed to impair social skills in autism are considered in light of the proposed integrated framework. Three central questions are addressed in this chapter:

(1) Given that the evolution of human social skills can be inferred from evidence for increasing complexity in social organization and brain structure, what are the forces that drove such genetic evolution?
(2) Are human social behaviours determined by brain systems specialized for social skills or by neural mechanisms serving both social and nonsocial human skills?
(3) What is the relation between known neural dysfunctions and social impairments in autism?

The goal of the chapter is to answer these questions in a manner that may shed light on the underlying deficits in autism.

QUESTION 1: WHAT GENERATED THE EVOLUTION OF HUMAN SOCIAL BEHAVIOURS?

Humans are social animals. Three million years ago we lived in sex divided social groups of 30–50 hunter-gatherers. At present, although small groups of humans still hunt and gather in South America, Africa, Indonesia, the Philippines and the South Pacific, the majority of humans live in or near towns and cities that range from a few hundred people to 25 million individuals. We seek social contact and group cohesion (Durham, 1991; Soltis et al., 1995), and agriculture, metal working, division of labour and industrialization have permitted extremes of mass aggregation.

With the exception of the orangutan, all primates are social. De Waal (1996) has argued that nonhuman primates have exhibited the following prosocial traits: mother–child and male–female attachment; succorance or active care for another individual; emotional contagion and social mimicry; long term bonds of friendship; reciprocity in support and aggression; peace making; conflict avoidance; adjustment of behaviour toward and special care of disabled individuals and helpless infants; active maintenance of social bonds; play and teasing; monitoring of the social interaction of pairs and groups of other individuals; social teaching; and the accommodation of differing needs through active negotiation. Povinelli & Eddy (1996) have reported that in addition to self-recognition in mirrors, chimpanzees 'display mutual gaze in affiliative contexts, unlike many other primate species for whom direct eye contact is an aversive stimulus' (1996: 129) and display 'very robust evidence of gaze following' (1996: 134).

De Waal identified the limitations of the social nonhuman hominoid primates (gorillas, bonobos, chimpanzees) as follows:

utterances of language-trained apes . . . show little if any evidence of grammar. The transmission of knowledge from one generation to the next is rarely, if ever, achieved through active teaching. And it is still ambiguous how much planning and foresight, if any, go into the social careers of monkeys and apes. (De Waal, 1996: 211).

Povinelli & Eddy (1996) have proposed that 'despite the remarkable sophistication of the chimpanzees' deployment of the gaze following response, it is possible that a dissociation between gaze following and understanding the mental state of attention behind gaze (i.e. having a theory of mind) may

243

still exist within their species (and possibly our own as well) (1996: 134).

Findings in ethological study of apes thus suggest that social apes have extremely elaborate social networks of shifting alliances, dominance hierarchies and group formation, as well as many varied caring, sharing, joint attention and interactive regulatory behaviours without the benefit of the exchange of detailed and situationally varying information that syntax would provide, without the benefit of information transfer across generations, and without the benefit of the production and exchange of complex plans. In sum, apes have sophisticated social cognition without sophisticated cognitive skills.

The social skills of our primate relations are likely to represent preadapted complexity that emerged from the fitness of genetic ensembles supporting central nervous system governance of patterns of social behaviours. A subset of ape social behaviours, however, are likely to represent adaptive complexity resulting from the innate preadapted ability to learn and create new behaviour patterns. 'With behavioral plasticity (available through learning) the possibilities of integrating a social group in important and intricate ways become that much greater' (Bonner, 1988: 235–6).

Mechanisms of evolution

Both preadapted complexity (built in behaviour patterns that have increased human fitness) and adaptive complexity (the ability to learn and create new adaptive behaviours during the course of an organism's lifespan) have been interpreted to be the result of one of five possible mechanisms: (1) religious providentialism, (2) Lamarckian instructionism, (3) Darwinian selectionism, (4) generative complexity plus selectionism (Kauffman, 1993), or (5) 'spandrelism' – the adaptive reconfiguration of byproducts of selection (Gould & Lewontin, 1979). The first mechanism, providentialism, is the argument by design. It posits that because all living and nonliving elements of the world are both complex in make up and suitable for our use, in the same manner that we design complex technological for our use, a greater Designer has provided all living and nonliving things in the world. In this view human social behaviour has been designed for our use.

Instructionism is the now discounted theory of Lamarck that the learned traits and skills of a parent can become part of the genetic inheritance of the child. In Lamarckian evolution a parent's improved social skills would be part of a child's genome. Selectionism is Darwin's proposal that blind variation gives rise to traits that are selected for if and when they increase an individual's fitness, measured by the successful production of relatively more offspring. In Darwinian terms, complex social skills must have increased the fitness of individuals (Cziko, 1995).

Generative complexity plus selectionism alters and augments Darwin's original thesis concerning selection. Proposed by Kauffman (1993), this model claims that organisms and their constitutive internal systems (e.g. the brain, the immune system) will self-generate greater and greater systemic complexity through internal biophysical replicating forces. In Kauffman's view biological systems are kept from complexifying into the chaos of disorganization precisely by means of environmental selection pressures. For Darwin selection was the vehicle for the increase of beneficent variation within species, and the source of speciation itself. In Kauffman's model, however, variation and speciation are spontaneously and continuously occurring self-generated biophysical events, and it is selection that provides system stasis by conserving orderly patterns in complex systems within and across species over time. Generative complexity means that 'if optimal networks, both in terms of complexity of task performed, and in terms of capacity to adapt lie in the ordered regime at the edge of chaos, then selection must hold networks in this poised ensemble . . . Insofar as selection tunes the ensemble explored but is unable to avoid its generic properties, those quasi universal features may be expected to shine through across the aeons and across phyla' (1993: 535). Thus a Kauffman model interpretation of the evolution of human social skills would look for conservation of neural and behavioural function across species and across time within species.

Spandrelism (Gould & Lewontin, 1979) has been argued to be the source of many complex and adaptive behaviours. A spandrel literally is an architectural term describing the space left between the outer curve of an arch and the rectangular frame around the arch. Metaphorically it has been proposed as a label for an unintended effect. The arch is intended, the rectangular framework is intended, but the two triangular spaces between the left and right sides of the arch and frame are the unintended result of the interaction of two intended (the arch and the frame) designs. For Gould & Lewontin (1979) much of human complex social behaviour could be the result of the 'spandrel' of increased brain size. If brain size were adapted for the need to remember how to find raw materials for tools, and adapted for the planning sequencing skills to make and effectively use tools (Calvin, 1994), the increased brain tissue, as a spandrel, became available to be adapted for social skills. Conversely, it has been argued by Humphrey

(1976) and Ingold (1994) that brain size increased to support the fitness provided by the complexity of human social behaviour and then as a spandrel, such increased neural tissue was available to support the development of other complex cognitive skills, such as tool making.

Evolved sources of human social behaviour

The three viable theoretical models proposing mechanisms for evolutionary processes – spandrelism, selectionism and generative complexity plus selectionist stasis – offer a means to organize a variety of models of the cardinal point or points of origin of human social behaviours. Eleven current theoretical frameworks that hold promise for understanding the social impairments in autism are reviewed here. These 11 models can be categorized by (1) the proposed evolved core point of origin of the behaviour, and (2) the associated evolutionary mechanism. This dual categorization yields three neural system spandrel models, three neural system quasi spandrel models, two neural system selectionist models and three neural–cultural generative complexity models.

Three neural system spandrel models

(1) OXYTOCIN

There is now evidence that oxytocin and vasopressin contribute to a mammalian neurotransmitter system that governs social affiliation and elaborated imprinting (Insel, 1992; Carter et al., 1995; Landgraf, 1995). Oxytocin now appears to be an essential base for social attachment and elaborated imprinting: the drive for proximity to individuals eliciting affiliative states in mammals (Landgraf, 1995). Insel and Carter and others have developed animal models demonstrating that oxytocin release and uptake in the mammalian brain is associated with reproductive acts, parental care, infant attachment and affiliative behaviours (Insel, 1992; Carter et al., 1995).

Carter (reviewed in Angier, 1996) has suggested that while oxytocin's first function in mammals was to support the development of mother–infant attachment, the neuropeptide's ability to regulate brain–behaviour relations may have been coopted to serve other affiliative goals including alliances and partnerships. For Carter, if oxytocin is a basis for all social affiliation, it is a spandrel reconfiguration of maternal pair bonding. Moreover, Carter has argued that oxytocin's reconfiguration for social alliances beyond maternal–offspring pair bonding provided the spandrel opening for the evolution of advanced nonsocial cognitive skills (Angier, 1996).

(2) POLYVAGAL SYSTEM AND SOCIABILITY

As reviewed in Angier (1996), Porges has argued that the ability to affiliate in mammals is a byproduct of the efficiency of a high powered internal temperature maintaining metabolism. Porges's 'polyvagal theory' identifies a spandrel unfolding of the tripartite vagal nerve system as the basis of sociability. The first role of the primitive vagal nerve in fish was to limit oxygen consumption, thus adaptively reducing metabolism when necessary. The primitive vagal nerve elaborated into both a metabolic slowdown and a metabolic speed-up system. The speed-up system triggers the sympathetic nervous system permitting an animal to use more oxygen in order to support the evolved fight or flight response. The 'spandrel' of this dual vagal nerve system then supported the development of a third function. The third and newest element in the vagal system controls facial expressions and vocalizations, regulates heart rate and inhibits the flight or flight response. Thus the newest reconfiguration of the vagal system engenders human sociability because, according to Porges, it enables humans to interact with others while being 'fully engaged in our surroundings, without major metabolic demands or challenges' (Angier, 1996: C11). Only in crises do we shift to the most primitive near-death state of extreme metabolic slowing.

(3) PAIN, EMOTIONS AND COMMUNICATION

Panksepp & Sahley (1987) have theorized that components of the pain system evolved into the basis for human social interaction. They proposed that the neurophysiological basis for pain responses came to serve mammalian social attachment which then, in humans, emerged in communication functions. They have hypothesized that 'from an evolutionary perspective, higher order behavioural processes, such as the capacity for social attachment, may have arisen from existing neural systems that mediate pain, thus helping decrease the incidence of destruction to members of a species' (Sahley & Panksepp, 1987: 362).

Sahley and Panksepp proposed that because attachment and language have evolved out of the opioid based pain system, therefore damage to the opioid system will impair social attachment and language functions. The Panksepp–Sahley model is a spandrel argument: social skills are an evolved byproduct of the pain experience: cries of distress become linked to attachment, calls of attachment are the spandrel basis for social interaction and communication.

Three neural system quasi spandrel models

(1) ATTENTION AND SOCIAL BEHAVIOURS

Courchesne et al. (1994) have identified cerebellar abnormalities as the key neural deficit in autism and have reported findings for larger and smaller than normal cerebellar structures in autism. In the Courchesne et al. model of social skills (1994, 1995) the cerebellum determines the rapid voluntary shifting of attention which, in turn, determines the ability to engage in joint social attention, which in turn serves as the central core of social functioning.

This model can be construed as a quasi spandrel model because all social behaviour is assumed to be an extrapolated byproduct of mobilization of attentional resources via joint attention. The theory does not propose evolved reconfiguration of the cerebellum but does propose deployment of elementary behaviours in more complex assemblies.

(2) EXECUTIVE FUNCTIONS AND SOCIAL BEHAVIOURS

Lesions of the prefrontal cortex can result in impaired social rule use, shallow affect, and deficits in executive function, the organization and planning of voluntary behaviours. Ozonoff et al. (1991) found evidence for executive deficits in high functioning autistics and proposed that 'prefrontal impairment is the underlying deficit in autism, capable of explaining both cognitive and social symptoms of the disorder' (1991: 1100).

The thesis that frontal lobe functions determine human social functioning is a quasi spandrel model in that the full range of social behaviours are posited to be extrapolated from planning skills and affect expression. Damasio's related model of executive functions and affect, the somatic marker theory (1994), is also a quasi spandrel model in that social decision-making based on affect coding is the cornerstone of complex sociality.

(3) IMAGINATION, INTENTIONAL RELATIONS AND SOCIAL UNDERSTANDING

Barresi & Moore (1996) have developed an evolutionary model of social understanding. They postulate that there are two essential capacities of the human conceptual system for social understanding: (1) the conceptual system must be able to represent the activities of agents that are directed at objects (e.g. intentional relations), and (2) the conceptual system must be able to represent our own activities and the activities of others (1996: 107). From this spandrel basis of representation all social comprehension is proposed to develop.

Two neural system implicit selectionist models

(1) ATTACHMENT AND WARMTH

MacDonald (1992) has separated warmth and attachment as two innate and elementary social systems. He has offered five arguments for the separation of these two systems. First, 'positive feelings of affection and warmth appear to result from a different biological system than do negative emotions such as fear, distress and anxiety, which are so central to attachment research' (1992: 754). Second, attachment is found in all primates; however, 'there is no reason to suppose that there has been evolution of intimate relationships, pair bonding or affection' (1992: 755) in primates. Third, 'attachment appears to be compatible with lack of warmth, and even maltreatment' (1992: 755). Fourth, there is no sex difference in attachment, but there is a sex difference in warmth. Fifth, attachment is relevant for infant security, but reciprocated positive social interaction is crucial to childhood and adult relationships.

MacDonald (1992) has stressed the adaptive value of these two systems in development. Warmth and attachment can be viewed as having evolved via selection because they have increased individual fitness as tested by natural selection. Moreover, individuals vary in the degree of warmth and degree of attachment in infancy suggesting the active effects of ongoing selection pressures for sociability in the human population.

(2) APPROACH–AVOIDANCE: BOLD AND SHY

Kagan (1994) has identified innate approach–avoidance dimensions of social interaction. He has grouped children who are high, low and normal (mid-range) in reactivity as infants. Kagan found that inhibited children showed greater activation in the right than left frontal lobe region, a finding associated in other samples with negative affect and anxiety (Davidson, 1994). Kagan has proposed that 'because inhibited children are sympathetically reactive, afferent feedback from the heart, circulatory vessels and other sympathetic targets to the amygdala should be greater in inhibited children' (1994: 158). He also proposed that the amygdala feed forward to the cortex could desynchronize alpha wave activity in inhibited children, and that because there is greater reciprocal activity in their right hemisphere amygdala–frontal activation loop, the affect expression of inhibited children is similar to the patterns of anxiety expressed by people who are not happy.

Kagan (1994) identified a range of characteristics of inhibited children including reluctance to initiate social interaction, absence of spontaneous smiles with unfamiliar people, excessive fears, high muscle tension and the inability to relax in new situations (1994: 165). Conversely, Kagan's longitudinal study findings suggest that uninhibited children develop strong patterns of sociability, spontaneous smiles, lack of fear, relaxed muscle tone and the ability to take pleasure in new situations.

The pattern of Kagan's findings suggest that the three variant temperaments (inhibited, normal and uninhibited) are on a continuum. The continuum itself is an index of the presence of selection. Newly emerging and disappearing traits in a species generally are more variable than stable traits in a species. Incoming traits are variable because selection pressures are relatively new and fitness stabilization for the trait has not yet been achieved. Conversely, disappearing traits are variable because now no selection pressures exist to maintain that trait and in the absence of selection pressures random variation may result. It may be inferred that complex social interaction skills are evolutionarily new and therefore 'incoming' traits. If so, then uninhibited prosocial individuals may exhibit greater fitness.

Three neural–cultural implicit generative complexity models

(1) PERSONALITY GENETIC ARCHITECTURE

Cloninger et al. (1996) reported that four discrete domains of dimensional traits – Novelty Seeking, Harm Avoidance, Reward Dependence and Persistence – were identified in large samples of twins in the USA and Australia. Cloninger et al. (1996) have proposed that these four gene-based traits together regulate internal states governing an individual's social interactions and interactions with the environment.

The Cloninger model proposes that human temperament 'has a simple genetic architecture, but weak correlations among a network of multiple heritable dimensions produces complex nonlinear dynamics because each person responds to experience with multiple motivations, which sometimes conflict' (Cloninger et al., 1996: 3).

In the Cloninger model individuals at the extremes of one or more of the four dimensions are likely to form a specific focal adaptive or maladaptive social character stabilization. The dimensional range of novelty seeking interacting with the ranges of harm avoidance, persistence and reward dependence are theorized to 'produce self-organization with a stage like development toward quasi stable multidimensional configurations, which are called the attractors of a complex system' (1996: 3). In Cloninger's model these stabilized states are distinct personality types. For example, someone high in novelty seeking (restless, curious, exploring and information seeking), low in harm avoidance (optimistic), high in reward dependence (sociable) and high in persistence will be likely to be a mature, creative extrovert. Someone high in novelty seeking, low in reward dependence (aloof, pessimistic and anxious) and average in harm avoidance and persistence is likely to become disorganized and schizotypal (Cloninger et al., 1996: 3).

The Cloninger model can be viewed as a generative complexity with selectionism, i.e. Kauffman's model. Genetic variation is produced as the dimensions of each stable, universal, heritable domain, and extremes of dimensions are formed into ordered regimes of specific personality types by environmental selection pressures of social interaction in modern culture.

(2) FOUR SOCIAL PATTERNS

Fiske (1992) has argued that there are only four systems, two innate and two learned, governing all human social interaction behaviour. In Fiske's model, the first pattern is innately determined communal sharing wherein all group members give all that they have to the group without reserve and the group supports all members. This provides a tight altruistic regulation of social and work behaviour in that members of a group must share food, effort and information completely or risk being ostracized from the group. Every member, including the group's leader, shares the social role of group commitment. The second pattern proposed by Fiske is authority ranking wherein an innate hierarchical pecking order determines the roles and rules for the regulation of an individual's behaviour. Rules vary by rank and power. Those with more power have greater social role variation. The third pattern proposed is equality matching which Fiske defines as learned turntaking regulation of the behaviour of individuals. The fourth pattern is market pricing. In market pricing, items of information/goods/services are learned to have different values depending on their judged relevance to an individual's needs, and this value of information/goods/services must be computed by some means. Those individuals who offer more valued information/goods/services will be accorded greater value in the society.

In Fiske's model these four patterns are not mutually exclusive. Fiske would say that a given complex human event can involve altruistic behaviour, exhibitions of authority ranking, evidence of turntaking regulation of behaviour and signs that cost-benefit analysis has guided interaction behaviour. Fiske also posited that the first two patterns (altruism and pecking order regulation) are innate and occur in other animals. He proposed, however, that the last two (turntaking and cost-benefit analysis) are not innate, and require central nervous system information processing beyond the capabilities of any creatures other than ourselves. This thesis is reasonable because turntaking and cost-benefit analysis must require more complex representations to be held in working memory in order to compute turns and values.

Fiske's model can be interpreted in terms of generative complexity and selectionism. The first two patterns represent stabilizing solutions to group organization wherein the complexity of individual group members' variation in food and safety needs, and individual differences in power and problem solving skills are group regulated by stable internal individual neural regulation. The second two patterns represent cultural memes (gene like units of cultural innovation that are replicable across cultures) that extend the organizational complexity of the first two patterns, serving to coregulate individual needs for goods, services and safety with the group's need for stable patterns of coregulation.

(3) COREGULATORY MECHANISMS OF SOCIAL BEHAVIOUR

Waterhouse (1988) proposed that human social interaction depends on a series of three increasingly open means of coregulation of one individual's behaviour by another. The first proposed was pair bonding, with physical contact, co-thermoregulation, coregulation of a range of internal body states and the vital transmission of body fluids in the coregulatory processes of sexual intercourse and maternal breast feeding of infants. The second was motor imitation in face to face interaction, with consequent coregulatory effects of emotional contagion (Ekman, 1993) and coregulatory joint attention through mimesis of directed attention. The third, most open coregulatory process proposed was message exchange, verbal and nonverbal communication in face to face interaction, in signals and calls from a great distance and through symbols across time and through space (Waterhouse, 1988).

All three systems are proposed as adaptive. The coregulation involved in the mother–child nursing, bonding, attachment process ensures the physical and emotional survival of the infant (Insel, 1992; Carter, reported in Angier, 1996). Motor synchrony or motor imitation provides a basis for learning (Meltzoff & Gopnik, 1993) and also contributes to pair and group social cohesion by reducing the threat valence that the novel motor behaviours of others may generate (Meltzoff & Gopnik, 1993). Message exchange supports the activity of more than one person and allows the accumulation of information across individuals and generations (Sperber & Wilson, 1986; Clark, 1992).

Although the three coregulatory processes are normally supportively intertwined throughout life, they unfold in sequence: babies nursed at birth, begin development of motor synchrony in interaction patterns with their mothers in the first weeks of life and will express elementary forms of the behavioural sequences of intentional message interaction even before they can speak single words (Field et al., 1982).

Each coregulatory system involves requisite behavioural sequences and subordinate skills. The infant's role in pair bonding requires an initial sucking reflex, the ability to obtain endogenous central nervous system reward from the process of nursing, and the ability to be calmed by touch (Blass, 1992). Motor synchrony requires intact gross and fine motor functions, near normal vision, attention to social behaviour of another and, presumably, the normal functioning of an innate programme which governs nonlearned imitation (Meltzoff & Gopnik, 1993). Intentional message exchange involves many subordinate processes including: (1) selective attention to others and nonconscious assignment of reward value to others, (2) percept generation of (a) faces, (b) utterances, and (c) the whole other individual in context, (3) holding these percepts in working memory, (4) judgement of the novelty, salience and significance of these working memory percepts in terms of stored memory, (5) interpretation of the gist or message of a communication from another, (6) recognition of one's own message associated emotions or feeling states, (7) evaluation of the emotions, motives and plans of the other interactant, (8) the motivation or intention to generate a response, (9) generation of appropriate content for the message, (10) motor expression of a coordinated (a) vocal, (b) facial, (c) gestural, and (d) postural response containing a responsively appropriate message, (11) monitoring the reaction of the other interactant, and (12) modifying the ongoing response in attunement to the reaction of the other interactant (Sperber & Wilson, 1986; Leech, 1990; Clark, 1992).

This model fits Kauffman's generative complexity with the selection model. Two interacting individuals each have innate universal programmes of behaviour with a range of possibilities for individual variation in the expression of these programmes. The variability of each interactant's individual behaviour is coregulated by the behaviour of the other individual. Thus individual variability in the innately shaped neural programmes for social behaviour is tightly constrained by environmental selection pressure. The environmental selection pressure, however, is not temperature or predators or the presence of limited food: the interaction selection pressure consists of the behaviours produced by the cointeractant.

Thus increasing complexity and variability in social behaviours expressed by one individual is stabilized and limited by the 'environment' of the social behaviours expressed by his or her cointeractant(s). In this way, through coregulatory social interaction we provide one another with forces that help to keep our generated behaviours back from the edge of maladaptive complexity and chaotic dysfunction. In addition to the neural programmes we carry innately, we have the ability to learn further constraints for our social behaviour in the form of pragmatics (rules for the social use of language), social manners (as in introductions, signs of respect), and the social rituals such as greetings, small talk, toasts and jokes. In this way our learned cultural rules support the constraints inherent in the interactive process. The assumed adaptive goal is an effective, relevant, affiliating and nondisruptive exchange of information.

Table 9.1. *Evolved human traits and behaviour that support social behaviour in face to face interaction*

Individual traits for social dispositions and social comprehension
Novelty seeking
Reward dependence (warmth)
Persistence
Harm avoidance   Inhibited (third vagal (parasympathetic) < normal)
                Normal (third vagal system = normal)
                Uninhibited (third vagal system > normal)
Cognitive skill for representing intentional relations

Paired and group shared coregulatory interactive behaviours
Pair bonding (oxytocin based attachment)
  Infants and mothers; sex partners
Imitation (emotional contagion, joint attention, motor acts)
Message exchange   Predator-distress (pain and fear communication)
                Food discovery (communal sharing)
                Rank and territory (authority ranking)
                Equality matching
                Market pricing

Integrative model of the source of human social behaviour

Can these models of social behaviour be integrated into a single meta-model? Table 9.1 outlines a new proposal for a meta-model based on two groups of gene based behavioural regulatory systems. The first group includes individual traits that influence social (and nonsocial) reactive directedness of behaviour. The second group includes behaviours that coregulate the interaction of two or more individuals. The first group of five traits is based on Cloninger and colleagues' model of the four domains of dimensional dispositions with the addition of Barresi and Moore's social interpretation skill evolved conceptual trait where attention (Courchesne) and planning (Rogers and colleagues executive functions) are considered to be necessary to social interpretation.

Kagan's reactive temperament types have been embedded in the Cloninger trait of harm avoidance. This would not, however, be acceptable to Kagan (1994: 44–5) who has argued that the use of questionnaires, application of factor analyses and the inference of overly broad domains (e.g. harm avoidance) in trait research are all problematic. Nonetheless, behavioural inhibition is a key feature of harm avoidance, and the absence of behavioural inhibition is associated with risk taking.

In the proposed meta-model, the Porges polyvagal theory of reactivity is tagged to Kagan's reactivity types. Inhibited individuals are too easily aroused by environmental stimuli; uninhibited individuals are often insensitive to environmental stimuli.

MacDonald's (1992) concept of warmth has been embedded in the Cloninger trait of reward dependence. MacDonald proposed that warmth be identified as an expression of the Positive Social Reward (PSR) system, and based his conceptualization of PSR on the notion of reward dependence (1992: 759). MacDonald has posited that warmth represents the 'attraction to the rewards of intimacy and affection' and that warmth had adaptive evolutionary value because it 'functions to facilitate within family transfer of resources' (1992: 759), and may be a 'generalized system underlying human family functioning' (1992: 760).

The three level coregulatory model of social interaction (Waterhouse, 1988) has been embedded with the oxytocin model (Insel, 1992; Carter et al., 1995) and MacDonald's model of attachment as constituents of the first level pair bonding. Fiske's model of four interaction patterns has been embedded in message exchange, and the Panksepp–Sahley model, in turn, has been embedded as a constituent of the distress message. In addition, three specific message domains have been identified: predator-distress, food discovery, rank and territory. These three messages, along with (a) the message domain associated with maternal pair bonding and mating, and (b) the message domain associated with imitative group cohesion, represent the five basic domains of primate and mammalian communication content (Quiatt & Reynolds, 1995).

Waterhouse et al. (1997) proposed that there are two adaptive goals of all social interaction: an affiliative goal (desiring physical proximity and enjoying being with another person) and a strategic goal (hoping to obtain some advantage or benefit by means of interaction with the other person). At all levels of coregulation, however, essential communication can be viewed as affiliation for the individual and strategic for the species. In sex partner and mother–child bonding interactions, the affiliative goals of the individuals ensure the strategic species goals of reproduction and survival of offspring. In group member imitation, the behavioural copying affiliates individuals in emotional contagion, conjoint attention and motor behaviours, all of which serve the strategic goal of survival of the group. In message exchange, sharing relevant information affiliates individuals and supports their survival.

In humans and social apes, however, Machiavellian strategic communication has developed (Byrne & Whiten, 1988; Byrne, 1995). There are many Machiavellian strategic aspects of the control of message exchange. There is societal regulation of information flow in a hierarchical pattern within and outside of institutions. There is the societal assignment of specific roles in conversation which will have a strategic focus. Within the individual, there is the assessment of what constitutes equal sharing of information, and the assessment of the costs versus the benefits of the interaction. An individual or group of individuals can engage in message exchange that is, in fact, disaffiliative and strategic. Some of the forms of such Machiavellian communication strategies include mini-max game playing (seeking to give the least in exchange for the most relevant benefit to oneself), selective sharing or withholding of valued information, and the creation of false information for exchange (i.e. lying). These strategies are disaffiliative because one or both interactants seek to gain an informational advantage at the expense of the other.

Machiavellian strategies in message exchange are likely to involve greater individual variation because they are evolutionarily new and appear to require both effective imagination and well functioning working memory. Moreover, patterns of normal individual variation may develop differently in strategic skills than in affiliative processes. There are powerful negative sanctions against deceptive communication in most cultures, except where specifically prescribed by social manners (Goffman, 1974; Sperber & Wilson, 1986; Clark, 1992).

QUESTION 2: HOW MANY NEURAL MECHANISMS GOVERN HUMAN SOCIAL BEHAVIOURS?

The range of expressed human behaviour depends on evolved behavioural neural control systems that include:

(1) innate universal autonomic and reflex programmes that govern breathing, yawning, sneezing and blinking (Shepherd, 1994)
(2) innate categorical and continuum dispositional programmes for behaviours such as reactive temperament (Kagan, 1994; Cloninger et al., 1996)
(3) innate 'starter' parameter setting programmes for specific forms of learning such a phobias, words (categorization of content), images of faces, food aversions (Pinker, 1994; Plotkin , 1994; Shepherd, 1994) and,
(4) innate individually varying potentiatable frameworks for learning complex motor skills, learning real world knowledge and for constructing novel skills, artefacts, plans and theories (Shepherd, 1994).

Cloninger's four reactive temperament types are theorized to depend on four distinct gene based neurotransmitter cascades that induce specific dispositional states, thus focusing and patterning behavioural selection choices. For example, the neuropeptide oxytocin and beta endorphins have been found to be involved in social reward dependence, and dopamine is theorized to be the underlying element of novelty seeking. Harm avoidance is hypothesized to be based on arousal and de-arousal systems involving the neurotransmitters epinephrine (adrenaline) and norepinephrine (noradrenaline) and gamma amino butyric acid (GABA).

The neural basis for representations of intentional relations is unclear. Although Barresi and Moore argue that 'in human beings there has evolved a capacity to enter into shared intentional relations with another and associated intentional schema to integrate first and third person information about these intentional relations' (1996: 122), they provide little in the way of a neural mechanism for this evolved skill, other than to argue that it may depend on the ability to pay attention and to integrate sensory information from several modalities into a representation (1996: 121). Such a representation system must operate on social and nonsocial objects and events, so the special abilities claimed by Barresi & Moore (1996) must depend on an as yet unspecified further elaboration of sensory integration and imagination.

The behaviours and related neurotransmitters hypothesized to be involved in pair bonding are likely to predate the specific individually varying dispositional states induced by the neurotransmitter cascades that form temperament. Pair bonding involves specific reflexes and innate releasing mechanisms with associated fixed patterns of behaviour that coregulate motor actions and internal states in order that successful mating can take place, and in order that infants can be breast fed. Imitation, in turn, depends on cross modal integration in the hippocampus, along with an innate limbic system mechanism hypothesized to direct nonconscious mimicry. This function too may be assumed to predate individual variation in temperament.

As described earlier, conversation and nonverbal message exchange depends on a wide variety of central nervous system functions that involve attention, judgement, working memory, assessment of novelty, recall of prior information in long term memory, ability to determine the general meaning of what is being said, as well as a flexible sense of the emotions or feeling states of the other interactant.

Clearly, the neural control of conversation is complex. Knowledge of language, and comprehension of words and sentence patterns, and of the expressive signals of others is required. Moreover, the normal pragmatic rules of conversation require the constant internal review of and external reconsideration of ideas in sentence fragments that appeared earlier (Leech,

1990; Clark, 1992) in the interaction. Shared contents of working memory is called 'common ground' (Clark, 1992). Repeating elements of common ground in the conversation support the maintenance of the episode in working memory, and this supports topic control within the continuing conversation. When conversational partners re-activate elements of common ground they also enhance the long term memory of information of that conversation. The process of flexible redirection between working memory and long term memory is crucial for conversation because retrieval of information from long term memory is a necessary component in establishing the conversational common ground.

In terms of the neural systems involved in conversation, it is known that the frontal cortex sends projections to the hippocampal complex, exerting modulatory control of the amygdala and hippocampus, and reciprocal projections between the hippocampal complex and frontal cortex serve to link the internal state of the individual to knowledge of external stimuli. Projections from the hippocampus and amygdala are crucial to frontal processes of behavioural planning and initiation because they provide the frontal cortex with integrated sensory records, and linked to assignment of affective significance – what can be termed an associatively unified assessment of the individual's current perceptions and feelings. Furthermore, normal frontal symbiotic cortex projections to the hippocampus modulate hippocampal function, and similarly symbiotic frontal projections to the amygdala modulate affective computations. Thus successful, fluid conversation is a very powerful test of the network integrity of a wide range of individual neural functions.

In fact, the greatest concurrent information processing load imposed on humans is found in social interaction (Quiatt & Reynolds, 1995). As so many varied neural systems can contribute to the complexity of social interaction behaviour, and because social interaction requires flexible and complex sequences of behaviour, therefore, despite the built in supports that have evolved to trigger and maintain social interaction, engaging in social interaction is likely to be a good test of the state of an individual's central nervous system function. Equally important is the fact that social learning is a vehicle for acquisition of complex interaction sequences of behaviours (Plotkin, 1988, 1994). Social learning requires focal attention to others, and to the interactions of others. Human innate dispositions, reflexes, triggered skills, parameter setting mechanisms and frameworks for acquisition all contribute to reducing the learning load by providing innate species knowledge. So much information and so many regulatory rules must be learned, however, that interaction remains a complex task for the human central nervous system.

QUESTION 3: WHAT CONNECTS NEURAL DYSFUNCTION AND SOCIAL IMPAIRMENT IN AUTISM?

Neural dysfunctions

Many brain deficits have been proposed as the source of autism including brainstem, reticular activating system, cerebellum, thalamus, locus ceruleus, limbic system, hippocampus, amygdala, temporal and parietal lobe white matter, association cortex and frontal lobes (Waterhouse et al., 1996a). Tying proposed brain deficits to specific abnormalities in autism has not been successful, however. The current standard diagnosis of autism (*Diagnostic and Statistical Manual of Mental Disorders* (DSM-IV), American Psychiatric Association, 1994) requires the presence of (1) impaired reciprocal social interaction, (2) absent, odd or severely delayed language skill, and (3) a restricted repertoire of interests and activities.

Some researchers have assumed that social impairment actually represents a more basic functional impairment. Information processing (Minshew, 1994), executive function (Ozonoff et al., 1991), memory (DeLong, 1992) and theory of mind (Happé & Frith, 1995) each have been proposed as the source of autistic social impairment.

Waterhouse et al. (1996a) have proposed a model that outlines four systemically related neural dysfunctions that theorized conjointly generate diagnostic and nondiagnostic autistic symptoms. These four dysfunctions are: (1) canalaesthesia, in which hippocampal system dysfunction 'canalizes' sensory records, disrupting integration of information, (2) impaired assignment of the affective significance of stimuli, in which amygdaloid system dysfunction disrupts affect association, (3) asociality, in which oxytocin system dysfunction flattens social bonding and affiliativeness, and (4) extended selective attention, in which developmental malorganization of temporal and parietal polysensory regions yields abnormal overprocessing of first order unisensory representations.

They also reviewed 41 studies providing separate evidence for each of these four dysfunctions in 484 cases of autism, and concluded that if all four were studied conjointly in a single sample, 51–70% of cases of autism would be found to have all four proposed dysfunctions (Waterhouse et al., 1996a).

Social impairment

The social dysfunctions of autism are severe (Fein et al., 1986). The key diagnostic behaviours in autism are those indexing social impairment: impaired use of nonverbal behaviours to regulate social behaviours, lack of friends, does not seek others to share an experience, lack of social or emotional reciprocity, and lack of social imitative or pretend play (DSM-IV, APA, 1994).

In an epidemiological study, Wing & Gould (1979) categorized social impairment in autism into three groups. The three are: (1) aloof and indifferent to other people, (2) passive and controllable but lacks any social initiative, and (3) actively makes odd approaches to others. These groups have been validated in a variety of studies (Waterhouse et al., 1996b). The subgroup of autistic children labelled Aloof have no affiliative drive and no interaction skills. The subgroup of autistic children labelled Passive may express limited affiliative drive and minimal interaction skills. The subgroup of autistic children categorized as Active but Odd are affiliative in a uniquely intrusive and persistent way, and have no skill for establishing or maintaining normal interactions.

None of the three subtypes of autism – Aloof, Passive and Active but Odd – expresses normal personalities. Most autistic individuals appear to lack social reward dependence. Aloof individuals appear to obtain no reward from social interaction, Passive individuals do not seek others but accept the attention of others at times, and Active but Odd individuals do seek interaction with others but only to deliver pestering repetitive monologues about favourite obsessive interests.

Many autistic individuals show unusual fears but are unable to behave in a harm avoidant way; they often seem unaware of dangers. In avoiding social interaction, however, they may be expressing acute harm avoidance as if social interaction were the source of harm. Few autistic individuals show novelty seeking, and only Active but Odd high functioning autistic individuals show persistence. Their persistence is extreme and abnormally focused on trivial or meaningless items of information. Finally, only a few extremely high functioning autistic individuals are able to conceptualize intentional relations across individuals.

Surprisingly, many autistic individuals do show attachment to their mothers or carers (Rogers et al., 1993). This attachment may be abnormally fixated or unstable, but a majority of autistic individuals do show evidence of attachment. Similarly, except for the most aloof individuals, most autistic individuals show some evidence of imitation of the motor behaviour of others (Smith & Bryson, 1994). Although nearly half of all autistic children have little or no language skill, by the time of adolescence a majority of autistic individuals have some language, and a large subgroup have a reasonable vocabulary, basic syntactic skill in the creation of sentences and some ability to conduct brief interactions.

In sum, we would suggest that the majority of autistic individuals do not express the normal traits of personality as outlined in the four element Cloninger model. More specifically, the majority of autistic individuals do not exhibit harm avoidance, novelty seeking, persistence or social reward dependence. It is possible that autistic individuals may have some central disruption in transmitter cascades, or disruption for receptors for transmitters, or both, that underpin these four personality traits. Given that autistic individuals are able to learn, albeit slowly, they must have the neurotransmitter and neuroananatomcial systems necessary for the acquisition of knowledge, but these systems are insufficiently developed to enable them to conceptualize complex schema for intentional relationships. Therefore in addition to aberrantly limited personality development, they are limited in learning the social roles that in normal individuals overlay and proscribe the expression of essential reactive personality traits.

Conversely, a majority of autistic individuals show evidence of the three proposed levels of coregulatory behaviours. They show attachment (however abnormal), ability in nonconscious imitation of the behaviours of others and a majority develop the ability to engage in brief interactions by the time of puberty. Thus we might conclude that the neural mechanisms that underwrite social coregulation are evolutionarily older and neurologically more robust than those defined as generating individual traits of personality and complex conceptualization.

Modahl et al. (1992) hypothesized that autistic individuals have abnormal oxytocin functioning, with impairment to oxytocin receptors in the amygdala and hippocampus, and subsequently they found that oxytocin functioning is abnormal in autistic individuals (Modahl et al., in press). This, they suggested, would account for disruptions in maternal–child pair bonding, and would also account for lack of social reward, as the same neurotransmitters posited to be part of the reward dependence participate in the pair bonding mechanism. They also proposed that the amygdala and hippocampal systems are disrupted by abnormal neurodevelopmental overgrowth in autism, and that temporal and parietal association tissues are malorganized (Waterhouse et al., 1996a). These neural disruptions would limit complex conceptualizations and would also interfere with novelty seeking and harm avoidance. Without normal hippocampal and amygdala function and a normal temporal/parietal association cortex the ability to discern harm would be sharply limited, and the ability to identify novel objects and novel events would also be curtailed. Normal persistence would also be affected by the attentional abnormalities created by these disruptions.

Waterhouse and Fein hypothesize that the dimensional personality traits are relatively more fragile constructs: several hundred thousand years 'new' in the evolutionary history of humans. They are much newer than the 75 million year old basic mechanisms of mammalian pair bonding and the more than 200 million year old core patterns of invertebrate nonconscious motor imitation and communicative signalling systems. Although the neurodevelopmental disorders that give rise to autism compromise social personality traits, social comprehension skills and basic coregulatory pair and group mechanisms for adaptive acts and social cohesion, the newest and most fragile traits are most easily disrupted, regardless of the fact that they may employ some of the same neurotransmitter systems as are employed by basic interactive mechanisms.

CONCLUSION AND COMMENT

Special training programmes for the development of social skills in autism are themselves dependent on simple and repetitive social interaction in the form of behaviour modification programmes. Such programmes have been shown to be effective when they are introduced early in the child's development.

The difficultly with intense training in social skills is that the trained social skills often appear stiff, halting and overly formal. An autistic young adult had learned to say 'Hello, how are you?' He said this at every point of greeting with everyone he would see during a day. He had not been taught the rule for offering a reduced greeting (nod, brief smile, grunt or other acknowledgment of another person) after the first full scale greeting of the day, because he is unable to learn the complex notion that repetition of the same greeting carries the additional meaning of possible disregard for the other individual, and he is unable flexibly to alter his responses in slightly variant contexts.

Maurice, writing about her successful training of her autistic daughter and autistic son (Maurice, 1993), has suggested that behaviour modification is simply common sense applied consistently:

teaching kids by breaking down tasks into small, manageable units . . . spelling out expectations . . . praising good behaviour . . . physically prompting through a behaviour . . . walking a child through a task . . . having certain consequences (yes aversives!) for disobeying the rules. (Maurice, 1993: 257–58)

Maurice was worried that some autistic like behaviour may have remained, even though an evaluation of her children suggested only very mild residual effects.

Significant improvement remains rare in autism. Even with intense behaviour modification programmes at home and at school, very few autistic individuals will have a fully normal outcome. Social skills training in autism is a relatively recent application of behaviour modification (Koegel & Koegel, 1995; Lord, 1995). It began as efforts to teach everyday living skills, and then was extended in order to teach autistic children basic cognitive skills. Until effective preventive, genetic and pharmacological treatments are developed, behaviour modification will remain the most important treatment available. In terms of individuation of personality and temperament, however, it is unclear whether social skills training will induce a slightly more social version of an autistic persona (less Aloof, less Passive, Active-but-less-Odd), or whether social skills training can reveal greater individual variation in personality and temperament. Scarr (1992) has argued that twin studies reveal that the temperaments or personalities of normally developing individuals become more defined and more true to the individual's genome as individuals move into adolescence. In adolescence we move into a wider range of social environments in which we also have greater choice of selection of the social environment. Selection of environments (i.e. friends and activities) by the individual permits better expression of the variation in the genotype in the social acts of the phenotype (Scarr, 1992) through more varying, more fluid and more complex patterns of social interaction. If more varying, more fluid and more complex patterns of social interaction can be taught through systems of behaviour modification (Maurice, 1993), will successful autistic individuals be able to develop distinct personalities and unique reactive temperaments?

REFERENCES

Angier, N. (1996). Illuminating how bodies are built for sociability. *New York Times*, April 30, pp. C1 and C11.
Barresi, J. & Moore, C. (1996). Intentional relations and social understanding. *Behavioral and Brain Sciences*, **19**, 107–54.
Blass, E. M. (1992). The ontogeny of motivation: opioid bases of energy conservation and lasting affective change in rat and human infants. *Current Directions in Psycho-*

logical Science, **1**, 116–20.

Bonner, J. T. (1988). *The Evolution of Complexity by Means of Natural Selection.* Princeton, NJ: Princeton University Press.

Byrne, R. W. (1995). *The Thinking Ape.* Oxford: Oxford University Press.

Byrne, R. W. & Whiten, A. (1988). *Machiavellian Intelligence: Social Expertise and the Evolution of Intellect in Monkeys, Apes and Humans.* Oxford: Oxford University Press.

Calvin, W. H. (1994). The unitary hypothesis: a common neural circuitry for novel manipulations, language, plan-ahead, and throwing. In *Tools, Language and Cognition in Human Evolution,* ed. K. R. Gibson & T. Ingold, pp. 429–45. New York: Cambridge University Press.

Carter, C. S., DeVries, A. C. & Getz, L. L. (1995). Physiological substrates of mammalian monogamy: the prairie vole model. *Neuroscience Biobehavioral Reviews,* **19**, 303–14.

Clark, H. (1992). *Arenas of Language Use.* Chicago: University of Chicago Press.

Cloninger, C. R., Adolfsson, R. & Svrakic, N. M. (1996). Mapping genes for human personality. *Nature Genetics,* **12**, 3–4.

Courchesne, E. (1995). New evidence of cerebellar and brainstem hypoplasia in autistic infants, children, and adolescents: the MR imaging study by Hashimoto and colleagues. *Journal of Autism and Developmental Disorders,* **25**, 19–22.

Courchesne, E., Townsend, J., Akshoomoff, N. A., Yeung-Courchesne, R., Murakami, G. A. & Lincoln, A. (1994). A new finding in autism: impairment in shifting attention. In *Atypical Cognitive Deficits in Developmental Disorders: Implications for Brain Function,* ed. S. H. Broman & J. Grafman, pp. 101–38. Hillsdale, NJ: Erlbaum.

Cziko, G. (1995). *Without Miracles: Universal Selection Theory and the Second Darwinian Revolution.* Cambridge, MA: MIT Press.

Damasio, A. (1994). *Descartes's Error.* New York: Grosset/Putnam.

Davidson, R. (1994). Complexities in the search for emotion-specific physiology. In *The Nature of Emotions,* ed. P. Ekman & R. J. Davidson, pp. 237–42. New York: Oxford University Press.

DeLong, R. G. (1992). Autism, amnesia, hippocampus and learning. *Neuroscience and Biobehavioral Review,* **16**, 63–70.

De Waal, F. (1996). *Good Natured: The Origins of Right and Wrong in Humans and Other Animals.* Cambridge, MA: Harvard University Press.

Durham, W. H. (1991). *Coevolution.* Stanford, CA: Stanford University Press.

Ekman, P. (1993). Facial expression and emotion. *American Psychologist,* **48**, 384–92.

Fein, D., Pennington, B., Markowitz, P., Braverman, M. & Waterhouse, L. (1986). Toward a neuropsychological model of infantile autism: are the social deficits primary? *Journal of the American Academy of Adolescent Psychiatry,* **25**, 198–212.

Field, T. M., Woodson, R. & Greenberg, R. (1982). Discrimination and imitation of facial expressions by neonates. *Science,* **218**, 179–81.

Fiske, A. (1992). The four elementary forms of sociality: framework for a unified theory of social relations. *Psychological Review,* **99**, 689–723.

Goffman, E. (1974). *Frame Analysis.* Cambridge, MA: Harvard University Press.

Gould, S. J. & Lewontin, R. C. (1979). The spandrels of San Marco and the Panglossian paradigm: a critique of the adaptionist programme. *Proceeding of the Royal Society of London,* **285**, 281–8.

Happé, F. G. E. & Frith, U. (1995). Theory of mind in autism. In *Learning and Cognition in Autism,* ed. E. Schopler & G. B. Mesibov, pp. 177–98. New York: Plenum Press.

Humphrey, N. (1976). The social function of intellect. In *Growing Points in Ethology,* ed. P. P. G. Bateson & R. A. Hinde, pp. 303–17. Cambridge: Cambridge University Press.

Ingold, T. (1994). Tool-use, sociality and intelligence. In *Tools, Language and Cognition in Human Evolution,* ed. K. R. Gibson & T. Ingold, pp. 429–45. New York: Cambridge University Press.

Lynn Waterhouse and Deborah Fein

Insel, T. R. (1992). Oxytocin – a neuropeptide for affiliation: evidence from behavioral, receptor autoradiographic, and comparative studies. *Psychoneuroendocrinolog*, **17**, 3–35.

Kagan, J. (1994). *Galen's Prophecy*. New York: Basic Books.

Kauffman, S. (1993). *The Origins of Order*. New York: Oxford University Press.

Koegel, L. K. & Koegel, R. L. (1995). Motivating communication in children with autism. In *Learning and Cognition in Autism*, ed. E. Schopler & G. B. Mesibov, pp. 73–88. New York: Plenum Press.

Landgraf, R. (1995). Morton Jones Memorial Lecture. Intracerebrally released vasopressin and oxytocin: measurement, mechanisms and behavioral consequences. *Journal of Neuroendocrinology*, **7**, 243–53.

Leech, G. (1990). *Principles of Pragmatics*. New York: Longman.

Lord, C. (1995). Facilitating social inclusion: examples from peer intervention programs. In *Learning and Cognition in Autism*, ed. E. Schopler & G. B. Mesibov, pp. 221–42. New York: Plenum Press.

MacDonald, K. (1992). Warmth as a developmental construct: an evolutionary analysis. *Child Development*, **63**, 753–73.

Maurice, C. (1993). *Let Me Hear Your Voice; A Family's Triumph Over Autism*. New York: Fawcett Columbine.

Meltzoff, A. N. & Gopnik, A. (1993). The role of imitation in understanding persons and developing a theory of mind. In *Understanding Other Minds*, ed. S. Baron-Cohen, H. Tager-Flusberg & D. J. Cohen, pp. 335–66. New York: Oxford University Press.

Meltzoff, A. N. & Moore, M. K. (1977). Imitation of facial and manual gestures by human neonates. *Science*, **198**, 75–8.

Minshew, N. J. & Dombrowksi, S. M. (1994). In vivo neuroanatomy of autism: neuroimaging studies. In *The Neurobiology of Autism*, ed. M. L. Bauman & T. L. Kemper, pp. 66–85. Baltimore, MD: The Johns Hopkins University Press.

Modahl, C., Fein, D., Waterhouse, L. & Newton, N. (1992). Does oxytocin deficiency mediate social deficits in autism? *Journal of Autism and Developmental Disorders*, **24**, 449–51.

Modahl, C., Green, L., Fein, D., Morris, M., Waterhouse, L., Feinstein, C. & Levin, H. (1998). Plasma oxytocin levels in autistic children. *Biological Psychiatry*. (In press.)

Ozonoff, S., Pennington, B. F. & Rogers, S. J. (1991). Executive function deficits in high-functioning autistic individuals: relationship to theory of mind. *Journal of Child Psychology and Psychiatry*, **32**, 1081–105.

Panksepp, J. & Sahley, T. L. (1987). Possible brain opioid involvement in disrupted social intent and language development of autism. In *Neurobiological Issues in Autism*, ed. E. Schopler & G. Mesibov, pp. 357–72. New York: Plenum Press.

Pinker, S. (1994). *The Language Instinct*. New York: William Morrow.

Plotkin, H. C. (1988). *The Role of Behavior in Evolution*. Cambridge, MA: MIT Press.

Plotkin, H. C. (1994). *Darwin Machines and the Nature of Knowledge*. Cambridge, MA: Harvard University Press.

Povinelli, D. J. & Eddy, T. J. (1996). Chimpanzees: joint visual attention. *Psychological Science*, **7**, 129–35.

Quiatt, D. & Reynolds, V. (1995). *Primate Behaviour*. Cambridge, England: Cambridge University Press.

Rogers, S. J., Ozonoff, S. & Maslin-Cole, C. (1993). Developmental aspects of attachment behavior in young children with pervasive developmental disorders. *Journal of the American Academy of Child and Adolescent Psychiatry*, **32**, 1274–82.

Sahley, T. L. & Panksepp, J. (1987). Brain opioids and autism: an updated analysis of possible linkages. *Journal of Autism and Developmental Disorders*, **17**, 201–16.

Scarr, S. (1992). Developmental theories for the 1990s: development and individual differences. *Child Development*, **63**, 1–19.

Shepherd, G. (1994). *Neurobiology*, 3rd edn. New York: Oxford University Press.

Smith, I. M. & Bryson, S. E. (1994). Imitation and action in autism: a critical review. *Psychological Bulletin*, **116**, 259–73.

Soltis, J., Boyd, R. & Richerson, P. J. (1995). Can group-functional behaviors evolve by group selection? *Cultural Anthropology*, **36**, 473–94.

Sperber, D. & Wilson, D. (1986). *Relevance: Communication and Cognition*. Cambridge, MA: Harvard University Press.

Waterhouse, L. (1988). Aspects of the evolutionary history of human social behaviour. In *Aspects of Autism: Biological Research*, ed. L. Wing, pp. 102–14. London, England: Gaskell.

Waterhouse, L., Fein, D. & Modahl, C. (1996a). Neurofunctional mechanisms in autism. *Psychological Review*, **103**, 457–89.

Waterhouse, L. & Fein, D. (1997). Perspectives on social impairment. In *Autism and Developmental Disorders: a Handbook*, ed. D. Cohen & F. R. Volkmar, pp. 909–19. New York: John Wiley.

Waterhouse, L., Morris, R., Allen, D., Dunn, M., Fein, D. & Feinstein, C. (1996b). Diagnosis and classification in autism. *Journal of Autism and Developmental Disorders*, **26**, 59–86.

Wing, L. & Gould, J. (1979). Severe impairments of social interaction and associated abnormalities in children: epidemiology and classification. *Journal of Autism and Developmental Disorders*, **9**, 11–30.

Index

Note: page numbers in *italics* refer to figures and tables

Index